# Cholesterol in Atherosclerosis and Coronary Heart Disease

For permission to use material from this book please contact us:
Telephone 631-231-7269; Fax 631-231-8175
Web Site: http://www.novapublishers.com



**Library of Congress Cataloging-in-Publication Data**

Cholesterol in atherosclerosis and coronary heart disease / Jean P. Kovala, (editor).
p. ; cm.
Includes bibliographical references and index.
ISBN 1-59454-302-X (hardcover)
1. Coronary heart disease. 2. Atherosclerosis. 3. Hypercholesteremia. 4. Cholesterol--Pathophysiology.
[DNLM: 1. Hypercholesterolemia--complications. 2. Cardiovascular Diseases--etiology. 3. Coronary Arteriosclerosis--etiology. ] I. Kovala, Jean P.
RC685.C6C47 2005
616.1'23071--dc22

2005002278

*Published by Nova Science Publishers, Inc. ✣ New York*

# Contents

# Preface

High-density lipoproteins mediate a variety of antiatherogenic effects. These include reverse cholesterol transport, reversal of endothelial dysfunction, and reduction of inflammation, among others. A large corpus of epidemiologic data has consistently demonstrated that high levels of HDL protect against the development of atherosclerotic disease, while low levels of this lipoprotein substantially increase risk for MI, stroke, sudden death, and restenosis after angioplasty. There is substantial clinical trial based support for treating patients with low HDL with pharmacotherapy. In the primary and secondary prevention settings, such statin trials as AFCAPs/TexCAPs, LCAS, and HATS demonstrate significant risk reduction when treating patients with low HDL and average or elevated LDL levels ($\geq$ 130 mg/dL). Numerous new therapies for raising HDL and treating CAD in patients with low HDL are under active investigation. CETP inhibitors, a vaccine against CETP, an edible form of HDL comprised of D-amino acids, and bioengineered HDLs will be entering endpoint-driven, large-scale clinical trials. The results of these studies, as described in Chapter 1, will help to more poignantly delineate the role of HDL in the prevention and treatment of atherosclerotic disease. In the meantime, the treatment of patients with low HDL with statins, fibrates, and niacin yields significant reductions in risk for cardiovascular morbidity and mortality and has also been shown to decrease the rate of progression of atheromatous plaques in patients with CAD.

As reported in Chapter 2, during inflammation, several cell types synthesize and secrete phospholipase $A_2$ that catalyses lipid oxidation in LDL. Myeloperoxidase, a heme protein secreted by activated phagocytes, oxidizes L-tyrosine to a tyrosyl radical that is a physiological catalyst for the initiation of lipid oxidation in LDL. Lipid oxidation results in the generation of aldehydes that substitute lysine residues in the apolipoprotein B-100 moiety. Lipid together with protein oxidation in LDL results in the generation of oxidized LDL.

The authors, among others, have demonstrated an association between coronary heart disease (CHD) and increased plasma levels of oxidized LDL. Recently, we have demonstrated a higher prevalence of elevated oxidized LDL in persons with high-calculated CHD risk prior to events. Elevated oxidized LDL in persons with high-calculated CHD risk predicted future myocardial infarction even after adjusting for age, gender, race, smoking, and the metabolic syndrome. The effect of oxidized LDL on myocardial infarction can be explained by its effects on endothelial cells, monocyte infiltration and foam cell formation, and on smooth-muscle cell migration and apoptosis.

In Chapter 3, the authors report about our experience with LDL apheresis over more than 13 years. A total of 32 patients (19 males, 13 females; mean age at starting apheresis 50 years) were treated with different procedures (HELP, DALI, immunoadsorption, lipid filtration) for in the mean 80 months (6 to 161 months). According to the official rules an elevated atherosclerotic risk is a prerequisite for the indication of LDL apheresis. The intervals between two procedures were determined individually on the basis of LDL-C levels before procedures. 21 patients had a positive family history for either lipid disorders or coronary heart disease. The majority of patients suffered from a heterozygous form of hypercholesterolemia, in two patients a familial defective apolipoprotein B was found, in 9 patients a concomitant elevation of lipoprotein(a) was observed. 21 patients had also elevated triglyceride levels, at least temporarily. Before starting treatment with LDL apheresis in 25 patients an angiographically documented coronary atherosclerosis was found. 10 patients had suffered from a myocardial infarction, in 3 patients a PTCA was performed, 11 patients underwent a cardiac bypass operation. 5 patients were after a heart transplantation. In 6 patients a peripheral arterial occlusive disease was known. Only 3 patients were obese (Body Mass Index >= 30 kg/m$^2$). In 24 patients an accompanying hypertension and in 11 patients a diabetes mellitus was present. All patients were treated with a statin (atorvastatin, pravastatin, simvastatin, fluvastatin), in some patients (n = 14) ezetimibe was added recently. All LDL apheresis methods induced a reduction of LDL-C of at least 60 %. Lipoprotein(a) was reduced in the same range. Comparing the different LDL apheresis methods, in our hands the immunoadsorption and the DALI methods appeared to be the most effective ones. In no patient who was treated with LDL apheresis at our department a new myocardial infarction had developed. 5 patients underwent a PTCA and 3 patients a cardiac bypass surgery. One patient had died. In conclusion, it appears that LDL apheresis presents an effective tool in improving the prognosis in these high-risk patients.

Both a high plasma low-density lipoprotein (LDL) cholesterol level and a low plasma high-density lipoprotein (HDL) cholesterol level are critical risk factors for atherosclerosis and coronary heart disease. Therefore, increasing the plasma HDL cholesterol level is the next target for the treatment of atherosclerosis and coronary heart disease. Although statins, fibrates, and niacin can be used to improve low plasma HDL cholesterol levels, the effect of such drugs is limited. Agents that achieve better elevation of plasma HDL cholesterol levels are therefore needed. Among the many methods that may be used to raise the plasma HDL cholesterol level, Chapter 4 focuses on cholesteryl ester transfer protein (CETP) inhibitors, including JTT-705 and torcetrapib.

In a number of epidemiological studies, the high density lipoprotein (HDL) cholesterol has been identified as a powerful independent negative risk factor for coronary artery disease. Therefore, the increase of serum HDL cholesterol recently became a therapeutic target, in addition to low density lipoprotein (LDL) cholesterol. It has already been reported that the recommended lipid lowering diet reduces not only total cholesterol but HDL cholesterol levels as well. However, we have reported in a previous study, that in patients with baseline HDL cholesterol < 39 mg/dl, the hypolipidemic diet decreased total cholesterol and triglyceride levels, and increased HDL cholesterol, while in patients with HDL cholesterol ≥

39 mg/dl the decrease of LDL cholesterol and triglyceride levels was followed by a decrease of HDL cholesterol. As an extension of this study, in another study, including a double number of patients, the decrease of HDL cholesterol levels in patients with baseline HDL cholesterol $\geq$ 39 mg/dl, after hypolipidemic diet, was again documented. Moreover, dyslipidemic individuals do not show uniform HDL response to the hypolipidemic drug treatment. Fibrates, nicotinic acid or its analogue may result in the decrease of total cholesterol, LDL cholesterol and triglyceride levels without a parallel decrease in HDL cholesterol. On the other hand, statins may decrease total cholesterol, LDL cholesterol and triglyceride levels with a concomitant significant decrease of HDL cholesterol levels. It seems that when the baseline HDL cholesterol level is taken into account, a better selection of the optimal therapy could be made. In Chapter 5, besides the HDL metabolism and its pleiotropic effects, the results of the studies regarding the response of HDL cholesterol to hypolipidemic treatment will be analyzed.

Hyperlipidemia is a common and important risk factor after solid organ transplantation, mainly heart transplantation. Graft coronary vasculopathy is an accelerated form of atherosclerosis in transplanted hearts and has proven to be one of the most important late complications of heart transplantation and is the most limiting factor for long-term survival.

The most important factors favoring the development of hyperlipidemia after heart transplantation are inappropriate diet in combination with reduced physical activity, adverse effects of immunosuppressive therapy, such as steroids and cyclosporine, and polygenic hypercholesteremia in combination with ischemic cardiomyopathy.

Treatment of hyperlipidemia in heart transplant recipients results in a variety of complications and side effects. To note, interactions between lipid-lowering drugs and immunosuppressive therapy. The use of HMG-CoA reductase inhibitors (statins) achieved significant reduction in cholesterol levels. Use of these substances has resulted in significantly extended long-term survival times, significantly less graft coronary disease, and less severe graft rejection.

Blocking the cholesterol biosynthesis by statins resulted in lower levels of Coenzyme Q10, which plays an important role as a redox carrier in the mammalian respiratory transport chain, having a direct regulatory role on succinyl and reduced nicotinamide adenine dinucleotide (NADH) dehydrogenases. Enhancing the dietary uptake with Q10 may reduce the detrimental effect of statins therapy.

Chapter 6 will review the common immunosuppressive drugs in clinical use, hyperlipidemia post transplantation and the current management therapies.

In Chapter 7, Prolonged postprandial lipemia (PPL) has been associated with changes in the lipoprotein profile and increased risk for atherosclerosis. Individuals with hypertriglyceridemia tend to have an exaggerated PPL. Evidence suggests that patients with PPL are more susceptible to cardiovascular disease. The syndrome of PPL in the presence of low concentration of high-density lipoprotein cholesterol (HDL-Chol) and high concentration of low-density lipoprotein (LDL)-Chol has been considered as a combined marker of cardiovascular disease. Dietary triglyceride (TG) is carried by chylomicrons and very low density lipoproteins (VLDL) in the blood stream. Lipoprotein lipase (LPL) cleaves the TG to fatty acid from these lipoproteins. There is growing evidence that physical exercise and omega-3 fatty acid (n-3FA) supplementation and are excellent non-pharmaceutical remedies for the treatment of hypertriglyceridemia and PPL. However, the mechanism of how physical activity attenuates PPL still remains unclear. It has been proposed that exercise-induced attenuation of PPL is due to either the elevation of LPL activity or the reduction of VLDL-TG synthesis. The attenuation of PPL by n-3FA supplementation appears to be due to a decrease in chylomicron and VLDL-TG secretion and possibly an increase in fasting LPL activity. This review summarizes the effect of exercise and n-3FA supplementation on plasma lipid metabolism and PPL.

As reported in Chapter 8, LLD use was low in the beginning of the nineties in the general population but has increased substantially over the period 1993-1998. The use of statins has increased nearly exponentially and now makes up more than 90% of the lipid-lowering drugs used. After publication of especially the 4S study in 1994, utilisation has at least quantitatively approached a level corresponding to the number of people in the general population, who need treatment according to current recommendations. The majority of patients treated with LLDs had drug indicators of cardiovascular risk factors. General practitioners issued 73% of the total number of LLD prescriptions. The study has shown good compliance with statin treatment in a Danish population measured by persistence as well as by continuity. However, a high percentage of the youngest group of patients without drug indicators of cardiac disease or diabetes discontinued treatment before obtaining the full benefit in terms of decreased risk of coronary heart morbidity and mortality. Contrary to Denmark, LLD use in Italy was characterised by high consumption, prevalence and incidence but low persistence in the period 1994 to 1996. Among patients with a history of myocardial infarction who met the criteria for LLD reimbursement, far too few were actually treated. Therefore, more attention is needed to initiate treatment in these patients.

In Chapter 9, products enriched with plant sterols and plant stanols either in its esterified or unesterified form have demonstrated to be effective in cholesterol lowering. This paper presents a review of literature on cholesterol lowering effects of plant sterols and plant stanols. Dosages of 1.5-2.5 per day reduce total cholesterol up to 10% and LDL cholesterol up to 16%. The mean reduction in LDL cholesterol is about 10% which on a population basis may result in a 20% risk reduction for coronary heart disease. Sterols and stanols seem to be equally effective. Factors possibly influencing the magnitude of the cholesterol lowering effect being esterification, food matrix, composition of the background diet, moment of consumption and blood cholesterol concentration are addressed. Plant sterols and stanols are not only effective in normo- and mildly hypercholesterolaemic subjects, but also in hypercholesterolaemic subjects receiving cholesterol lowering therapies. No effects are observed on HDL cholesterol and triacylglycerol level. Plant sterols and stanols are poorly absorbed and plasma concentrations are low, except in subjects with a rare inherited disorder phytosterolaemia. Safety of plant sterols and stanols has been extensively tested and no adverse effects seem to be present, although there is a lack of chronic exposure data. Consumption of plant sterols and stanols results in a substantial reduction of carotenoid levels. The implication of this reduction for human health on the long term is not clear. With the growing number of enriched products entering the market the consumption of plant sterols and stanols should be monitored. An intake not exceeding 1-3 g per day is adviced. A follow-up of samples from the general population eating plant sterol and stanol enriched foods by post marketing surveillance techniques is important to evaluate both the beneficial as well as the adverse effects on the very long term.

As reported in Chapter 10, homocysteine is a sulphydryl-containing aminoacid derived from demethylation of methionine and is metabolized either by remethylation or by transsulfuration. Nutritional deficiencies in the vitamin cofactors (folate, vitamin B12, and vitamin B6) required for homocysteine metabolism may promote hyperhomocysteinemia.

The prevalence of hyperhomocysteinaemia has been estimated to be about 5% in the general population, and 13-47% among patients with symptomatic atherosclerotic vascular disease. Multiple prospective and case-control studies suggested that a moderately elevated plasma homocysteine concentration is an independent risk factor for atherothrombotic vascular disease. Homocysteine concentrations are consistently higher in patients with peripheral, cerebrovascular, and coronary artery disease than in those without such diseases. Homocysteine seems to promote atherothrombogenesis by a variety of mechanisms; however, it is not yet clear whether homocysteine itself or a related metabolite or cofactor is primarily responsible for the atherothrombogenic effects of hyperhomocysteinemia in vivo. Before advocating widespread screening of patients with atherosclerotic vascular disease, we must have a clearer understanding of the clinical efficacy of potential therapeutic interventions. Vitamin supplementation decreases or even normalizes plasma homocysteine concentrations in most cases. Prospective, randomized clinical trials, however, will be necessary to determine the effect of vitamin supplementation on cardiovascular morbidity and mortality. The use of pills containing low dose B vitamins as a primary or secondary preventive measure against vascular disease remains unproved, although they are definitely cheap, probably innocuous, and may help prevent acute vascular episodes.

In Chapter 11, one of the earliest steps in the development of atherosclerosis involves a complex interaction between the vascular endothelium and various circulating components such as inflammatory cells, acute-phase proteins, and proatherogenic lipids. This initiates a cascade of endothelial injury and response-to-injury events, which, perhaps depending on the genetic vulnerability and the burden of risk factors, could have important implications for the clinical outcome of the vascular disease. Mounting epidemiological, experimental and microbiological evidence suggests that a wide spectrum of microbes could modulate the interaction between lipids & inflammation and the vascular endothelium, and influence the development of atherosclerosis. Accumulating studies support the view that pediatric population might represent a more fertile ground for the noxious effects of infection, possibly, in part, due to more sustained inflammatory and lipid-related mechanisms set by infection. In light of the multifactorial etiology of atherosclerosis, an interdisciplinary approach is important when establishing strategies aimed to retard atherosclerosis in order to attain gratifying benefit on the clinical outcome later in life.

In: Cholesterol in Atherosclerosis and Coronary Heart Disease ISBN 1-59454-302-X
Editor: Jean P. Kovala, pp.1-28 

*Chapter I*

# The Emerging Role of High-density Lipoprotein in the Management of Cardiovascular Disease

***Peter P. Toth****
University of Illinois School of Medicine, Peoria, Illinois

## Abstract

High density lipoproteins mediate a variety of antiatherogenic effects. These include reverse cholesterol transport, reversal of endothelial dysfunction, and reduction of inflammation, among others. A large corpus of epidemiologic data has consistently demonstrated that high levels of HDL protect against the development of atherosclerotic disease, while low levels of this lipoprotein substantially increase risk for MI, stroke, sudden death, and restenosis after angioplasty. There is substantial clinical trial based support for treating patients with low HDL with pharmacotherapy. In the primary and secondary prevention settings, such statin trials as AFCAPs/TexCAPs, LCAS, and HATS demonstrate significant risk reduction when treating patients with low HDL and average or elevated LDL levels (≥ 130 mg/dL). Numerous new therapies for raising HDL and treating CAD in patients with low HDL are under active investigation. CETP inhibitors, a vaccine against CETP, an edible form of HDL comprised of D-amino acids, and bioengineered HDLs will be entering endpoint-driven, large-scale clinical trials. The results of these studies will help to more poignantly delineate the role of HDL in the prevention and treatment of atherosclerotic disease. In the meantime, the treatment of patients with low HDL with statins, fibrates, and niacin yields significant reductions in risk for cardiovascular morbidity and mortality and has also been shown to decrease the rate of progression of atheromatous plaques in patients with CAD.

---

* M.D., Ph.D., FAAFP, FICA, FACC, Director of Preventive Cardiology, Sterling Rock Falls Clinic, Sterling, Illinois, University of Illinois School of Medicine, Peoria, Illinois. Email: peter.toth@srfc.com; Tel: (815) 632-5093; Fax: (815) 626-5947.

# Introduction

Derangements in lipoprotein metabolism play a pivotal role in the development of atherosclerotic disease. A large number of clinical trials have clearly demonstrated that lowering serum levels of low-density lipoproteins (LDL) is associated with significant reductions in cardiovascular morbidity and mortality [1-5] and rates of coronary atheroma plaque progression [6]. Other lipoproteins such as chylomicron and very low-density lipoprotein (VLDL) remnant particles are also believed to be atherogenic [7]. Based on the analysis of a large number of prospective epidemiologic studies and clinical intervention trials using a variety of pharmacologic agents, the National Cholesterol Education Program (NCEP) has articulated clearly defined goals for LDL and non-high-density lipoprotein (non-HDL) cholesterol based on global cardiovascular risk [8]. There is increasing recognition that, in addition to LDL and non-HDL, serum levels of high-density lipoprotein (HDL) also play a role in the determination of risk for atherosclerotic disease.

The NCEP has defined a serum HDL level < 40 mg/dL as a categorical risk factor for the development of coronary artery disease (CAD; 8). High serum levels of HDL are generally protective against the development of atherosclerotic disease. In Framingham risk scoring, an HDL > 60 mg/dL is a negative risk factor and is assigned a value of "-1." The Framingham Study showed that for every 20% increase in HDL, risk for CAD decreases 50% (Figure 1; 9]. Low serum levels of HDL strongly predispose patients to the development of CAD. In the Quebec Cardiovascular Study every 10% drop in HDL was associated with a 13% elevation in risk for CAD [10]. In the Kuipio Ischemic Heart Disease Risk Factor Study, an HDL < 42 mg/dL increased risk for a myocardial infarction (MI) 3.3-fold [11]. The Tromso Heart Study, a case-control study of 6595 men aged 20-49 years of age, showed that patients who developed CAD had HDL levels 35% lower than controls and that a low HDL increased the risk for CAD three-fold more than elevated LDL [12].

Low serum concentrations of HDL are the most common lipid abnormality in patients with CAD and occur in approximately 63% of these patients [13,14]. Low HDL is an important characteristic of the metabolic syndrome and is associated with increased risk for myocardial infarction [15], carotid artery disease [16], stroke and disability in the elderly [17,18], sudden death [19], restenosis after angioplasty [20] and severe atherosclerotic disease in the proximal left main coronary artery [21].

Low HDL is highly prevalent in the United States and occurs in approximately 15% of women and 35% of men [22]. The incidence of low HDL is expected to rise dramatically as the number of people afflicted with obesity, metabolic syndrome, and diabetes mellitus increases. The Western Collaborative Group Study, Cooperative Lipoprotein Phenotyping Study, Framingham Offspring Study, Israeli Ischemic Heart Disease Study, Honolulu Heart Study, and the Poland and United States Collaborative Study on Cardiovascular Epidemiology, among other studies, have all demonstrated that HDL is an independent risk factor for atherosclerotic disease [23-28]. Some clinicians believe that low HDL is associated with increased risk for CAD because it is a marker of hypertriglyceridemia and increased serum remnant particle concentrations. The Prospective Cardiovascular Munster Study [29]

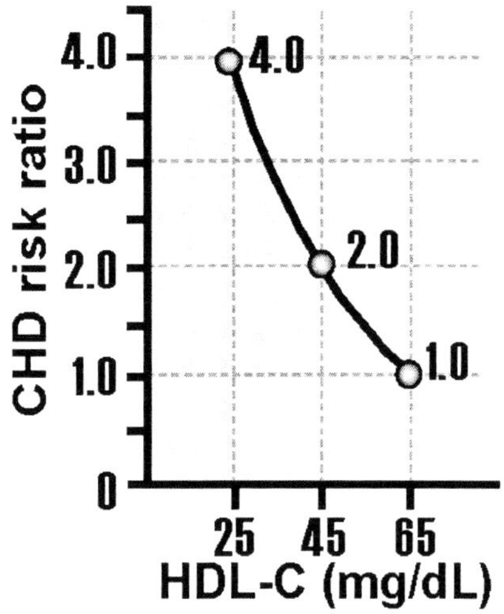


Figure 1. The relationship between risk for coronary heart disease and serum HDL in the Framingham Study. (Based on Kannel WB. High-density lipoproteins: epidemiologic profile and risks of coronary artery disease. *Am J Cardiol.* 1983;52:9B–12B.)

and ten-year follow-up data from the Caerphilly and Speedwell cohorts showed that the increased risk for CAD associated with low HDL is independent of serum triglyceride concentrations [30].

Despite the plethora of data correlating low HDL with increased risk for CAD, few physicians target this lipoprotein for therapeutic elevation. There are a number of reasons for this. First, raising HDL can pose a formidable challenge and often requires the use of intensive lifestyle modification and multiple drugs in order for it to be successful. Long-term compliance with such regimens is frequently low. Second, there are no currently no drugs available which specifically induce HDL elevation and leave other lipid fractions unchanged. This leaves open the question as to whether increasing HDL truly modulates risk for CAD independent of other lipoprotein fractions. Multivariate analysis of data from both the LIPID [31] and 4S [32] trials suggest that raising HDL with statin therapy does contribute to overall cardiovascular risk reduction. Third, the NCEP did not specify a target level to which HDL should be raised. More specific guidance has been promulgated for high risk groups. The Expert Group on HDL advocates a target value for HDL of 40 mg/dL or more in patients with CAD, CAD risk equivalents (diabetes mellitus, carotid artery disease, peripheral vascular disease, abdominal aortic aneurysm), metabolic syndrome, and patients with a 10-year Framingham risk that exceeds 20% [33]. Among diabetic patients, the American Diabetes Association defines an HDL $\geq$ 40 mg/dL as optimal [34]. In a multivariate analysis of macrovascular disease prevention in diabetic patients, the most important risk factor to address after LDL reduction is HDL elevation [35]. The American Heart Association (AHA) acknowledges that among women HDL $<$ 50 mg/dL is abnormal [36]. The AHA advocates the use of lifestyle modification and pharmacologic intervention to raise HDL above this threshold in women.

# Atheroprotective Effects of HDL

## Reverse Cholesterol Transport

Considerable clinical and basic scientific investigation have revealed some of the molecular mechanisms by which HDL inhibits atherogenesis. The most important of these mechanisms is reverse cholesterol transport (RCT), a series of reactions by which HDL is able to extract cholesterol from macrophages and fibroblasts resident within the subendothelial space of blood vessel walls and deliver it back to the liver for disposal as bile salts or biliary cholesterol or to steroidogenic organs for conversion into steroid hormones (Figure 2; 37]. The ability of HDL to increase the systemic clearance of cholesterol has been experimentally verified in human subjects [38]. If a patient has a reduced capacity to drive RCT secondary to decreased hepatic expression of apoprotein A-I, changes in enzyme activities, or low levels of HDL receptor expression, there will be progressive accumulation of cholesterol in the vessel wall. In contrast, recent investigations have shown that patients with increased capacity to export cholesterol out of blood vessel walls have decreased risk for atherosclerosis [39].

Reverse cholesterol transport involves a complex series of reactions. These are detailed in sequence below.

### *Apoprotein A-I*

Apoproteins A-I (apoA-I) and A-II (apoA-II) are the predominant apoprotein constituents of HDL. ApoA-I is produced by both the intestine and liver and can be secreted into plasma in its free form, as a component of HDL secreted by the liver, or as an apoprotein constituent of VLDL and chylomicra. ApoA-I can interact with macrophages and induce the concurrent extracellular translocation of phospholipid and cholesterol [40]. ApoA-I interacts with externalized cholesterol and phospholipid in the extracellular space to form nascent discoidal HDL (ndHDL; Figure 2). Because apoA-I is such an efficient acceptor of free cholesterol, the intravenous injection of apoA-I [41] and the transgenic overexpression of ApoA-I [42] in a variety of animal models is associated with reduced risk for atherosclerotic disease and can induce some degree of atheromatous plaque regression.

Low serum levels of apoA-I [43,44] and some mutations in this apoprotein are highly correlated with increased risk for atherosclerotic disease. Twenty three different mutations in apoA-I are associated with low HDL [i.e., hypoalphalipoproteinemia; 45]. Patients with ApoA-$I_{Zavalla}$ ($Leu_{159}$→Pro) experience a 4-fold reduction in serum HDL and have increased risk for CAD [46]. It is important to point out that not all apoA-I mutations associated with low HDL elevate risk for CAD. Patients who express ApoA-$I_{Milano}$ ($Arg_{173}$→Cys) have marked hypoalphalipoproteinemia (HDL 15-25 mg/dL) and manifest resistance to CAD. This apparent contradiction is largely attributable to the observations that ApoA-$I_{Milano}$ can inhibit platelet aggregation [47] and appears to have augmented capacity for stimulating the extracellular translocation of cholesterol from macrophages [48]. The treatment of mice with ApoA-$I_{Milano}$ infusions reduces the cholesterol content of fatty streaks [49] and atheromatous plaque [50]. The weekly intravenous infusion of ApoA-$I_{Milano}$ liposomes into humans with

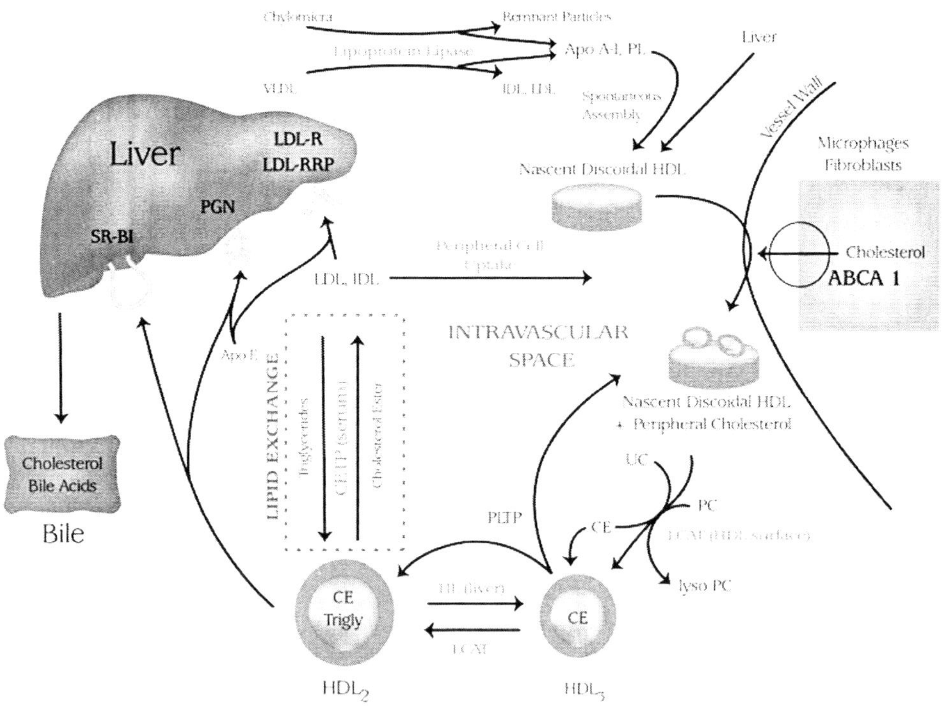


Figure 2. Molecular apparatus for reverse cholesterol transport. In order to deliver peripheral cholesterol back to the liver or steroidogenic organs such as the adrenal glands or ovaries, HDL interacts with cells such as macrophages within blood vessel walls. The HDL undergoes a series of cell receptor- and serum enzyme-dependent maturation reactions (i.e., “HDL speciation”). Abbreviations: ABCA1, ATP-binding membrane cassette transporter A1; Apo A-I, apoprotein A-I; ApoE, apoprotein E; CE, cholesteryl ester; CETP, cholesterol ester transfer protein; HL, hepatic lipase; IDL, intermediate-density lipoprotein; LCAT, lecithin:cholesterol acyltransferase, LDL, low-density lipoprotein; LDL-R, low-density lipoprotein receptor; LDL-RRP, low-density lipoprotein receptor-related protein; lysoPC, lysophosphatidylcholine; PC, phosphatidylcholine; PGN, proteoglycans; PL, phospholipid; PLTP, phospholipid transfer protein; SR-BI, scavenger receptor BI; Trigly, triglyceride; UC, unesterified cholesterol; VLDL, very low-density lipoprotein. (Reprinted with permission from *Toth PP. High-density lipoprotein: epidemiology, metabolism, and antiatherogenic effects. Disease-A-Month 2001; 47(8): 365-416.)*

CAD and a recent history of an acute coronary syndrome decreased plaque volume by 4.2% after only 5 weeks of therapy as determined by intravascular ultrasonography [51]. Given these results, there is understandably much excitement surrounding the possibility that HDL mimetics may radically transform the management of CAD.

### *ABCA1*

The ATP-binding membrane cassette transport protein A1 (ABCA1) mediates the transport of cholesterol into the extracellular space. Mutations in this transporter are responsible for the low serum levels of HDL in patients with Tangier's disease and familial hypoalphalipoproteinemia [52]. ABCA1 initiates the first step in RCT. ABCA1 transports cholesterol and phospholipid into the extracellular space using adenosine triphosphate as an energy source [53]. If ABCA1 is functionally impaired, apoA-I cannot be appropriately lipidated and it is more rapidly catabolized and cleared from serum. This can result in hypoalphalipoproteinemia. ApoA-I interacts directly with ABCA1 [54]. The amino acid residues at positions 220-231 in apoA-I promote specific binding to ABCA1 and result in the efflux of cellular lipid and ndHDL formation.

ABCA1 activity affects serum levels of HDL, the capacity for RCT, and risk for atherosclerotic disease. Two different studies with transgenic mice overexpressing human ABCA1 provide strong experimental support for these conclusions. These mice experience elevations in serum levels of apoA-I and HDL, increased rates of cholesterol and phospholipid externalization, increased RCT as demonstrated by increased biliary cholesterol excretion, and decreased risk for atheroslcerotic disease [55,56]. In the Regression Growth Evaluation Statin Study, Dutch men with the R219K form of ABCA1 have higher HDL, lower triglyceride, slower progression of CAD, and lower risk for acute coronary events [57]. Patients heterozygous for ABCA1 mutations with reduced capacity for lipid externalization have decreased serum HDL, increased triglycerides, and a three-fold higher risk for CAD with earlier onset compared to family members without these mutations [58]. Among the subjects in this study, every 8% change in ABCA1-mediated cholesterol efflux gave rise to a 0.1 mmol/L change in serum HDL. Another example of an ABCA1 variant is $ABCA1_{Alabama}$ (C254→T), a mutation associated with hypoalphalipoproteinemia and increased risk for premature CAD [59].

### *LCAT*

The enzyme lecithin:cholesterol acyltransferase (LCAT) esterifies cholesterol on the surface of HDL. The *sn*-2 fatty acid of phosphatidylcholine is used as an acyl chain donor. Esterified cholesterol partitions into the hydrophobic core of HDL particles. The esterification of externalized cholesterol establishes a local concentration gradient for free cholesterol out of peripheral cells. As the esterified cholesterol content of the HDL particle increases, it becomes rounder and larger, leading to the successive formation of two distinct HDL species, $HDL_3$ and $HDL_2$ (Figure 2).

Multiple mutations are known to affect LCAT activity. Familial LCAT deficiency is attributable to such mutations as $Lys_{209}$→Pro and $Met_{252}$→Ile. Patients who are homozygous for these mutations have complete or nearly complete loss of LCAT activity. The mutation ($Pro_{260}$→Stop) is associated with low serum HDL and apoA-I [60]. This is because patients with impairments in LCAT function have reduced capacity for cholesterol ester formation and increased catabolic rates and renal clearance of serum apoA-I and ndHDL. Despite the hypoalphalipoproteinemia found in these patients, there is no clear relationship between the severity of LCAT deficiency and risk for atherosclerotic disease. There are no known mutations that result in human LCAT overexpression. In one rabbit model, the overexpression of LCAT decreased risk for atherosclerotic disease [61].

LCAT is activated by apoA-I. The interaction between apoA-I and LCAT is dependent on three strictly conserved arginine residues (positions 149, 153, and 160) found within the α-helical repeat formed by amino acid residues 143-164 [62]. $ApoA\text{-}I_{Mallorca}$ has a decreased capacity to activate LCAT, reduced ability to promote intracellular cholesterol mobilization, and is associated with familial hypoalphalipoproteinemia [63].

### *PLTP*

Phospholipid transfer protein (PLTP) catalyzes the transfer of phospholipids from apoB100-containing lipoproteins into HDL particles. PLTP can remodel HDL into larger and smaller lipoprotein particles in a process termed "HDL conversion" [64]. During HDL conversion, two molecules of $HDL_3$ can fuse and then spontaneously split, thereby forming $HDL_2$ and ndHDL (Figure 2). Because ndHDL functions as an important acceptor of peripheral cholesterol, it has been suggested that PLTP overexperession might be antiatherogenic by promoting RCT [65]. No human polymorphisms resulting in PLTP overexpression are currently known. In a transgenic mouse model engineered to overexpress human PLTP, there is a 30-40% decrease in plasma HDL and a 2- to 3-fold increase in ndHDL compared to wild-type mice [66]. In support of this hypothesis, macrophages incubated with the plasma of these transgenic mice accumulate less LDL-derived cholesteryl esters than macrophages incubated with wild-type murine plasma. More recent *in vivo* investigations with transgenic mice have, however, refuted this hypothesis. As the magnitude of PLTP overexpression is varied 2- to 9-fold in mice fed a high fat and high cholesterol diet, serum HDL levels progressively decrease and the severity of aortic atheromatous plaque increases compared to wild-type mice [67]. The reductions in serum HDL and appear to strongly overshadow any elevation in ndHDL formation that PLTP overexpression may induce [68].

### *CETP*

Cholesterol ester transfer protein (CETP) facilitates the equimolar exchange of cholesteryl esters in HDL for triglycerides in apoB100-containing lipoproteins. The cholesteryl esters incorporated into these apoB lipoproteins can then be partitioned into multiple physiologic compartments, which include: (1) transfer to the liver via the LDL receptor and the LDL receptor-related protein (indirect RCT); and (2) transfer to such peripheral tissues as macrophages resident in blood vessel walls (Figure 2). Cholesterol delivered to the liver can either be excreted into bile or repackaged into apoB100-containing lipoproteins secreted into the circulation.

A number of polymorphisms in the CETP gene result in CETP deficiency and elevated serum HDL levels. These polymorphisms are the focus of considerable investigation. CETP deficiency is most intensively characterized in the Japanese. People in the Omagari region of Japan have a relatively high incidence of total CETP deficiency. This is attributable to homozygosity for a G→A mutation in the 5' splice donor site of intron 14 of the CETP gene. The HDL of affected individuals can be elevated 3- to 4-fold relative to individuals without this polymorphism. The mutation $D_{442}$→G in exon 15 decreases CETP activity by 30% and increases HDL levels 1- to 2-fold.

Some studies have shown reduced capacity for HDL mediated macrophage lipid extraction and increased risk for CAD in patients with near total CETP deficiency [69], though this issue remains unsettled. Patients who are heterozygous for CETP mutations and have some residual CETP activity appear to have decreased risk for CAD. Japanese-

American men enrolled in the Honolulu Heart Program with the $D_{442}$→G mutation and HDL levels > 60 mg/dL have a lower risk for coronary events relative to those participants whose HDL < 60 mg/dL [70]. In a seven-year follow-up study of 2,340 men aged 71-93 years enrolled in the Honolulu Heart Program, CETP deficiency states were associated with higher mean serum HDL and lower risk for CAD [71]. In another study evaluating Japanese men living in Kochi Prefecture, the $D_{442}$→G or Int14 +1 G→A mutations are associated with significantly fewer CAD-related events [72]. In the VA-HIT trial, the *Taq*I B2B2 genotype was associated with decreased CETP activity, increased baseline HDL levels, and a 48% lower risk for CHD compared to patients homozygous for the B1 allele [73]. An example of a CETP mutation that decreases HDL and increases risk for CAD is *EcoN*1 G/G [74].

Currently available pharmacologic interventions have relatively limited ability to increase low baseline levels of HDL. The modulation of HDL levels by therapeutic CETP inhibition has become an intense focus of investigation. Rabbits vaccinated with anti-CETP sera have a significant reduction in CETP activity, elevation in serum HDL levels, and decreased aortic atherosclerosis [75]. In a small pilot study, the injection of anti-CETP sera in humans was well tolerated and 53% of subjects developed autoantibodies after two injections [76]. The effects of vaccination on lipoprotein metabolism and whether or not a booster vaccinations will be necessary to sustain CETP inhibition are issues that require further exploration. Another approach to the modulation of CETP activity is to use inhibitors of this enzyme. Two such inhibitors are currently being investigated. JTT-705 inhibits CETP, raises serum HDL, and reduces aortic atherosclerosis by 70% in rabbits [77]. JTT-705 has demonstrated short-term safety in humans and can raise HDL up to 37% in a dose-dependent fashion after 1 month of therapy [78]. Torcetrapib administered at a dose of 120 mg twice daily can increase HDL in humans in a dose-dependent manner by up to 91% [79] and 106% [80]. Long-term outcome trials will have to be performed with each of these approaches in order to establish whether or not they produce sustained elevations in serum HDL, augment RCT, and decrease coronary morbidity and mortality [81].

### *Hepatic Lipase*

Hepatic lipase (HL) is produced by hepatocytes and plays an important role in HDL metabolism. HL is associated with the heparan sulfate proteoglycans of hepatocytes in the space of Disse and the endothelium lining hepatic sinusoids. HL hydrolyzes phospholipids and triglycerides during the conversion of $HDL_2$ to $HDL_3$ and of large buoyant to small dense LDL (Figure 2). A number of studies have examined the impact of HL polymorphisms on serum HDL levels. It is estimated that allelic variation in the gene for HL generates 25% of the variation in HDL levels in humans [82]. The overexpression of HL is associated with a high incidence of low HDL among Turkish men (53%) and women (26%) [83], which likely contributes to the high rate of premature CAD in this population. Mutations in the promoter region of the HL gene such as $G_{250}$→A and $C_{514}$→T correlate with increased serum HDL and decreased HL activity. Some studies suggest that when low HL activity is combined with CETP deficiency, risk for CAD increases [84].

Elevated HL activity appears to be detrimental in patients with insulin resistance and hypertriglyceridemia. In the Familial Atherosclerosis Treatment Study, the inhibition of HL with antilipidemic medications in patients with CAD and hypertriglyceridemia induced net coronary artery plaque regression [85]. Patients with insulin resistance frequently have both increased HL activity and hypertriglyceridemia. The hypertriglyceridemia develops secondary to increased free fatty acid flux into the liver and increased VLDL secretion. In these patients, CETP enriches HDL and LDL particles with triglycerides. The elevated triglyceride content of these lipoprotein particles makes them better substrates for HL, resulting in accelerated catabolism of HDL and increased production of small dense LDL [86]. This significantly worsens the intensity of the atherogenic milieu of these patients.

### *Endothelial Lipase*

Endothelial lipase (EL) is produced and secreted by endothelial cells and hydrolyzes acyl chains at the *sn*-1 position of phospholipids. Two groups of investigators have demonstrated that when EL is inhibited in mice either by polyclonal antibody inhibition [87] or inactivation by gene targeting [88], serum HDL levels increase significantly (25-60%). The precise roles of EL in human HDL metabolism and RCT have yet to be fully defined. The physiologic regulation of this enzyme and the effects of EL gene polymorphisms on risk for atherosclerotic disease require additional investigation. The therapeutic modulation of EL activity may provide a potentially important means of increasing serum HDL levels in the future.

### *Hepatic HDL Receptors*

The net movement of cholesteryl esters to the liver for elimination as biliary cholesterol or conversion into bile salts is the ultimate objective of RCT. Scavenger receptor class B type I (SR-BI) is located on the surface of hepatocytes [89]. SR-BI is a high-affinity receptor for HDL and mediates selective cholesteryl ester uptake into the liver [90]. In mice SR-BI deficiency decreases biliary cholesterol, increases the concentration of cholesteryl ester in HDL, and increases risk for atherosclerotic disease [91]. The overexpression of SR-BI in mice increases biliary cholesterol, decreases serum HDL, and reduces the risk for atherogenesis [92]. These findings support the concept that it is not the absolute level of HDL that determines risk for atherosclerotic disease. Rather, it is the RCT pathway' capacity to drive sufficient extraction and translocation of excess cholesterol from the periphery back to the liver for disposal.

The process of cholesteryl ester delivery and disposal by hepatic parenchyma is complex. HDL interacts with SR-BI via multiple α-helical segments in apoA-I [93]. The targeted disruption of these α-helical segments reduces lipid transfer from HDL [94]. SR-BI facilitates the trafficking of HDL through the endocytic compartment [95]. HDL undergoes transcytosis, with the secretion of HDL-derived cholesterol across the hepatocyte's apical membrane, while the delipidated HDL particle is secreted across the basal cell surface, where it reenters the central circulation. Cholesteryl esters transported into the hepatocyte by SR-BI are channeled to a membrane compartment where they are hydrolyzed to free cholesterol and fatty acids by a neutral cholesteryl ester hydrolase [96].

Additional hepatocyte HDL receptors have been identified. The β-chain of the mitochondrial F1-ATP synthetase is expressed on the hepatocyte surface and serves as a high-affinity HDL receptor [97]. HDL interacts with this receptor via apoA-I and undergoes holoparticle endocytosis in a reaction that hydrolyzes ATP. Glycosylphosphatidylinositol-anchored HDL-binding protein 1 binds HDL with high-affinity and mediates selective cholesteryl ester uptake in mice [98]. HDL metabolism and RCT are clearly quite complex phenomena. Future investigation will likely explore the intimate molecular details of how hepatocytes determine whether cholesterol will ultimately be eliminated or recycled into apoB100 containing lipoproteins and resecreted into the circulation. Additional work will also have to be performed to determine whether other hepatic HDL receptors exist and how, if at all, they interact to coordinate hepatic lipid uptake and metabolism.

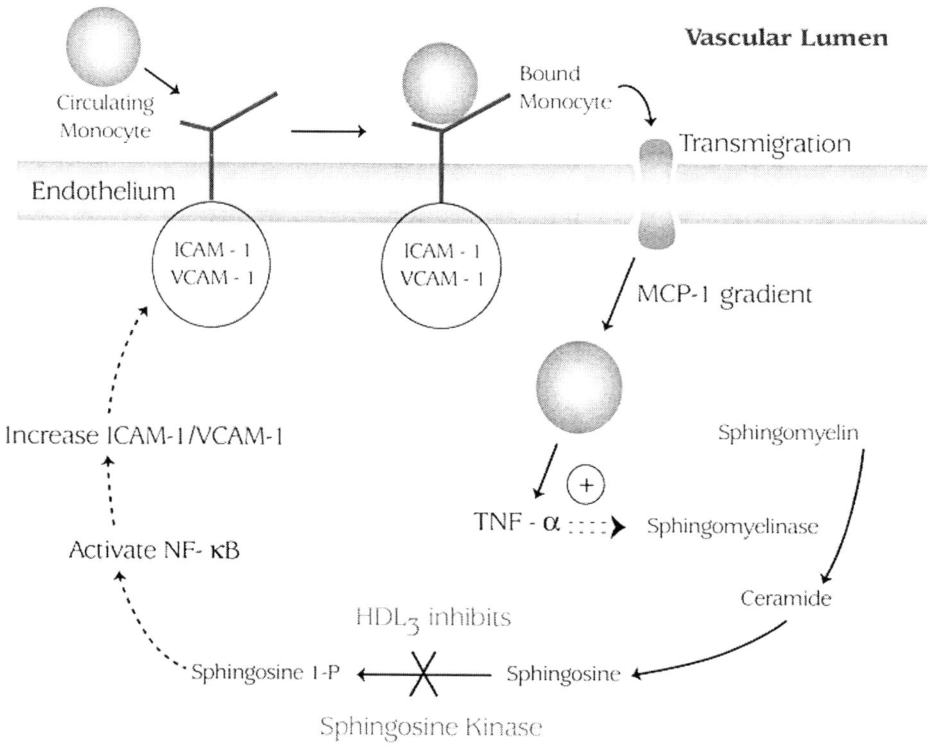


Figure 3. Inhibition of endothelial cell adhesion molecule expression by HDL. Adhesion molecules such as ICAM-1 and VCAM-1 facilitate the binding of monocytes to the luminal surface of endothelial cells. Once bound to the endothelium, monocytes can migrate into the subendothelial space by following a gradient of MCP-1. Activated monocytes can release TNF-α. TNF-α stimulates endothelial cell sphingomyelinase, an enzyme which catalyzes the production of ceramide, the precursor of sphingosine. Sphingosine is converted to sphingosine-1-phosphate by sphingosine kinase. Rising intracellular sphingosine 1-P levels activate nuclear factor κB, which increases the transcription and surface expression of a variety of inflammatory mediators, including ICAM-1 and VCAM-1. HDL attenuates endothelial cell adhesion molecule expression by inhibiting sphingosine kinase. Abbreviations: *ICAM-1*, intercellular adhesion molecule-1; *MCP-1*, monocyte chemoattractant-1; *NF-κB*, nuclear factor κB; *sphingosine 1-P*, sphingosine-1-phosphate; *TNF-α*; tumor necrosis factor-α; *VCAM-1*, vascular cell adhesion molecule-1. *(Based on work by Professor Phillip Barter, personal communication. Reprinted with permission from Toth PP. High-density lipoprotein: epidemiology, metabolism, and antiatherogenic effects. Disease-A-Month 2001; 47(8): 365-416.)*

## Additional Antiatherogenic Mechanisms

HDL exerts a number of other antiatherogenic effects. The fatty acids in LDL particles can be oxidized to reactive peroxides and hydroperoxides by transition metal cations and such enzymes as myeloperoxidase and lipoxygenase. Oxidized LDLs stimulate the expression of scavenger receptors (e.g., CD36) on the surface of macrophages resident within the subendothelial space. Scavenger receptors promote cellular cholesterol uptake and facilitate the formation of foam cells, fatty streaks, and atheromatous plaques [99]. HDLs can reduce oxidized lipids in LDL by three distinct antioxidant activities which they carry: platelet-activating factor acetylhydrolase, paraoxonase, and a variety of redox-active methionine residues contained within apoprotein A-I. HDL thereby reduces the toxicity and atherogenicity of LDL.

HDL decreases the expression of endothelial cell adhesion molecules such as ICAM-1 and VCAM-1 by inhibiting the formation of sphingosine-1-phosphate (Figure 3; 100) This decreases the binding of inflammatory white blood cells (e.g., monocytes and neutrophils) to the endothelial surface and reduces the likelihood that they will be able to transmigrate into the subendothelial space. HDL stimulates vasodilatation by stimulating endothelial cell nitric oxide (Figure 4; [101]) and prostacyclin production [102]. HDL exerts antithrombotic effects by potentiating the activities of proteins C and S [103], decreasing platelet reactivity and aggregability [104], and reducing thromboxane A2 production [105]. HDL stimulates endothelial cell mitosis along denuded areas of blood vessels [106] and inhibits endothelial cell apoptosis by delivering sphingosylphosphorylcholine and lysosulfatide, which block the activation of caspases 3 and 9 [107].

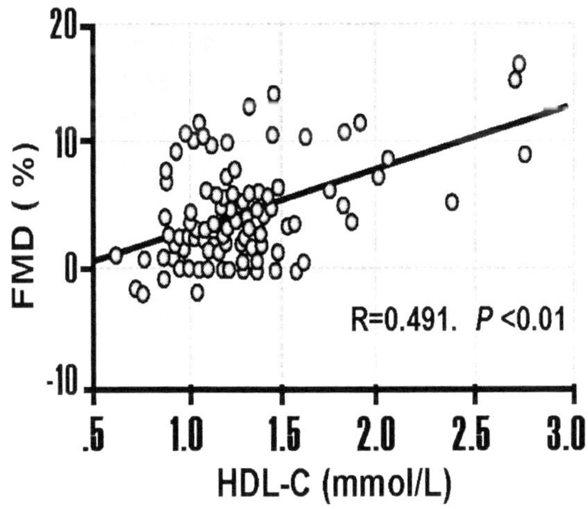


Figure 4. Effect of increasing serum HDL concentrations on brachial artery flow-mediated vasodilatation (r=0.491, p<0.01). (Reprinted with permission from *Li XP et al. Protective effect of high density lipoprotein on endothelium-dependent vasodilatation. Intn'l J Cardiol 2000; 73: 231-236.*)

Clearly, HDL can carry out a broad range of protective, antiatherogenic functions. These studies provide mechanistic insights into why epidemiologic studies consistently demonstrate that, with few exceptions, high levels of HDL reduce risk for cardiovascular morbidity and mortality, while low levels of this lipoprotein predispose patients to the development of atherosclerosis.

## Pharmacotherapy for Low HDL

A meta-analysis of data from the Framingham Study, the Multiple Risk Factor Intervention Trial, the Lipid Research Clinics Coronary Primary Prevention Trial, and the Lipid Research Clinics Prevalence Mortality Follow-up Study, demonstrated that for every 1 mg/dL rise in serum HDL for men and women, risk for future cardiovascular events decreases 2% and 3%, respectively [108]. In a cohort of 6408 Japanese men living in Osaka, for every 1 mg/dL elevation in HDL, risk for CAD and myocardial infarction decreased 5.7% and 6.4%, respectively [109]. HDL elevation is an important determinant of CAD risk reduction.

### Statins

The statins (3-hydroxy-3-methylglutaryl coenzyme A inhibitors) stimulate elevations in serum HDL by increasing rates of hepatic apoA-I expression and modestly inhibiting CETP. The various statins increase serum HDL levels to different degrees in a dose-dependent fashion (2-10%; [110]. In contrast to the other statins, atorvastatin has tendency to reduce serum HDL levels as the dose of this drug is increased. The patients with the lowest baseline levels of HDL experience relatively larger percent elevations in HDL in response to statin therapy when compared to patients with higher baseline HDL concentrations. Patients with hypertriglyceridemia can experience the most substantial elevations in HDL when treated with statins. For example, simvastatin at 40-80 mg/day can increase HDL 14-18% [111] while rosuvastatin at 20-40 mg/day can increase HDL 17-22% [112].

A number of intervention trials have confirmed the clinical efficacy statin therapy in patients with low HDL. The Air Force/Texas Coronary Atherosclerosis Prevention Study was a primary prevention trial that compared treatment with lovastatin to placebo in women and men with "average" risk for CAD (mean HDL 37 mg/dL, LDL 150 mg/dL). Patients with baseline HDL levels $< 40$ mg/dL experienced a three-fold (45% vs 15%) larger reduction in risk for first-time CAD related events compared to patients whose HDL $\geq 40$ mg/dL [113]. Consistent with these findings from AFCAPs/TexCAPs, the Heart Protection Study demonstrated a trend toward increasing benefit with simvastatin therapy as baseline HDL progressively declined [114]. One interpretation of these findings is that statin therapy significantly attenuates the excess risk associated with low HDL.

An analysis of angiographic data from the Lipoprotein Coronary Atherosclerosis Study (LCAS) showed that fluvastatin decreased rates of CAD progression significantly more in patients with baseline HDL $< 35$ mg/dL compared to those patients with HDL $\geq 35$ mg/dL ($p=0.01$; 115]. Among patients 70-82 years of age randomized to pravastatin therapy or placebo in the Prospective Study of Pravastatin in the Elderly at Risk trial, the only group with a statistically significant reduction in the primary endpoint (nonfatal MI, stroke, and coronary death) when treated with pravastatin was the one with a baseline HDL < 43 mg/dL [116]. In one study of Japanese patients with CAD, the ability of pravastatin to increase HDL levels was strongly correlated with reductions in atheromatous plaque volume as determined by intravascular ultrasound measurements, whereas reductions in total cholesterol and LDL were not [117].

Statin therapy disproportionately reduces cardiovascular morbidity and mortality as well as rates of atheromatous plaque progression in patients with low HDL. These observations may be partly explained by the fact that many of the pleiotropic effects exerted by statins (reversing endothelial cell dysfunction, augmenting nitric oxide and prostacyclin production, decreasing inflammation) can also be mediated by HDL. Statins should be the initial therapy of choice in dyslipidemic patients with a combination of low HDL and an LDL level above NCEP targets (Figure 5).

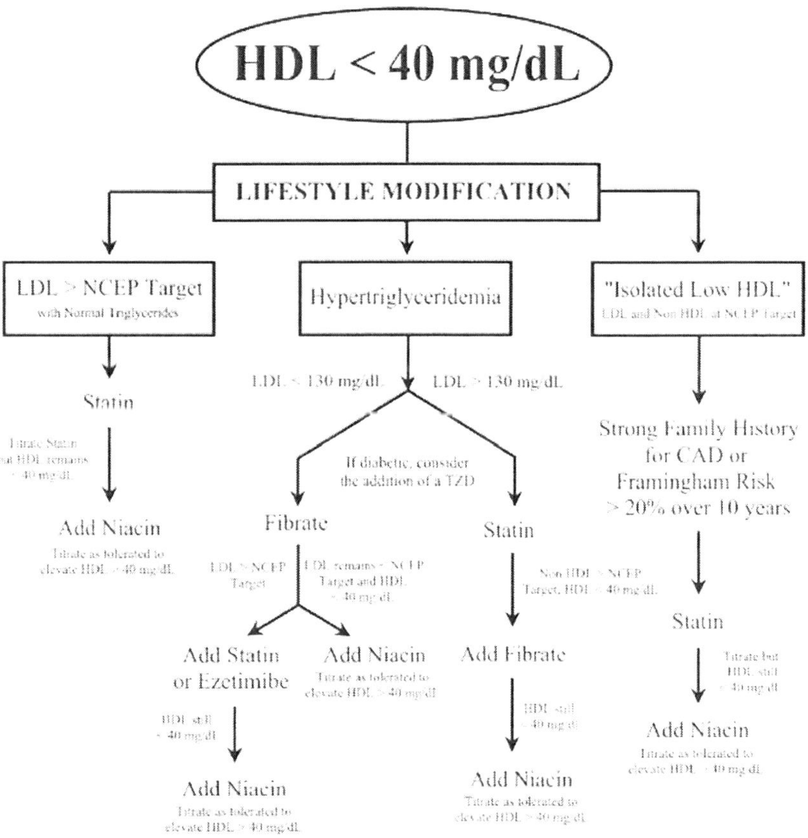


Figure 5. Flow chart depicting the management of low HDL under a variety of clinical circumstances. TZD: thiazolidinedione. (Reprinted with permission from *Toth PP. High-density lipoprotein and cardiovascular risk. Circulation 2004: 109: 1809-1812.)*

## Fibrate Therapy

Fibric acid derivatives are PPAR-α agonists with demonstrated clinical efficacy for treating patients with a combination of hypertriglyceridemia and low HDL. Fibrates stimulate HDL biosynthesis 6-20% by augmenting hepatic apoA-I expression and serum lipoprotein lipase activity. The activation of lipoprotein lipase allows for the catabolism of triacylglycerols in chylomicra and VLDL. As these large lipoproteins are hydrolyzed they release surface coat components that can be used to assimilate HDL in serum. Patients with insulin resistance are prone to low lipoprotein lipase activity due to increased production of apoCIII.

A number of fibrate intervention trials have demonstrated the efficacy of these drugs for reducing cardiovascular morbidity and mortality among patients with high serum triglycerides and low HDL (Figure 6). The Helsinki Heart Study (HHS) was a primary prevention trial which compared gemfibrozil therapy to placebo in 4081 men aged 40-55 years with dyslipidemia [118]. Among patients with baseline triglycerides > 200 mg/dL and HDL < 42 mg/dL, there was a 66% reduction in first-time cardiovascular events. The Veterans Affairs High-Density Lipoprotein Intervention Trial (VA-HIT) evaluated gemfibrozil therapy in men with CAD and mean LDL 111 mg/dL, HDL 31 mg/dL, and triglyceride 161 mg/dL over a 5 year follow-up period. The treatment group experienced a 6% elevation in HDL, no change in LDL, and a 31% reduction in triglycerides [119]. Gemfibrozil therapy reduced the composite endpoint of all-cause mortality and nonfatal MI by 22% (p=0.006) and the risk for stroke and transient ischemic attacks by 31% (p=0.036) and 59% (p<0.001), respectively. The diabetic patients enrolled in VA-HIT benefited even more from gemfibrozil therapy, with reductions of 32% (p=0.004) in the composite endpoint, 40% in stroke (p=0.046), and 41% (p=0.02) in CHD death [120]. VA-HIT was the first dyslipidemia trial to demonstrate a reduction in cardiovascular and cerebrovascular events independent of changes in serum levels of LDL. Most of the benefit of fibrate therapy was attributed to HDL elevation and the pleiotropic effects exerted by gemfibrozil. The Bezafibrate Infarction Prevention (BIP) trial was a secondary prevention trial which compared therapy with bezafibrate (400 mg/d) to placebo in 3,122 men and women with established CAD [121]. Among patients with a baseline serum triglyceride > 200 mg/dL and HDL <35 mg/dL, post-hoc analysis revealed that bezafibrate therapy decreased the composite endpoint of fatal/nonfatal MI and sudden death by 41% (p = 0.02).

Fibrates should be initial therapy in patients with hypertriglyceridemia, low HDL, and LDL < 130 mg/dL (Figure 6). Patients with such a lipid profile should also be evaluated for the metabolic syndrome and type 2 diabetes mellitus. Decreasing insulin resistance with exercise, weight loss, and thiazolidinedione (or rosiglitazone 4-8 mg daily or pioglitazone 15-45 mg daily) therapy can raise serum HDL levels.

Fibrates can be dosed as follows: (1) gemfibrozil 600 mg twice daily; or (2) fenofibrate 54 or 160 mg once daily. Fibrate therapy can induce a rise in serum LDL since these agents promote the conversion of VLDL to LDL via the activation of lipoprotein lipase in serum. If LDL levels exceed NCEP targets, then the addition of a statin or ezetimibe to the fibrate can be considered.

Gemfibrozil can decrease the elimination of statins by blocking their glucuronidation [122]. This can increase risk for hepatic and skeletal muscle toxicity. Fenofibrate does not block the glucuronidation of statins and is a safer choice when treating patients with combination therapy. No outcome trials using the combination of a fibrate and statin have yet been completed, though the Action to Control Cardiovascular Risk in Diabetes trial is underway and is evaluating the efficacy of simvastatin therapy alone to combination therapy with simvastatin and fenofibrate in 5800 diabetic patients. Fibrates can raise HDL in patients without concomitant hypertriglyceridemia.

## Niacin

Niacin raises serum HDL up to 35% by blocking its hepatic uptake and catabolism without adversely impacting cholesterol ester uptake by the liver. In the Coronary Drug Project, crystalline niacin (3000 mg daily vs placebo) given as monotherapy to men with established CAD reduced the risk for stroke and nonfatal MI by 24% and 27%, respectively, and also decreased the need for coronary bypass surgery by 47% (Figure 7; 123]. A primary prevention trial with niacin monotherapy has not yet been initiated. The combination of high-dose niacin and a statin can dramatically decrease CAD event rates and stabilize coronary plaque. In the High-Density Lipoprotein Atherosclerosis Treatment Study (HATS), patients with CAD and a mean HDL of 31 mg/dL, LDL 125 mg/dL, and triglyceride 213 mg/dL given simvastatin and 2-4 g of niacin daily experienced an 89% reduction in the composite endpoint of coronary death, MI, stroke, or the need for revascularization over three years of followup relative to placebo (Figure 8; 124]. In addition, patients given combination therapy with simvastatin and niacin experienced slight regression of atheromatous plaque volume (-0.4%). In contrast, among patients given placebo, atheromatous plaque volume increased 3.9% (Figure 9). The use of antioxidant supplements (vitamins E and C, selenium, and β-carotene) significantly attenuated the benefits of statin and niacin combination therapy in this trial.

Niacin adjuvant therapy should be used as tolerated to raise HDL above 40 mg/dL in high-risk patients who cannot achieve this threshold with statin or fibrate monotherapy (Figure 5). Crystalline niacin and Niaspan can be used at doses up to 3000 mg/day and 2000 mg/day, respectively. to raise HDL, particularly when statin or fibrate monotherapy does not raise HDL above 40 mg/dL in high-risk patients. The flushing associated with niacin usage is prostaglandin-mediated. Aspirin taken 1 hr before and avoiding fatty meals for 3-4 hrs prior to niacin dosing can help to attenuate the risk of flushing. Niacin can antagonize glycemic control, especially when administered at doses that exceed 1000 mg daily. Antiglycemic medications may have to be initiated in patients with impaired glucose tolerance or adjusted in patients with established diabetes mellitus. Niacin can provide substantial additional reductions in other lipid fractions, including LDL, triglycerides, and lipoprotein(a).

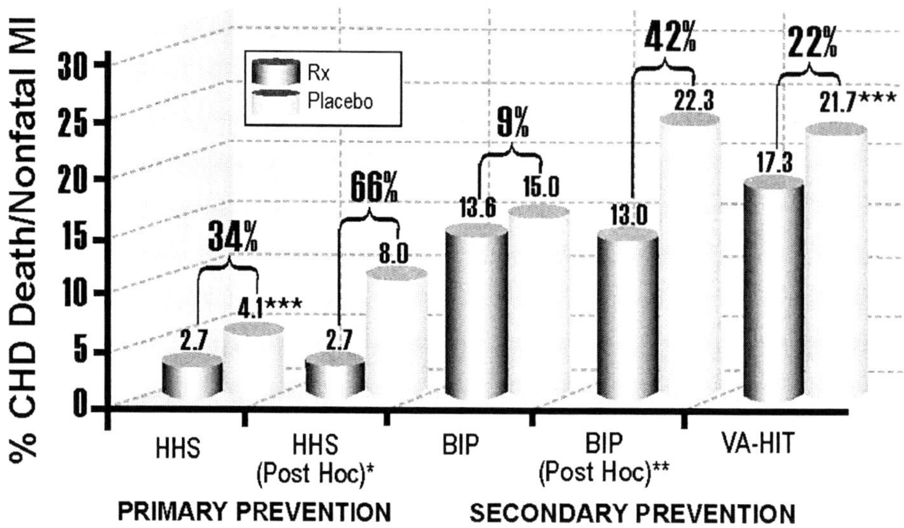


Figure 6. Effects of fibric acid derivatives on risk for primary and secondary acute coronary events. Abbreviations: Helsinki Heart Study (HHS); Veterans Affairs HDL Cholesterol Intervention Trial (VA-HIT); Bezafibrate Infarction Prevention (BIP) study. HHS "post-hoc" is for the patient sub-group with triglycerides > 200mg/dL and HDL < 42 mg/dL. BIP "post-hoc" is for the patient subgroup with triglycerides > 200 mg/dL and HDL < 35 mg/dL. (Figure obtained from LipidsOnline.org. Downloaded on 15 April 2004. Reprinted with permission).

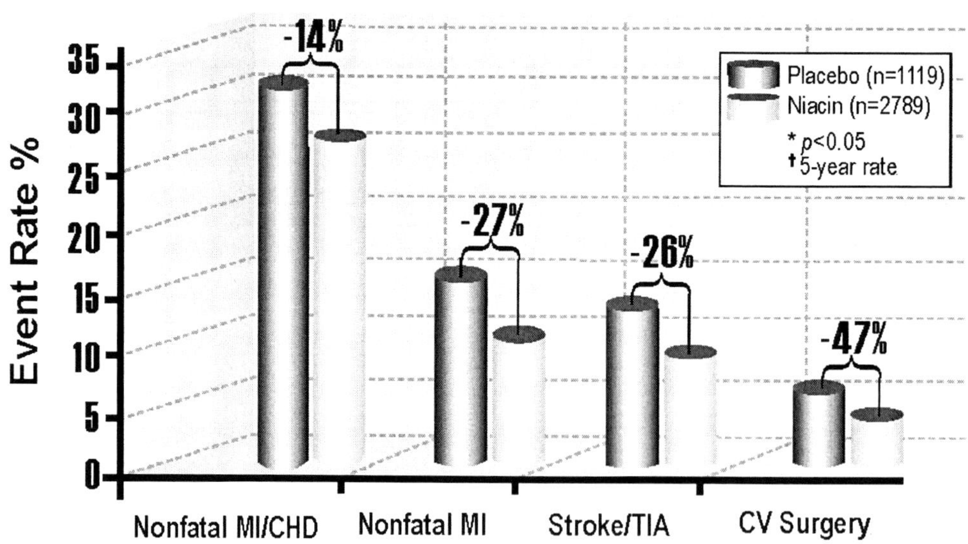


Figure 7. Effect of high-dose niacin (3.0 g/day) therapy *versus* placebo on cardiovascular outcomes in the Coronary Drug Project. (Based on *The Coronary Drug Project Research Group. Clofibrate and niacin in coronary heart disease. JAMA 1975; 231: 360-381.)*

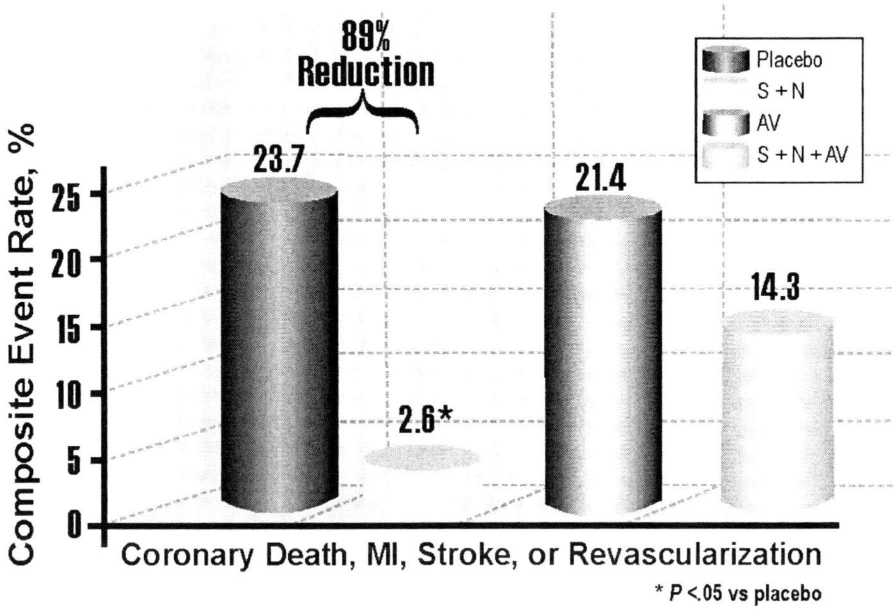


Figure 8. The effect of various treatments on the composite endpoint of coronary death, myocardial infarction (MI), stroke, and the need for revascularization in the HATS trial. Abbreviations: S+N, Simvastatin and niacin; AV, antioxidants including vitamins E and C, selenium, and beta-carotene. (Based on *Brown BG, Zhao XQ, Chait A, et al. Simvastatin and niacin, antioxidant vitamins, or the combination for the prevention of coronary disease. N Engl J Med 2001; 345: 1583-92.)*

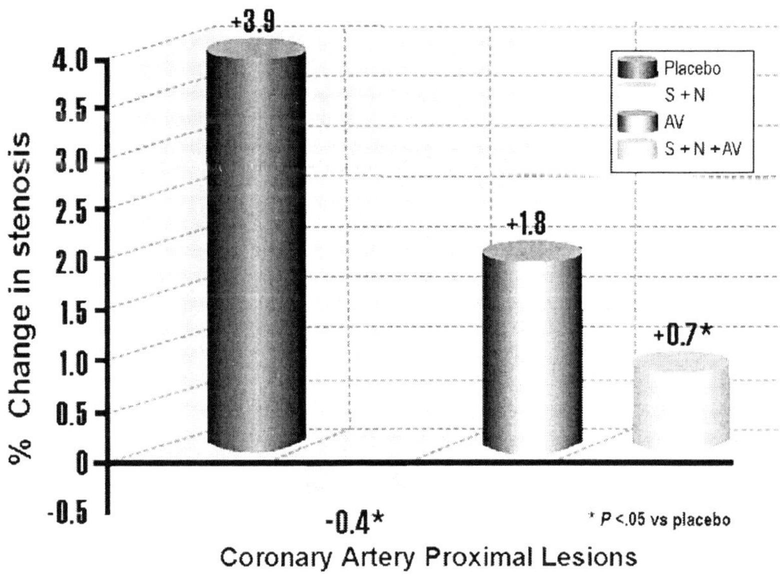


Figure 9. The effect of various treatments on percentage change in stenosis of proximal coronary arterial atheromatous lesions in the HATS trial. Abbreviations: S+N, Simvastatin and niacin; AV, antioxidants including vitamins E and C, selenium, and beta-carotene. (Based on *Brown BG, Zhao XQ, Chait A, et al. Simvastatin and niacin, antioxidant vitamins, or the combination for the prevention of coronary disease. N Engl J Med 2001; 345: 1583-92.)*

# Lifestyle Modification

The NCEP stresses the importance lifestyle modification for patients with lipoprotein concentrations that lie outside its specified target ranges. Serum HDL is decreased by cigarette smoking [125; Figure 10). However, smoking cessation can increase HDL by up to 20% over a period of months [126]. As shown in the Framingham Offspring Study, HDL correlates negatively with rising body mass index [127; Figure 11). Weight loss (1 mg/dL per 3 kg) and aerobic exercise can raise HDL, especially in patients who are markedly obese or have insulin resistance. Moderate alcohol ingestion can significantly raise serum HDL by stimulating hepatic apo A-I expression and is associated with decreased risk for acute coronary events [128].

# Conclusion

High-density lipoproteins mediate a variety of antiatherogenic effects. These include reverse cholesterol transport, reversal of endothelial dysfunction, and reduction of inflammation, among others. A large corpus of epidemiologic data has consistently demonstrated that high levels of HDL protect against the development of atherosclerotic disease, while low levels of this lipoprotein substantially increase risk for MI, stroke, sudden death, and restenosis after angioplasty.

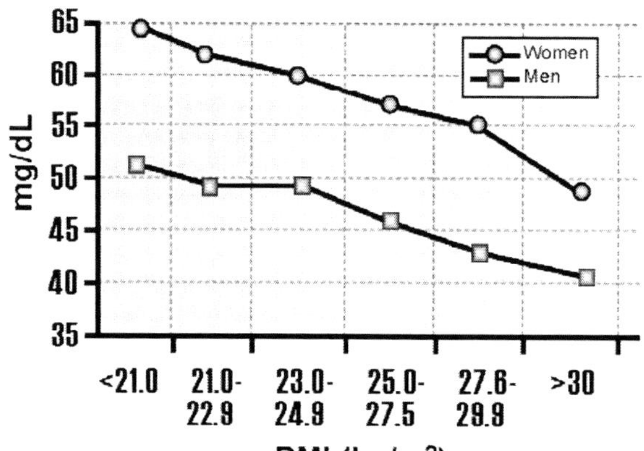


Figure 10. Mean serum HDL levels for men and women according to daily cigarette consumption in the Framingham Offspring Study. (Reprinted with permission from *Garrison RJ, Kannel WB, Feinleib M, et al. Cigarette smoking and HDL cholesterol: the Framingham Offspring Study. Atherosclerosis 1978; 30: 17-25*).

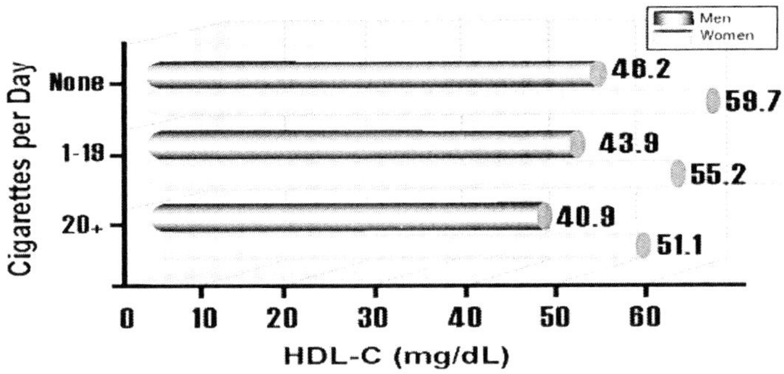


Figure 11. Mean serum HDL levels for men and women as a function of body mass index in the Framingham Offspring Study. (Figure kindly provided by Professor Peter W. F. Wilson, Director of the Framingham Offspring Study. Based on Lamon-Fava S, Wilson PWF, Schaefer EJ. Impact of body mass index on coronary heart disease risk factors in men and women. Arterioscler Thromb Vasc Biol 1996; 16: 1509-1515.)

There is substantial clinical trial based support for treating patients with low HDL with pharmacotherapy. In the primary and secondary prevention settings, such statin trials as AFCAPs/TexCAPs, LCAS, and HATS demonstrate significant risk reduction when treating patients with low HDL and average or elevated LDL levels ($\geq$ 130 mg/dL). The fibrate trials (HHS, VA-HIT, and BIP) support the treatment of patients with hypertriglyceridemia and low HDL. Patients with low HDL, normal triglycerides, and LDL $<$ 100 mg/dL comprise an equivocal group. In this clinical scenario, there is a paucity of clinical trial data to inform clinical decision making. It remains to be determined what LDL thresholds constitute high-risk for CAD at specific levels of HDL. If a patient has no other risk factors (e.g., hypertension, diabetes mellitus,, obesity, age considerations) other than an isolated low HDL but has a strong family history for premature CAD, then consideration should be given to treatment with a statin and niacin as indicated and lifestyle modification (Figure 5). If a patient presents with low HDL and has other risk factors but no evidence for CAD or a CAD risk equivalent, then calculation of the Framingham risk score is recommended. If the 10-yr risk $>$ 20%, then the patient is at high risk for CAD and should be treated with lifestyle modification and medication.

Numerous new therapies for raising HDL and treating CAD in patients with low HDL are under active investigation. CETP inhibitors [129], a vaccine against CETP [130], an edible form of HDL comprised of D-amino acids [131], and bioengineered HDLs will be entering endpoint-driven, large-scale clinical trials. The results of these studies will help to more poignantly delineate the role of HDL in the prevention and treatment of atherosclerotic disease. In the meantime, the treatment of patients with low HDL with statins, fibrates, and niacin yields significant reductions in risk for cardiovascular morbidity and mortality and has also been shown to decrease the rate of progression of atheromatous plaques in patients with CAD.

# References


[1] Sacks FM, Pfeffer MA, Moye LA, et al: The effect of Pravastatin on coronary events after myocardial infarction in patients with average cholesterol levels. *N Engl J Med* 335: 1001-1009, 1996.

[2] The LIPID Study Group: Prevention of cardiovascular events and death with pravastatin in patients with coronary heart disease and a broad range of initial cholesterol levels. *N Engl J Med* 339: 1349-1357, 1998.

[3] Scandinavian Simvastatin Survival Study Group: Randomized trial of cholesterol lowering in 4444 patients with coronary heart disease: the Scandinavian Simvastatin Survival Study (4S). *Lancet* 1999: 344; 1383-1389.

[4] Sever PS, Dahlof B, Poulter NR, et al. Prevention of coronary and stroke events with atorvastatin in hypertensive patients who have average or lower-than-average cholesterol concentrations, in the Anglo-Scandinavian Cardiac Outcomes Trial Lipid Lowering Arm (ASCOT-LLA): a mutlicentre randomised controlled trial. *Lancet* 2003;361: 1149-1157.

[5] Cannon CP, Braunwald E, McCabe CH, et al. Comparison of intensive and moderate lipid lowering with statins after acute coronary syndromes. *N Engl J Med* 2004; 350:

[6] Nissen SE, Tuzcu EM, Schoenhagen P, et al. Effect of intensive compared with moderate lipid-lowering therapy on progression of coronary atherosclerosis: a randomized controlled trial. *JAMA* 2004; 291: 1071-1080.

[7] Cullen P. Evidence that triglycerides are an independent coronary heart disease risk factor. *Am J Cardiol* 2000; 86: 943-949.

[8] Expert Panel on Detection, Evaluation, and Treatment of High Blood Cholesterol in Adults: Executive summary of the third report of the National Cholesterol Education Program (NCEP) Expert Panel on Detection, Evaluation, and Treatment of High Blood Cholesterol in Adults (Adult Treatment Panel III). *JAMA* 2001, 285: 2486-2497.

[9] Castelli WP, Garrison RJ, Wilson PWF, *et al.* Incidence of coronary heart disease and lipoprotein cholesterol levels: The Framingham Study. *JAMA* 1986; 256: 2835-8.

[10] Despres JP, Lemieux I, Dagenais GR, *et al.* HDL-cholesterol as a marker of coronary heart disease risk: the Quebec cardiovascular study. *Atherosclerosis* 2000; 153: 263-272.

[11] Salonen J, Salonen R, Seppanen K, *et al.* HDL, HDL2, and HDL3 subfractions, and the risk of acute myocardial infarction. *Circulation* 84: 129-139, 1991.

[12] Miller N, Forde O, Thelle D, *et al*: High-density lipoprotein and coronary heart disease: a prospective case-control study. *Lancet*: 965-968, 1977.

[13] Despres JP, Lemieux I, Dagenais GR, et al. HDL-cholesterol as a marker of coronary heart disease risk: the Quebec cardiovascular study. Atherosclerosis 2000; 153: 263-272.

[14] Rubins, HB, Robins SJ, Collins D, *et al.* Distribution of lipids in 8,500 men with coronary artery disease. Department of Veterans Affairs HDL Intervention Trial Study Group. *Am J Cardiol* 1995; 1196-1201.

[15] Goldbourt U, Yaari S, Medalic JH. Isolated low HDL cholesterol as a risk factor for coronary heart disease mortality: a 21-year follow-up of 8000 men. *Arterioscler Thromb Vasc Biol* 1997; 17: 107-113.

[16] Weverling-Rijnsburger AWE, Jonkers IJA, van Exel E, *et al.* High-density vs low-density lipoprotein cholesterol as the risk factor for coronary artery disease and stroke in old age. *Arch Intern Med* 2003; 163: 1549-1544.

[17] Corti MC, Guralnik JM, Silive ME, *et al*: HDL cholesterol predicts coronary heart disease mortality in older persons. *JAMA* 274: 539-544, 1995.

[18] Zuliani G, Romagnoni F, Bollini C, *et al*: Low levels of high-density lipoprotein cholesterol are a marker of disability in the elderly. *Gerontology* 45:317-322, 1999.

[19] Burke AP, Farb A, Malcom GT, *et al.* Plaque rupture and sudden death related to exertion in men with coronary artery disease. *JAMA* 1999; 281: 921-926.

[20] Shah P, Amin, J. Low high density lipoprotein level is associated with increased restenosis rate after coronary angioplasty. *Circulation* 1992; 85: 1279-1285.

[21] Pearson T, Bulkley B, Achuff S, *et al.* The association of low levels of HDL cholesterol and arteriographically defined coronary artery disease. *Am J Epidemiol* 1979; 109: 285-295.

[22] Johnson CL, Rifkind BM, Sempos CT, *et al.*: Declining serum total cholesterol levels among US adults: the National Health and Nutrition Examination Surveys. *JAMA* 1993, 269: 3002-3008.

[23] Rosenman R, Friedman M, Jenkins C, *et al*: Recurring and fatal myocardial infarction in the Western Collaborative Group Study. *Am J Cardiol* 19: 771-775, 1967.

[24] Goldbourt U, Medalie J: High density lipoprotein cholesterol and incidence of coronary heart disease: The Israeli ischemic heart disease study. *Am J Epidemiol* 109: 296-308, 1979.

[25] Wilson P, Garrison R, Castelli W, *et al*: Prevalence of coronary heart disease in the Framingham offspring study: role of lipoprotein cholesterols. *Am J Cardiol* 46: 649-654, 1980.

[26] Austin M, Rodriguez B, McKnight B, *et al*: Low-density lipoprotein particle size, triglycerides, and high-density lipoprotein cholesterol as risk factors for coronary heart disease in older Japanese-American men. *Am J Cardiol* 86: 412-416, 2000.

[27] Rywik S, Manolio T, Pajak,A, *et al*: Association of lipids and lipoprotein level with total mortality and mortality caused by cardiovascular and cancer diseases (Poland and United States collaborative study on cardiovascular epidemiology). *Am J Cardiol* 84: 540-548, 1999.

[28] Castelli W, Doyle J, Gordon T, *et al*: HDL cholesterol and other lipids in coronary heart disease. *Circulation* 55: 767-772, 1997.

[29] Assman G, and Schulte H: Relation of high-density lipoprotein cholesterol and triglycerides to incidence of atherosclerotic coronary disease (the PROCAM experience). *Am J Cardiol* 70: 733-737, 1992.

[30] Yarnell JW, Patterson CC, Sweetnam PM, *et al.* Do total and high density lipoprotein cholesterol and triglycerides act independently in the prediction of ischemic heart disease? *Arteroiscler Thromb Vasc Biol.* 2001; 21: 1340-1345.

[31] Simes, RJ, Merschner, IC, Hunt D, et al. Relationship between lipid levels and clinical outcomes in the Long-Term Intervention with Pravastatin in Ischemic Disease (LIPID) Trial. *Circulation* 2002; 105: 1162-1169.
[32] Pedersen TR, Olsson AG, Faergman O, et al. Lipoprotein changes and reduction in the incidence of major coronary events in the Scandinavian Simvastatin Survival Study. *Circulation* 1998; 97: 1453-1460.
[33] Sacks, FM and the Expert Group on HDL Cholesterol. The role of high-density lipoprotein (HDL) cholesterol in the prevention and treatment of coronary heart disease: expert group recommendations. *Am J Cardiol* 2002; 90: 139-143.
[34] American Diabetes Association. Management of dyslipidemia in adults with diabetes. *Diabetes Care* 2003; 26: S83-S86.
[35] Turner RC, Millns H, Neil HA, *et al.* Risk factors for coronary artery disease in non-insulin dependent diabetes mellitus (UKPDS 23). *BMJ* 1998; 316: 823-828.
[36] Mosca L, Appel LJ, Benjamin EJ, *et al.* Evidence-based guidelines for cardiovascular disease prevention in women. *Circulation* 2004;109:672-93.
[37] Toth PP. Reverse cholesterol transport: high-density lipoprotein's magnificent mile. *Curr Atheroscler Rep* 2003; 5: 386-393.
[38] Eriksson M, Carlson LA, Miettinen TA, et al. Stimulation of fecal steroid excretion after infusion of recombinant proapolipoprotein A-I. Potential reverse cholesterol transport in humans. *Circulation* 1999; 100: 594-8.
[39] Clee SM, Kastelein JP, van Dam M, *et al.*: Age and residual cholesterol efflux affect HDL cholesterol levels and coronary artery disease in ABCA1 heterozygotes. *J Clin Invest* 2000, 106: 1263-1270.
[40] Smith JD, Goff WL, Settle M, et al. ABCA1 mediates concurrent cholesterol and phospholipids efflux to apolipoprotein A-I. *J Lipid Res* 2004; 45:635-644.
[41] Miyazak A, Sakuma S, Morikawa W, *et al.* Intravenous injection of rabbit apolipoprotein A-I inhibits the progression of atherosclerosis in cholesterol-fed rabbits. *Arterioslcer Thromb Vasc Biol* 1995; 15: 1882-1888.
[42] Tangirala RK, Tsukamoto K, Chun SH, *et al.* Regression of atherosclerosis induced by liver-directed gene transfer of apolipoprotein A-I in mice. *Circulation* 1999; 100: 1816-1822.
[43] Downs JR, Clearfield M, Weis S, *et al.*: Primary prevention of acute coronary events with lovastatin in men and women with average cholesterol levels. Results of AFCAPS/TexCAPS. *JAMA* 1998, 279: 1615-1622.
[44] Assman G: Pro and con: high-density lipoprotein, triglycerides, and other lipid subfractions are the future of lipid management. *Am J Cardiol* 2000, 87(suppl): 2B-7B.
[45] Sorci-Thomas MG, Thomas MJ: The effects of altered apolipoprotein A-I structure on plasma HDL concentration. *Trends Cardiovasc Med* 2002, 12: 121-128.
[46] Miller M, Aiello D, Pritchard H, *et al.*: Apolipoprotein A-I Zavalla (Leu159→Pro): HDL cholesterol deficiency in a kindred associated with premature coronary artery disease. *Arterioscler Thromb Vasc Biol* 1998, 18: 1242-1247.
[47] Li D, Weng S, Yang B, *et al.*: Inhibition of arterial thrombus formation by apoA-I Milano. *Arterioscler Thromb Vasc Biol* 1999, 19: 378-383.

[48] Chiesa G, Sirtori CR. Apolipoprotein A-I Milano: current perspectives. *Curr Opin Lipidol* 2003; 14: 159-163.

[49] Chisea G, Monteggia E, Marchesi M, *et al.* Recombinant apolipoprotein A-I Milano infusion into rabbit carotid artery rapidly removes lipid from fatty streaks. *Circ Res* 2002; 90: 974-980.

[50] Shah PK, Yano J, Reyes O, *et al.* High-dose recombinant apolipoprotein A-I Milano mobilizes tissue cholesterol and rapidly reduces plaque lipid and macrophage content in apolipoprotein E-deficient mice: potential implications for acute plaque stabilization. *Circulation* 2001; 103: 3047-3050.

[51] Nissen SE, Tsunoda T, Tuzcu EM, *et al.* Effect of recombinant apoA-I Milano on coronary atherosclerosis in patients with acute coronary syndromes. A randomized controlled trial. *JAMA* 2003; 290: 2292-2300.

[52] Brooks-Wilson A, *et al.*: Mutations in ABCA1 in Tangier disease and familial high-density lipoprotein deficiency. *Nat Genet* 1999, 22: 336-345.

[53] Attie AD, Kastelein JP, Hayden MR: Pivotal role of ABCA1 in reverse cholesterol transport influencing HDL levels and susceptibility to atherosclerosis. *J Lipid Res* 2001, 42: 1717-1726.

[54] Chroni A, Liu T, Gorshkova I, *et al.*: The central helices of ApoA-I can promote ATP-binding cassette transporter A1 (ABCA1)-mediated lipid efflux. *J Biol Chem* 2003; 278(9): 6719-6730.

[55] Vaisman BL, Lambert G, Amar M, *et al.*: ABCA1 overexpression leads to hyperalphalipoproteinemia and increased biliary cholesterol excretion in transgenic mice. *J Clin Invest* 2001, 108: 303-309.

[56] Singaraja RR, Fiever C, Castro G, *et al.*: Increased ABCA1 activity protects against atherosclerosis. *J Clin Invest* 2002, 110: 35-42.

[57] Clee SM, Zwinderman AH, Engert JC, *et al.*: Common genetic variation in ABCA1 is associated with altered lipoprotein levels and a modified risk for coronary artery disease. *Circulation* 2001, 103: 1198-1205.

[58] Clee SM, Kastelein JP, van Dam M, *et al.*: Age and residual cholesterol efflux affect HDL cholesterol levels and coronary artery disease in ABCA1 heterozygotes. *J Clin Invest* 2000, 106: 1263-1270.

[59] Hong SH, Rhyne J, Zeller K, *et al.*: $ABCA1_{Alabama}$: a novel variant associated with HDL deficiency and premature coronary artery disease. *Atherosclerosis* 2002, 164: 245-250.

[60] Kasid A, Rhyne J, Zeller K, *et al.*: A novel TC deletion resulting in Pro260→Stop in the human LCAT gene is associated with a dominant effect on HDL-cholesterol. *Atherosclerosis* 2001, 156: 127-132.

[61] Hoeg J, Santamarina-Fojo S, Berard A, *et al.*: Overexpression of lecithin: cholesterol acyltransferase in transgenic rabbits prevents diet-induced atherosclerosis. *Proc Natl Acad Sci* 1996, 93: 11448-11453.

[62] Roosbeck S, Vanloo B, Duverger N, *et al.*: Three arginine residues in apolipoprotein A-I are critical for activation of lecithin:cholesterol acyltransferase. *J Lipid Res* 2001, 42: 31-40.

[63] Martin-Campos JM, Julve J, Escola JJ, *et al.*: ApoA-$I_{Mallorca}$ impairs LCAT activation and induces familial hypoalphalipoproteinemia. *J Lipid Res* 2002, 43: 115-123.
[64] Husskonen J, Olkkonen VM, Jauhiainen M, *et al.*: The impact of phospholipid transfer protein (PLTP) on HDL metabolism. *Atherosclerosis* 2001; 155: 269-281.
[65] Cheung M, Wolfbauer G, Brown B, *et al.*: Relationship between plasma phospholipid transfer protein activity and HDL subclasses among patients with low HDL and cardiovascular disease. *Atherosclerosis* 1999; 142: 201-205.
[66] van Haperen R, van Tol A, Vermeulen P, *et al.*: Human phospholipid transfer protein increases the antiatherogenic potential of high density lipoproteins in transgenic mice. *Arterioscler Thromb Vasc Biol* 2000; 20: 1082-1088.
[67] van Haperen R, van Tol A, van Gent T, *et al.*: Increased risk of atherosclerosis by elevated plasma levels of phospholipid transfer protein. *J Biol Chem* 2002; 277(50): 48938-48943.
[68] Lie J, Crom R, Gent T, et al. Elevation of plasma phospholipids transfer protein increases the risk of atherosclerosis despite lower apolipoprotein B-containing lipoproteins. *J Lipid Res* 2004; 45:805-811.
[69] Yamashita S, Maruyama T, Hirano K, *et al.*: Molecular mechanisms, lipoprotein abnormalities and atherogenicity of hyperalphalipoproteinemia. *Atherosclerosis* 2000; 152: 271-285.
[70] Tall A, Jiang X, Silver D.: George Lyman Duff memorial lecture: lipid transfer proteins, HDL metabolism, and atherogenesis. *Arterioscler Thromb Vasc Biol* 2000; 20: 1185-1188.
[71] Curb JD, Abbott RD, Rodriguez BL, et al. A prospective study of HDL-C and cholesteryl ester transfer protein gene mutations and the risk of coronary heart disease in the elderly. *J Lipid Res* 2004; 45:948-953.
[72] Moriyama Y, Okamura T, Inazu A, *et al.*: A low prevalence of coronary heart disease among subjects with increased high-density lipoprotein cholesterol levels, including those with plasma cholesteryl ester transfer protein deficiency. *Prev Med* 1998; 27; 659-667.
[73] Brousseau ME, O'Connor JJ, Ordovas JM, *et al.*: Cholesteryl ester transfer protein TaqI B2B2 genotype is associated with higher HDL cholesterol levels and lower risk of coronary heart disease endpoints in men with HDL deficiency. Veterans Affairs HDL Cholesterol Intervention Trial. *Arterioscler Thromb Vasc Biol* 2002; 22: 1148-1154.
[74] Wu JH, Lee YT, Hsu HC, *et al.*: Influence of CETP gene variation on plasma lipid levels and coronary heart disease: a survey in Taiwan. Atherosclerosis 2001; 159: 451-458.
[75] Rittershaus CW, Miller DP, Thomas LJ, *et al.*: Vaccine-induced antibodies inhibit CETP activity in vivo and reduce aortic lesions in a rabbit model of atherosclerosis. *Arterioscler Thromb Vasc Biol* 2000; 20: 2106-2112.
[76] Davidson MH, Maki K, Umporowicz D, *et al.*: The safety and immunogenicity of a CETP vaccine in healthy adults. *Atherosclerosis* 2003; 169: 113-120.
[77] Okamoto H, Yonemori F, Wakitani K, *et al.*: A cholesteryl ester transfer protein inhibitor attenuates atherosclerosis in rabbits. *Nature* 2000; 406: 203-207.

[78] de Grooth GJ, Kuivenhoven JA, Stalenhoef AF, *et al.*: Efficacy and safety of novel cholesteryl ester transfer protein inhibitor, JTT-705, in humans: a randomised phase II dose-response study. *Circulation* 2002; 105: 2159-2165.

[79] Clark RW, Sutfin TA, Ruggeri RB *et al.*: Raising high-density lipoprotein in humans through inhibition of cholesteryl ester transfer protein: an initial multidose study of torcetrapib. *Arterioscler Thromb Vasc Biol* 2004; 24: 490-497.

[80] Brousseau ME, Schaefer EJ, Wolfe ML, *et al.*: Effects of an inhibitor of cholesteryl ester transfer protein on HDL cholesterol. *N Engl J Med* 2004: 350: 1505-1515.

[81] Barter PJ, Brewer HB, Chapman MJ, *et al.*: Cholesteryl ester transfer protein. A novel target for raising HDL and inhibiting atherosclerosis. *Arterioscler Thromb Vasc Biol* 2003; 23: 160-167.

[82] Cohen J, Wand Z, Grundy S, et al.: Variation at the hepatic lipase and apolipoprotein AI/CIII/AIV loci is a major cause of genetically determined variation in plasma HDL cholesterol levels. *J Clin Invest* 1994; 94: 2377-84.

[83] Bersot TP, Vega GL, Grundy SM, *et al.*: Elevated hepatic lipase activity and low levels of high-density lipoprotein in a normotriglyceridemic, nonobese Turkish population. *J Lipid Res* 1999; 40: 432-438.

[84] Jansen H, Verhoeven AJ, Sijbrands EJ: Hepatic lipase: a pro- or anti-atherogenic protein? *J Lipid Res* 2002; 43: 1352-1362.

[85] Zambon A, Hokanson JE, Brown BG, *et al.*: Evidence for a new pathophysiological mechanism for coronary artery disease regression: hepatic lipase-mediated changes in LDL density. *Circulation* 1999; 99: 1959-1964.

[86] Ginsberg H: Insulin resistance and cardiovascular disease. *J Clin Invest* 2000; 106: 453-458.

[87] Jin W, Millar JS, Broedl U, *et al.*: Inhibition of endothelial lipase causes increased HDL cholesterol levels in vivo. *J Clin Invest* 2003; 111: 357-362.

[88] Ishida T, Choi S, Kundu RK, *et al.*: Endothelial lipase is a major determinant of HDL level. *J Clin Invest* 2003; 111: 347-355.

[89] Trigatti BL, Rigotti A, Braun A: Cellular and physiological roles of SR-BI, a lipoprotein receptor which mediates selective lipid uptake. *Biochim Biophys Acta* 2000; 1529: 276-286.

[90] Krieger M: Scavenger receptor class B type I is a multiligand HDL receptor that influences diverse physiologic systems. *J Clin Invest* 2001; 108: 793-797.

[91] Van Eck M, Twisk J, Hoekstra M, *et al.*: Differential effects of scavenger receptor BI deficiency on lipid metabolism in cells of the arterial wall and in the liver. *J Biol Chem* 2003; manuscript M211233200 in press.

[92] Kozarsky KF, Donahee MH, Glick JM, *et al.*: Gene transfer and hepatic overexpression of the HDL receptor SR-BI reduces atherosclerosis in the cholesterol-fed LDL receptor-deficient mouse. *Arterioscler Thromb Vasc Biol* 2000; 20: 721-727.

[93] Williams DL, Llera-Moya M, Thuahnai ST, *et al.*: Binding and cross-linking studies show that scavenger receptor BI interacts with multiple sites in apolipoprotein A-I and identifies the class A amphipathic α-helix as a recognition motif. *J Biol Chem* 2000; 275: 18897-18904.

[94] Liu T, Krieger M, Kan HY, *et al.*: The effects of mutations in helices 4 and 6 of apoA-I on scavenger receptor class B type I (SR-BI)-mediated cholesterol efflux suggest that formation of a productive complex between reconstituted high density lipoprotein and SR-BI is required for efficient lipid transport. *J Biol Chem* 2002; 277: 21576-21584.

[95] Silver DL, Wang N, Xiao X, *et al.*: High density lipoprotein (HDL) particle uptake mediated by scavenger receptor class B type I results in selective sorting of HDL cholesterol from protein and polarized cholesterol secretion. 2001; 276: 25287-25923.

[96] Connelly MA, Kellner-Weibel G, Rothblat GH, *et al.*: Scavenger receptor, Class B, type I (SR-BI)-directed HDL-cholesterol ester hydrolysis. *J Lipid Res* 2003; manuscript M200186-JLR200 in press.

[97] Martinez LO, Jacquet S, Esteve JP, *et al.*: Ectopic β-chain of ATP synthase is an apolipoprotein A-I receptor in hepatic HDL endocytosis. *Nature* 2003; 421: 75-79.

[98] Ioka RX, Kang MJ, Kamiyama S, *et al.*: Expression cloning and characterization of a novel glycosylphosphatidylinositol-anchored high density lipoprotein-binding protein, GPI-HBP-I. *J Biol Chem* 2003; 278: 7344-7349.

[99] Steinberg D, Gotto AM: Preventing coronary artery disease by lowering cholesterol levels. Fifty years from bench to bedside. *JAMA* 282: 2043-2050, 1999.

[100] Barter, P. Inhibition of endothelial cell adhesion molecule expression by high-density lipoproteins. *Clin Exp Pharmacol Physiol* 1997; 24: 286-287.

[101] Li X, Zhao S, Zhang S, et al. Protective effect of high-density lipoprotein on endothelium-dependent vasodilatation. *Int J Cardiol* 2000; 73: 231-6.

[102] Vinals M, Martinez-Gonzalez J, Badimon L. Regulatory effects of HDL on smooth muscle cell prostacyclin release. *Arterioscler Thromb Vasc Biol* 1999; 19: 2405-11.

[103] Griffin J, Kojima K, Banka C, *et al*: High-density lipoprotein enhancement of anticoagulant activities of plasma protein S and activated protein C. *J Clin Invest* 103: 219-227, 1999.

[104] Nofer J, Walter M, Kehrel B, et al. HDL3-mediated inhibition of thrombin-induced platelet aggregation and fibrinogen binding occurs via decreased production of phosphoinositide-derived second messengers 1,2-diacylglycerol and inositol 1,4,5-tris-phosphate. *Arterioscler Thromb Vasc Biol* 1998; 18: 861-869.

[105] Beitz J, Mest HJ: Thromboxane A2 formation by washed platelets under the influence of low and high density lipoproteins. *Prostaglandins Leukot Med* 23: 303-307, 1986.

[106] Tamagaki T, Sawada S, Imamura H, et al. Effects of high-density lipoproteins on intracellular pH and proliferation of human vascular endothelial cells. *Atherosclerosis* 1996; 123: 73-82.

[107] Nofer JR, Levkau B, Wolinska I, et al. Suppression of endothelial cell apoptosis by high-density lipoproteins and HDL-associated lysosphingolipids. *J Biol Chem* 2001; 276: 34480-5.

[108] Gordon D, Probstfield J, Garrison R, *et al.* High-density lipoproteins cholesterol and cardiovascular disease. *Circulation* 1989; 79: 8-15.

[109] Kitamura A, Iso H, Naito Y, *et al.* High-density lipoprotein cholesterol and premature coronary heart disease in urban Japanese men. *Circulation* 1994; 98: 2533-2539.

[110] Jones PH, Davidson MH, Stein, EA, *et al.* Comparison of the efficacy and safety of rosuvastatin versus atorvastatin, simvastatin, and pravastatin across doses (STELLAR Trial). *Am J Cardiol* 2003; 92: 152-160.
[111] Crouse J, Frohlich J, Ose L, *et al*: Effects of high doses of simvastatin and atorvastatin on high-density lipoprotein cholesterol and apolipoprotein A-I. *J Am Coll Cardiol* 1999: 83; 1476-1477.
[112] Hunninghaake DB, Stein EA, Bays HE, et al. Rosuvastatin improves the atherogenic and atheroprotective lipid profiles in patients with hypertriglyceridemia. *Coronary Artery Disease* 2004; 15: 115-123.
[113] Downs JR, Clearfield M, Weis, S, *et al.* Primary prevention of acute coronary events with Lovastatin in men and women with average cholesterol levels. Results of AFCAPS/TexCAPS. *JAMA* 1998; 279: 1615-1622.
[114] Heart Protection Study Group. MRC/BHF Heart Protection Study of cholesterol lowering with simvastatin in 20,536 high-risk individuals: a randomized placebo-controlled trial. *Lancet* 2002; 360: 7-22.
[115] Ballantyne C, Herd A, Ferlic L, *et al.* Influence of low HDL on progression of coronary artery disease and response to Fluvastatin therapy. *Circulation* 1999: 99; 736-743.
[116] Shepherd, J, Blauw GJ, Murphy MB, et al. Pravastatin in elderly individuals at risk of vascular disease (PROSPER): a randomised controlled trial. *Lancet* 2002; 360: 1623-30.
[117] Ishikawa K, Tani S, Watanabe I, et al. Effect of Pravastatin on Coronary Plaque volume. *Am J Cardiol* 2003; 92: 975-977.
[118] Manninen V, Elo MO, Frick MH, et al. Lipid alterations and the decline in incidence of coronary heart disease in the Helsinki Heart Study. *JAMA* 1988; 260: 641-51.
[119] Robins SJ, Collins D, Wittes JT, et al. VA-HIT Study Group. Veterans Affairs High-Density Lipoprotein Intervention Trial. Relation of gemfibrozil treatment and lipid levels with major coronary events. *JAMA* 2001; 285: 1586-1589.
[120] Rubins HB, Robins SJ, Collins D, *et al.* Diabetes, plasma insulin, and cardiovascular disease. *Arch Intern Med.* 2002; 162:2597-2604.
[121] The BIP Study Group: Secondary prevention by raising HDL cholesterol and reducing triglycerides in patients with coronary artery disease. The Bezafibrate Infarction Prevention Study. *Circulation* 2000; 102: 21-27.
[122] Prueksaritanont T, Zhao JJ, Ma B, *et al.* Mechanistic studies on metabolic interactions between gemfibrozil and statins. *J Pharmacol Exp Ther* 2002; 301:1042-1051.
[123] The Coronary Drug Project Research Group. Clofibrate and niacin in coronary heart disease. *JAMA* 1975; 231: 360-381.
[124] Brown BG, Zhao XQ, Chait A, et al. Simvastatin and niacin, antioxidant vitamins, or the combination for the prevention of coronary disease. *N Engl J Med* 2001; 345: 1583-92.
[125] Garrison RG, Kannel WB, Feinleib M, et al. Cigarette smoking and HDL cholesterol: the Framingham Offspring Study. *Atherosclerosis* 1978; 30: 17-25.
[126] Moffatt RJ. Effects of smoking on serum lipids and high-density lipoprotein cholesterol. *Atherosclerosis* 1988;74:85–89.

[127] Lamon-Fava S, Wilson PWF, Schaefer EJ. Impact of body mass index on coronary heart disease risk factors in men and women. The Framingham Offspring Study. *Arterioscler Thromb Vasc Biol* 1996; 16: 1509-1515.

[128] Pownall HJ. Alcohol and coronary heart disease. *Mediguide to Heart Diseases* 2000; 3: 1-7.

[129] Brousseau ME, Schaefer EJ, Wolfe ML, et al. Effects of an inhibitor of cholesteryl ester transfer protein on HDL cholesterol. *N Engl J Med* 2004; 350: 1505-15.

[130] Davidson, MH, Maki K, Umporowicz D, et al. The safety and immunogenicity of a CETP vaccine in healthy adults. *Atherosclerosis* 2003; 169: 113-120.

[131] Navab M, Anantharamaiah GM, Hama S, *et al.* Oral administration of an apo A-I mimetic peptide synthesized from D-amino acids dramatically reduces atherosclerosis in mice independent of plasma cholesterol. *Circulation* 2002; 105: 290-292.

In: Cholesterol in Atherosclerosis and Coronary Heart Disease ISBN 1-59454-302-X
Editor: Jean P. Kovala, pp.29-44 

*Chapter II*

# Oxidized LDL: Role in Cardiovascular Risk and Disease

***Paul Holvoet****

Center for Experimental Surgery and Anesthesiology, University of Leuven, Belgium

## Abstract

During inflammation, several cell types synthesize and secrete phospholipase A2 that catalyses lipid oxidation in LDL. Myeloperoxidase, a heme protein secreted by activated phagocytes, oxidizes L-tyrosine to a tyrosyl radical that is a physiological catalyst for the initiation of lipid oxidation in LDL. Lipid oxidation results in the generation of aldehydes that substitute lysine residues in the apolipoprotein B-100 moiety. Lipid together with protein oxidation in LDL results in the generation of oxidized LDL.

We, among others, have demonstrated an association between coronary heart disease (CHD) and increased plasma levels of oxidized LDL. Recently, we have demonstrated a higher prevalence of elevated oxidized LDL in persons with high-calculated CHD risk prior to events. Elevated oxidized LDL in persons with high-calculated CHD risk predicted future myocardial infarction even after adjusting for age, gender, race, smoking, and the metabolic syndrome. The effect of oxidized LDL on myocardial infarction can be explained by its effects on endothelial cells, monocyte infiltration and foam cell formation, and on smooth-muscle cell migration and apoptosis.

* Address of correspondence: P. HOLVOET, Center for Experimental Surgery and Anesthesiology, University of Leuven, Campus Gasthuisberg, O & N, Herestraat 49, B-3000 Leuven, Belgium. Tel 32-16-34.71.49; Fax 32-16-34.71.14; E-mail:paul.holvoet@med.kuleuven.ac.be

## Oxidative Modification of LDL

Endothelial cells, monocytes, macrophages, lymphocytes and smooth muscle cells are all capable of enhancing the rate of oxidation of LDL (for review: [1]). During inflammation, several cell types synthesize and secrete phospholipase $A_2$. Myeloperoxidase, a heme protein secreted by activated phagocytes, oxidizes L-tyrosine to a tyrosyl radical that is a physiological catalyst for the initiation of lipid oxidation in LDL. In striking contrast to other cell-mediated mechanisms for LDL oxidation, the myeloperoxidase-catalyzed reaction is independent of free metal ions. Lipid oxidation results in the generation of aldehydes that substitute lysine residues in the apo B-100 moiety of LDL thereby generating oxidized LDL.

We have isolated oxidized LDL from the plasma of CHD patients and have shown that it is only minimally to moderately oxidized. Indeed, only 60-90 lysine residues of a total of 356 per apoB-100 molecule were substituted. This rather low extent of oxidation explains why others and we could detect oxidized LDL in the blood [2]. As yet there is no data available about the relation between the plaque composition and the level of circulating oxidized LDL. It is however important to determine if elevated oxidized LDL is a marker of coronary plaques with high lipid and macrophage content that are believed to be prone to plaque rupture that leads to acute coronary syndromes.

## Oxidized as a Marker of Coronary Heart Disease

We have developed the first assay for circulating oxidized LDL. It is a mAb-4E6 based competition ELISA [2-4]. The monoclonal antibody mAb-4E6 is directed against a conformational epitope in the apoB-100 moiety of LDL that is generated as a consequence of substitution of at least 60 lysine residues of apoB-100 with aldehydes. This number of substituted lysine residues corresponds to the minimal number of substituted lysine residues required for scavenger-mediated uptake of oxidized LDL. Specificity of the assay is excellent, since the C50 values, i.e. concentrations that are required to obtain 50% inhibition of antibody binding in the ELISA, are 25 mg/dl for native LDL isolated by ultra centrifugation from the plasma of a healthy volunteer, and 0.025 mg/dl for oxidized LDL with at least 60 aldehyde-substituted lysine residues per apoB-100 obtained by copper-ion induced oxidation of the same LDL [3]. Therefore, 160 mg/dL LDL in a person's plasma would only contribute <0.2 mg/dL in the oxidized LDL assay. We have studied the association of oxidized LDL with stable angina and acute coronary syndromes.

Compared to healthy controls, plasma levels of oxidized LDL are significantly elevated in patients with stable angina pectoris, patients with unstable angina pectoris, and patients with acute myocardial infarction [4;5]. Circulating oxidized LDL did not discriminate between patients with stable angina and patients with acute coronary syndromes (unstable angina and AMI).

The Framingham Heart Study [6] has elucidated the quantitative relationship between cardiovascular risk factors -age gender, hypercholesterolemia, dyslipidemia, hypertension, diabetes, smoking- and CHD. It showed that these major risk factors are additive in predictive power. Accordingly, the total risk of a person can be estimated by a summing of the risk imparted by each of them. Recently, the American Heart Association and the American College of Cardiology issued a scientific statement that assessed the Global Risk Assessment Scoring (GRAS) as a guide to primary prevention [7]. GRAS is based on age, total cholesterol, HDL-cholesterol, systolic blood pressure, diabetes and smoking. Predisposing factors such as obesity, physical inactivity and family history of premature CHD are not included in GRAS.

Patients with established CHD had indeed high global risk assessment scores as well as high levels of circulating oxidized LDL. Receiver operating characteristic curve analysis revealed that the sensitivity of oxidized LDL for CHD was higher than that of GRAS (Figure 1). Overall, the receiver operating characteristic curve analysis revealed a sensitivity of oxidized LDL for CHD of 82%, with a specificity of 90%. Logistic regression analysis revealed that the diagnostic value of oxidized LDL for CHD was additive to that of GRAS ($p<0.001$): 94% of subjects with high (exceeding the $90^{th}$ percentile of distribution in controls) circulating oxidized LDL and high GRAS had CHD [5].

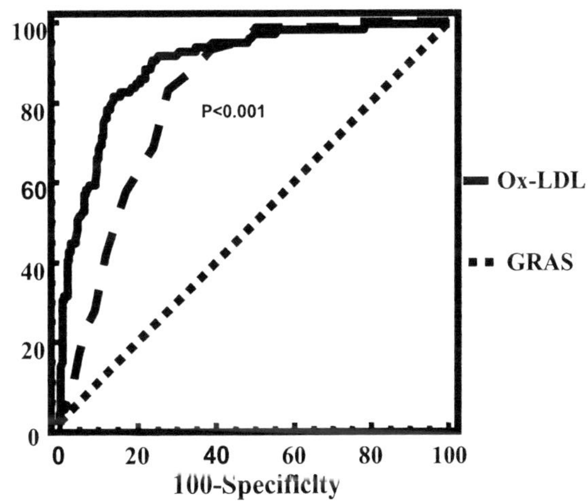


Figure 1. Representative receiver operating characteristic curves of circulating oxidized LDL (OxLDL) and the Global Risk Assessment score (GRAS) for CHD.

Other groups later confirmed the association between CHD and elevated levels of circulating oxidized LDL [8-10]. Although, some of those groups observed a slight temporal elevation of oxidized LDL shortly after AMI [8;10], they could not convincingly show that circulating oxidized LDL is a sensitive marker of acute coronary syndromes.

Recently, Hulthe and co-workers showed an association between sub-clinical atherosclerosis and circulating oxidized LDL that correlated with inflammatory cytokines [11;12] suggesting that increased oxidation of LDL occurs before CHD has developed. As yet it is unknown if coronary plaque composition correlates with levels of oxidized LDL. It is however important to know if a high lipid and macrophage content is associated with elevated oxidized LDL and thus to determine if oxidized LDL is a marker of plaque instability rather than of plaque load.

## Oxidized LDL as a Marker of a High Coronary Heart Disease Risk Status

The question remained whether a high CHD risk status prior to events is associated with a higher prevalence of elevated oxidized LDL. We studied this association in the Health ABC cohort. The study population contained 3,033 well functioning 70-79 year old persons in the Memphis, TN and the Pittsburgh, PA vicinities [13].

A useful concept introduced by the Third Report of the National Cholesterol Education Program Expert Panel on Detection, Evaluation, and Treatment of High Blood Cholesterol in Adults (ATP III) to assist in selection of patients at high CHD risk is that of the CHD risk equivalents [14]: a 10-year risk for CHD above 20% by Framingham scoring, diabetes and non-coronary forms of cardiovascular disease. In the Health ABC cohort, 385 persons had CHD and 1183 persons had CHD risk equivalents. The remaining 1535 participants were at low risk. The odds ratio for established CHD in the highest quintile of oxidized LDL was 2.3 (95% CI: 1.6-3.4) adjusting for age, gender, ethnicity, smoking, LDL-cholesterol and C-reactive protein. This finding thus further supported the value of oxidized LDL as a marker of CHD. A new and important finding was that the odds ratio for high CHD risk status in the highest quintile of oxidized LDL, compared to the lowest quintile and adjusting for age, gender, ethnicity, smoking, LDL-cholesterol, and C-reactive protein was 3.0 (95% CI: 2.3-4.0) (Figure 2). The odds ratio for elevated oxidized LDL among persons with high CHD risk prior to events was higher than that among persons with established CHD. A likely explanation is that once CHD has been diagnosed persons are frequently treated with a statin that is associated with lowering of LDL-cholesterol and oxidized LDL [13].

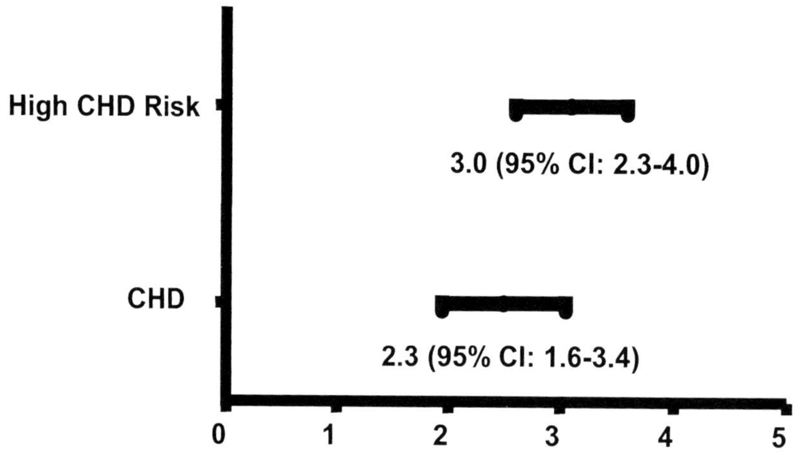


Figure 2. Prevalence of established CHD, respectively high CHD risk status, for persons in the highest quintile of oxidized LDL compared with those in the lowest quintile. The odds ratios were adjusted for age, gender, ethnicity, smoking, LDL-cholesterol, and C-reactive protein.

## The Metabolic Syndrome and Oxidation of LDL

Persons with the metabolic syndrome are at increased risk for developing CHD as well as increased mortality from CHD and all causes [15;16]. The Third Report of the National Cholesterol Education Program Expert Panel on Detection, Evaluation, and Treatment of High Blood Cholesterol in adults, draws attention to the importance of the metabolic syndrome and provides a working definition of this syndrome [14]. Metabolic syndrome components were defined as detailed in the ATPIII report: 1) waist circumference >102 cm in men and >88 cm in women; 2) fasting triglycerides >= 1.70 mmol/l (150 mg/dl); 3) HDL-cholesterol <1.03 mmol/l (40 mg/dl) in men and < 1.29 mmol/l (50 mg/dl) in women; 4) blood pressure $\geq$ 130/85 mmHg; 5) fasting-glucose $\geq$ 6.10 mmol/l (110 mg/dl). Persons with at least three of these components were defined as having the metabolic syndrome. Findings from the Third National Health and Nutrition Examination Survey showed that the metabolic syndrome is highly prevalent within the United States. The prevalence increased from 6.7% among participants aged 20 through 29 years to 43.5% and 42.0% for participants aged 60 through 69 years and aged at least 70 years, respectively [17].

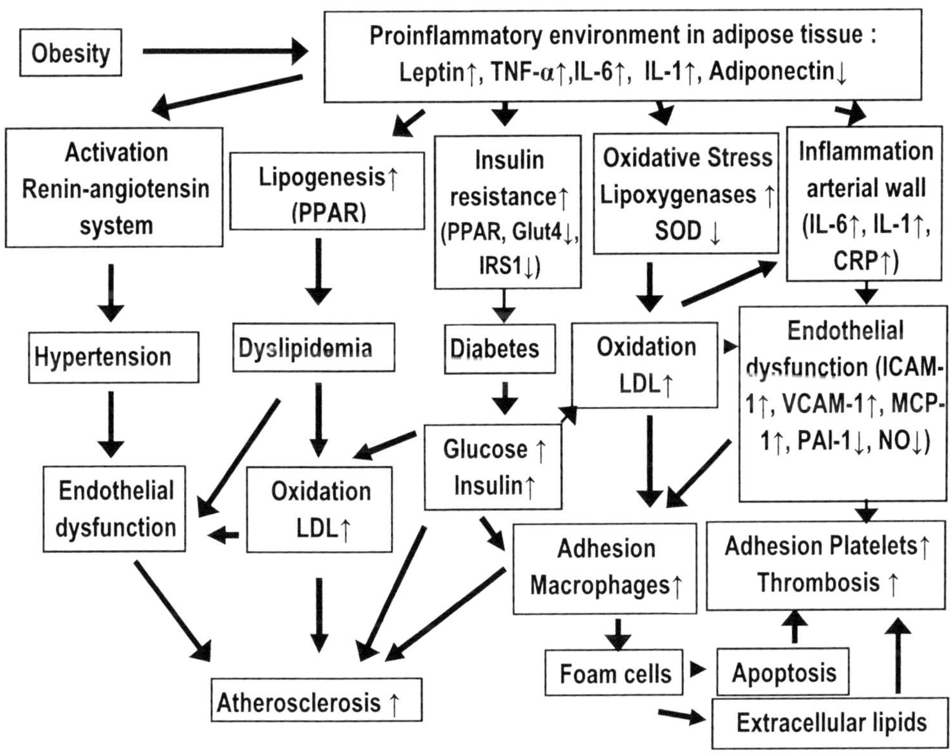


Figure 3. Interaction between the metabolic syndrome components obesity, hypertension, dyslipidemia and diabetes with inflammation, oxidation of LDL, endothelial dysfunction, atherosclerosis and thrombosis. CRP: C-reactive protein; GLUT4: glucose transporter 4; ICAM: intercellular adhesion molecule; IL: interleukin; IRS1: insulin receptor substrate-1; MCP-1: monocyte chemoattractant protein-1; NO: nitric oxide; PAI-1: plasminogen activator inhibitor; PPAR: peroxisome proliferator-activated receptor; SOD: superoxide dismutase; TNF: tumor necrosis factor; VCAM: vascular cell adhesion molecule.

The putative interaction between the metabolic syndrome components obesity, hypertension, dyslipidemia and diabetes with inflammation, oxidation of LDL, endothelial dysfunction, atherosclerosis and thrombosis is illustrated in Figure 3.

Because the metabolic syndrome is associated with high risk for CHD, a process that as discussed above involves LDL oxidation, we examined the relationship between metabolic syndrome components and circulating oxidized LDL in the Health ABC cohort. The prevalence of the metabolic syndrome was 38% i.e. similar to that in an age-matched cohort of the US population.

The metabolic syndrome was associated with higher levels of oxidized LDL due to a higher fraction of LDL that was oxidized, not to higher levels of LDL-cholesterol. Persons with the metabolic syndrome had twice the odds of having elevated oxidized LDL (>1.90 mg/dl) compared with persons without the metabolic syndrome, with adjustment for age, gender, race, smoking and LDL-cholesterol. The odds of having high oxidized LDL for persons with the metabolic syndrome was 2.6 when levels of oxidized LDL were expressed as a percentage of the LDL that was oxidized (Figure 4) [18].

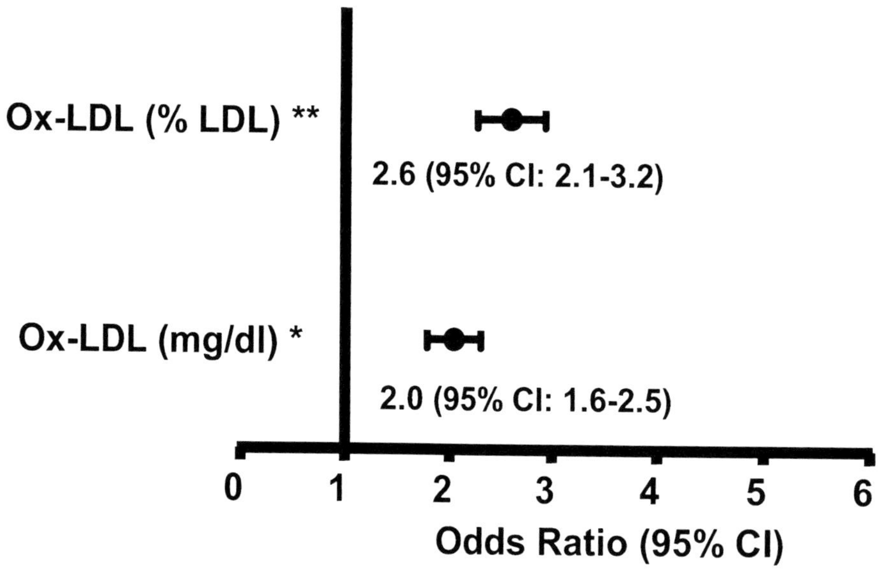


Figure 4. Prevalence of elevated oxidized LDL (higher than the 90th percentile of distribution in persons without the metabolic syndrome) for subjects with the metabolic syndrome compared with subjects without the metabolic syndrome. * Levels of oxidized LDL were expressed in mg/dL and the odds ratios were adjusted for age, sex, ethnicity, smoking and LDL-cholesterol. ** Levels of oxidized LDL were expressed as percentage of LDL that is oxidized and odds ratios were adjusted for age, sex, ethnicity, and smoking.

High triglycerides, low HDL-cholesterol, a high triglyceride-to-HDL-cholesterol ratio, high glucose and insulin, and high glycated hemoglobulin were all associated with a higher prevalence of elevated oxidized LDL [18]. In elders, three dominant factors have been identified in the relation between the metabolic syndrome and CHD: 1) the central metabolic factor comprising obesity, fasting and non-fasting insulin, dyslipidemia (HDL-cholesterol loading negative and triglycerides loading positive); 2) the glucose factor; and 3) the blood pressure factor [19;20]. Our study thus showed a strong association with two out of three of the metabolic syndrome factors: the central metabolic syndrome factor with obesity, dyslipidemia and insulin resistance, and the glucose factor. The association with these different factors suggests that oxidized LDL may be generated through several mechanisms (for review [1]) and that alternative therapeutic approaches, beyond cholesterol lowering, could reduce levels of circulating oxidized LDL. Importantly, we have demonstrated that poor glycemic control, even after adjusting for the metabolic syndrome components, is associated with increased oxidation of LDL.

## Oxidized LDL and Prediction of Cardiovascular Events

In the Health ABC cohort and in agreement with earlier reports, the metabolic syndrome increased the risk for incident myocardial infarction (Figure 5). A new and important finding was that oxidized LDL increased the risk of incident myocardial infarction. The incidence of myocardial infarction was 5.7% in the highest quintile of oxidized LDL compared to 2.6% ($P<0.01$) in the lowest quintile. The risk ratio for participants in the highest quintile, adjusted for age, sex, ethnicity, and smoking was 2.3 (95% CI, 1.2-4.2). After further adjusting for the metabolic syndrome, the risk ratio for participants in the highest quintile of oxidized LDL was 1.9 (1.1-3.5) (Figure 5). There was no significant interaction between the metabolic syndrome and oxidized LDL suggesting that the effect of oxidized LDL on myocardial infarction was independent of the metabolic syndrome [18]. Thus, our data not only further support the predictive value of the metabolic syndrome for CHD but also strongly suggest that baseline levels of oxidized LDL add prognostic information concerning future risk for myocardial infarction.

Earlier, we had already demonstrated that baseline plasma levels of oxidized LDL predicts the development of transplant CHD independent of pretransplant ischemic heart disease or dilated cardiomyopathy, time after transplantation, age and serum levels of LDL- and HDL-cholesterol [21].

## Biological Effects of Oxidized LDL

From the above can be concluded that oxidized LDL contributes to the pathogenesis of atherothrombotic disease. Studies in cell systems suggested that several mechanisms could be involved. Table 1 summarizes some of these putative mechanisms. As yet we are however not sure which of those mechanisms are relevant *in vivo*. Indeed, previous studies into the effect of *in vitro* oxidized LDL on vascular cell function did not determine the minimal amounts of oxidized LDL that are required to alter the redox state of vascular cells. These

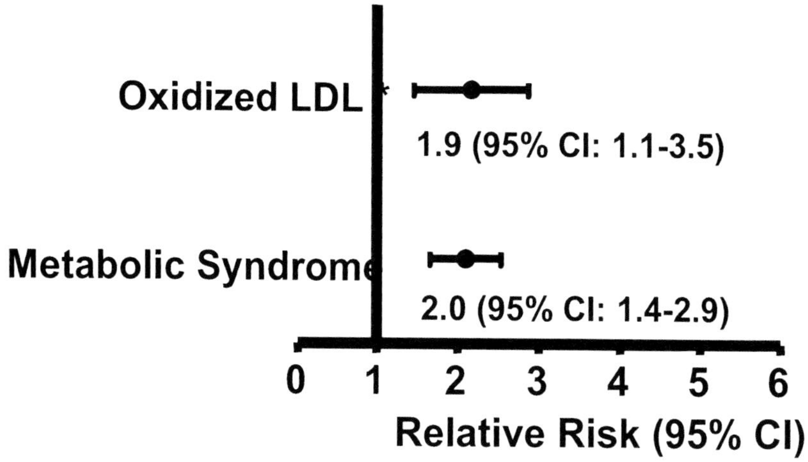


Figure 5. Relative risk of myocardial infarction in relation to the metabolic syndrome. The relative risk ratio for myocardial infarction for persons with the metabolic syndrome compared with persons without the metabolic syndrome was adjusted for age, sex, ethnicity, smoking, and LDL-cholesterol. Relative risk in relation to elevated oxidized LDL. The relative risk ratio for persons in the highest quintile of oxidized LDL compared to subjects in the lowest quintile of oxidized LDL was adjusted for age, sex, ethnicity, smoking, LDL-cholesterol, and the metabolic syndrome.

studies typically used concentrations of oxidized LDL that are 10-fold higher than those detected in the plasma. Furthermore, *in vitro* oxidized LDL applied to those cell systems typically was extensively oxidized. By contrast, *in vivo* oxidized LDL is minimally modified. This is an important matter because the concentration of various active components in oxidized LDL depends on the degree of oxidation of LDL. Putative biologically active components are: oxidized phospholipids, oxycholesterol, and protein oxidation products.

Minimally Modified-LDL (MM-LDL) induces endothelium to express adhesion molecules for monocytes, intercellular adhesion molecule 1 (ICAM-1) and vascular cell adhesion molecule (VCAM-1) [22]. Active compounds in MM-LDL are phospholipid auto-oxidation products such as 1-palmitoyl-2-(5-oxovaleroyl)-sn-glycero-3-phosphocholine (POVPC), 1-palmitoyl-2-glutaroyl-sn-glycero-3-phosphocholine (PGPC), and 1-palmitoyl-2-epoxyisoprostane E(2)-sn-glycero-3-phosphocholine (PEIPC) [23]. More advanced oxidation products have pro-apoptotic effects on endothelial cells, macrophages and smooth muscle cells. These effects could be attributed to oxidation products of phosphatidylcholine, or to oxysterols. Oxysterol mediated apoptosis involves activation of MAP and Jun/SAP kinases [24;25].

**Table 1. Biological Effects of Oxidized LDL**

**Effects on Endothelial Cells**

- Impaired Vasoreactivity:
  - NO-bioavailability ↓
  - Endothelin↑
- Procoagulation:
  - Platelet adhesion ↑ (NO↓, PGI↓)
  - Impaired fibrinolysis (tPA↓, PAI-1↑)
  - Pro-thrombosis (TF↑, TM↓)
- Recruitment of Monocytes:
  - Chemotaxis: MCP-1 ↑
  - Adhesion: VCAM-1 ↑
  - Proliferation: Growth factors ↑

**Effect on Monocytes – Macrophages:**

- *Direct effects:*
  - Macrophage retention: MIF
  - Foam Cell Formation: PF4
  - Apoptosis
  - Secretion of MMP's
- *Indirect effects:*
  - Chemotaxis - Adhesion - Proliferation

Effect on Smooth Muscle Cells

- ***Direct effects:***
  - Migration inhibition
  - Apoptosis
  - Foam cell formation
- *Indirect effects:*
  - Migration (PDGF)
  - Proliferation (bFGG)

bFGF: basic fibroblast growth factor; MCP-1: monocyte chemoattractant protein-1; MIF: macrophage migration inhibitory factor; MMP: matrix metalloproteinase: NO: nitric oxide; PAI-1: plasminogen activator inhibitor; PDGF: platelet-derived growth factor; PF4: platelet factor 4; PGI: prostacyclin; TM: thrombomodulin; TF: tissue factor; tPA: tissue plasminogen activator; VCAM: vascular cell adhesion molecule.

## Study of the Role of Oxidation of LDL in Cardiovascular Disease in a Mouse Model of the Metabolic Syndrome

Recently, we have described a mouse model of the metabolic syndrome [26]. We have obtained this model by crossing LDL-receptor deficient with leptin-deficient (ob/ob) mice. These mice (Figure 6) feature obesity, dyslipidemia, diabetes, and hypertension leading to accelerated atherosclerosis and impaired micro-vascular function.

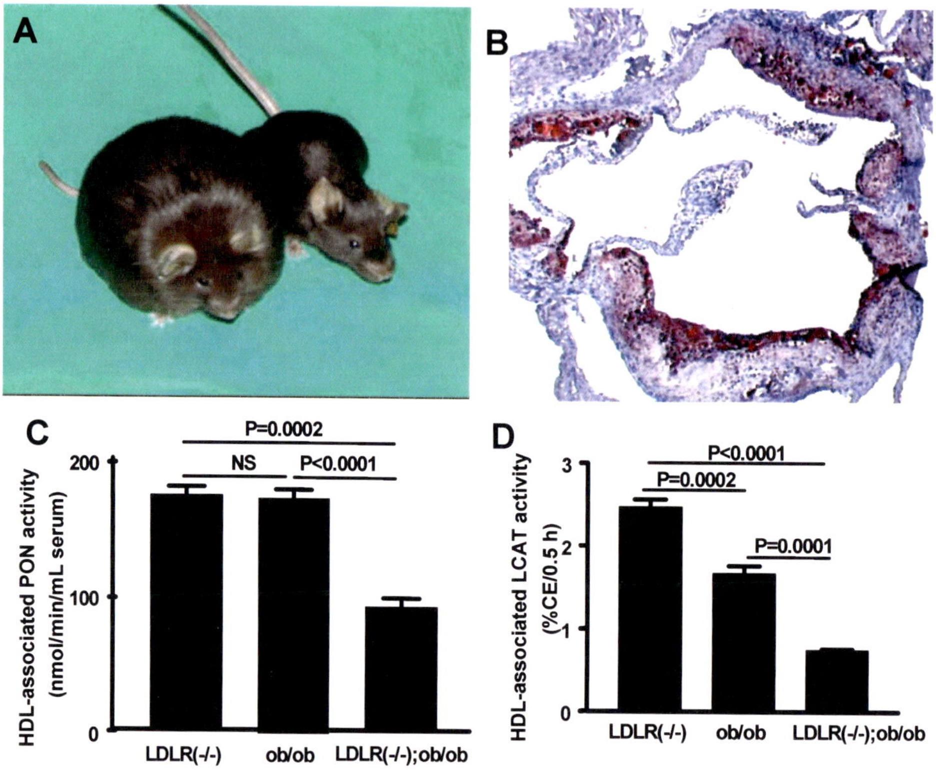


Figure 6. Mouse model of the metabolic syndrome. Mice with combined deficiency of the LDL-receptor and the leptin gene (LDLR(-/-);ob/ob) are obese (A; left mouse) and have complex lesions in their aortic arch at the age of 24 weeks (B). The HDL-associated anti-oxidant paraoxonase (PON) and lecithin:cholesterol transferase (LCAT) activity is lower compared to mice with the single LDL-receptor (LDLR-/-) or leptin (ob/ob) deficiency.

Accelerated atherosclerosis in those mice is due to a lower HDL-associated anti-oxidant paraoxonase and lecithin:cholesterol acyltransferease activity (Figure 6) that results in increased accumulation of oxidized LDL that induces monocyte infiltration and foam cell generation that in its turn results in increased expression of myeloperoxidase that oxidizes LDL [26]. Adenovirus-mediated overexpression of lecithin:cholesterol acyltransferease in those mice resulted in a significant reduction of atherosclerosis in the absence of a change in cholesterol and triglycerides and without improving glucose tolerance and insulin sensitivity. Earlier we had demonstrated that overexpression of apolipoprotein A-1, the predominant protein of HDL, and of PAF-acetylhydrolase, that degrades oxidized phospholipids and thereby renders them inactive, resulted in reduced oxidation of lipoproteins and atherosclerosis[27;28]. The protective mechanisms of HDL and HDL-associated anti-oxidant enzymes are summarized in Figure 7.

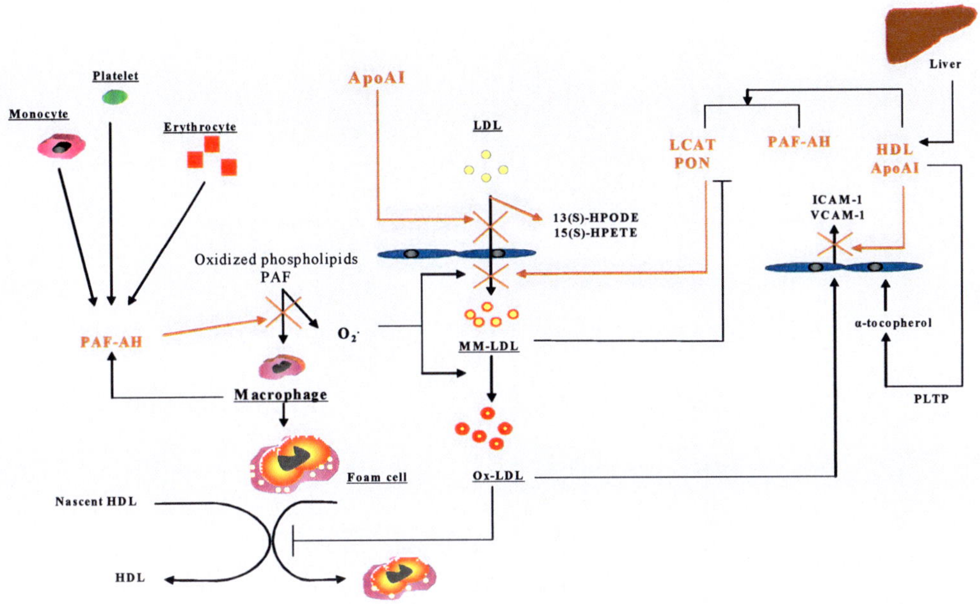


Figure 7. Anti-atherogenic mechanisms of HDL and HDL-associated anti-oxidant enzymes lecithin:cholesterol acyltransferase (LCAT), platelet activating factor-acetylhydrolase (PAF-AH), and paraoxonase (PON). HDL and apolipoprotein A-1 (apoAI) prevent the oxidized LDL-induced overexpression of the monocyte-specific adhesion molecules ICAM-1 and VCAM-1 thereby inhibiting monocyte infiltration. HDL-associated phospholipid transfer protein (PLTP) aids the transport of α-tocopherol into the arterial wall, thereby increasing the anti-oxidant activity. ApoAI, LCAT and PON prevent the oxidation of phospholipids in LDL. PAF-AH, that is not only associated with HDL but also produced by macrophages, neutralizes oxidized phospholipids and thereby renders them inactive. HDL also induces the reverse cholesterol transport from foam cells to the liver; LCAT is a key enzyme in this transport.

It has been shown that weight-loss in insulin-resistant, but not in insulin-sensitive, obese persons reduces their CHD risk [29]. It is however not known to what extent changes in the intra-abdominal adipose gene expression profile are important for the reduction of the risk [30]. To unravel the underlying mechanisms we have studied the effect of diet-restriction induced weight-loss on the prevalence of the metabolic syndrome components, atherosclerosis and heart function in the double deficient mice. Weight-loss induced an up-regulation of PPARα and PPARγ, and a change in the expression of genes that regulate the glucose transport and insulin sensitivity, lipid metabolism, oxidative stress and inflammation, most of which are under the transcriptional control of these PPARs. Changes in gene expression were associated with increased insulin-sensitivity, decreased hypertriglyceridemia, decreased oxidation of LDL and inflammation, reduced mean 24-hour blood pressure and heart rate, restored circadian variations of blood pressure and heart rate, increased ejection fraction, and reduced atherosclerosis. In short, weight-loss had an effect on most interactions between metabolic syndrome components and other cardiovascular risk factors in the pathogenesis of atherothrombosis that have been discussed above (Figure 3).

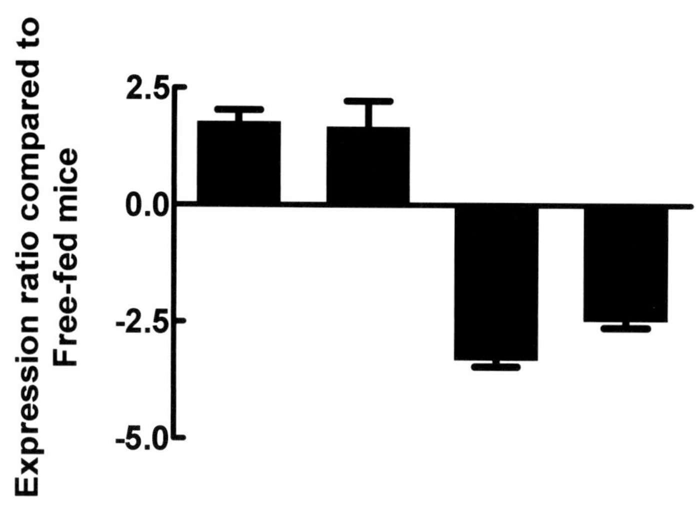


Figure 8. PPAR-related changes in gene expression that are in agreement with the reduced oxidative stress upon weight-loss. Weight-loss in obese, dyslipidemic and diabetic mice resulted in induction of PPARs in their adipose tissue that correlated with induction of glutathione peroxidase (GPx) and superoxide dismutase (SOD), two anti-oxidant enzymes, and down-regulation of arachidonate lipoxygenase-5 (Alox5 ap), that induces LDL oxidation, and of platelet factor 4 (PF-4) that enhances the uptake of oxidized LDL by macrophages and thereby induces foam cell generation.

Interestingly, we have now identified PPAR up-regulation in the adipose tissue, the heart and the arterial wall as a useful strategy to reduce oxidation of LDL and thereby reduce the 'cardiovascular risk'.

Weight-loss in the double deficient mice was associated with reduced atherosclerosis and improved cardiovascular function when food intake was restricted in 12-week old mice, i.e. when no atherosclerotic lesions were present in their aortic arch, or in 24-week old mice, i.e. when complex lesions had already developed. Translated to the human situation, these data indicate that diet restriction and weight control is important for both primary and secondary prevention. Figure 8 shows that PPAR induction in the adipose tissue resulted in an induction of the anti-oxidant enzymes glutathione peroxidase and super oxide dismutase, and down-regulation of the oxidative enzyme arachidonate lipoxygenase-5, and of platelet factor 4 that enhances the scavenger-receptor mediated uptake of oxidized LDL by macrophages and thereby enhances foam cell formation.

## Conclusions

Previously we, among others, had detected elevated levels of circulating oxidized LDL in the blood of middle-aged CHD patients. Two important questions remained to be answered: 1) are levels of circulating oxidized LDL elevated in persons at high CHD risk prior to CHD events; and 2) do levels of oxidized LDL predict CHD events?

We addressed those questions in the Health ABC study. We indeed demonstrated elevated levels of oxidized LDL in well-functioning elders that had CHD risk equivalents prior to CHD events. Importantly we showed for the first time in a population cohort that the metabolic syndrome is associated with a higher fraction of LDL that is oxidized and thus with higher levels of circulating oxidized LDL. This association was consistent across gender and race. Our data supported further the importance of identifying individuals with the metabolic syndrome as a high-risk group for the development of CHD.

Finally our study of the Health ABC cohort identified the oxidation of LDL as a potential mechanism explaining the increased risk for myocardial infarction among persons with the metabolic syndrome. The lack of interaction between the metabolic syndrome and oxidized LDL to predict the risk of myocardial infarction suggests that the mechanisms by which oxidized LDL could contribute to the increased risk are independent of the metabolic syndrome. We are however well aware that an epidemiological study does not give insight in the mechanisms by which the metabolic syndrome and oxidized LDL can contribute to the development of CHD or to plaque instability. Therefore, well-designed cellular and animal studies are required. Although several putative atherogenic mechanisms for oxidized LDL have been proposed on the basis of the findings of cellular studies, we have to keep in mind that those studies typically used concentrations of oxidized LDL that are 10-fold higher than those detected in the plasma. Also animal studies have their limitations because animal models usually do not allow studying the interaction between several cardiovascular risk factors that do generally occur in patients. To better address the role of those interactions we have used mice that are deficient in both the LDL-receptor and the leptin gene. This mouse model features several of the metabolic syndrome components: obesity, dyslipidemia, hypertension, and diabetes, that are associated with increased oxidative stress, accelerated atherosclerosis and impaired microvascular function in the heart.

Our prospective study in heart transplant patients showed that baseline levels of oxidized LDL predicted the development of transplant CHD independent of levels of LDL- and HDL-cholesterol and of pretransplant history of ischemic heart disease. Thus, the level of oxidized LDL in the blood was an independent predictor of the development of transplant CHD that was associated with a further increase of plasma levels of oxidized LDL. Although the study identified oxidized LDL as a prognostic marker of transplant CHD it did not prove that oxidized LDL has an active role in the development of CHD. Oxidized LDL could however contribute to the progression of atherosclerosis by enhancing endothelial injury, by inducing foam cell generation and smooth muscle apoptosis.

Intervention trials are required to evaluate the active role of oxidized LDL in the development of CHD in general. The recent findings that plasma levels of oxidized LDL are also increased in young obese persons before diabetes has developed but who are at increased risk for diabetes and CHD, and that those levels correlate with the intima-media thickness in their carotid artery suggest that this may be the case. The elevation of oxidized LDL in these patients could only partly be explained by the characteristic dyslipidemia. Beyond LDL-cholesterol lowering, those interventions may aim at increasing the levels of antioxidants in LDL and/or increasing HDL and/or HDL-associated antioxidant enzymes such as paraoxonase and lecithin:cholesterol acyltransferase, that prevent the oxidation of LDL, or PAF-acetylhydrolase that degrades oxidized phospholipids in LDL. Recently, we identified in mice the up-regulation of PPARs in the adipose tissue and the arterial wall as a putative therapeutic approach to reduce the oxidation of LDL in the arterial wall.

## Acknowledgements

Supported in part by the Interuniversity Attraction Poles Program – Belgian Science Policy (P5/02). We acknowledge collaboration with the departments of Cardiology and Endocrinology of the University of Leuven, Belgium, and the Health ABC study centers: the Sticht Center on Aging, Wake Forest University School of Medicine, Winston-Salem, NC; the Departments of Pathology and Biochemistry, University of Vermont, Burlington, VT; the University of California, Prevention Sciences Group, San Francisco, CA; the Vanderbilt University, Nashville, TN, USA; the Department of Medicine, University of Pittsburgh, PA; the Laboratory of Epidemiology, Demography and Biometry, National Institute on Aging, NIH, Bethesda.

## References

[1] Mertens A, Holvoet P. Oxidized LDL and HDL: antagonists in atherothrombosis. *FASEB J.* 2001;15:2073-84.

[2] Holvoet P, Stassen JM, Van Cleemput J, Collen D, Vanhaecke J. Oxidized low density lipoproteins in patients with transplant- associated coronary artery disease. *Arterioscler Thromb Vasc Biol.* 1998;18:100-107.

[3] Holvoet P, Donck J, Landeloos M, Brouwers E, Luijtens K, Arnout J et al. Correlation between oxidized low density lipoproteins and von Willebrand factor in chronic renal failure. *Thromb Haemost.* 1996;76:663-69.

[4] Holvoet P, Vanhaecke J, Janssens S, Van de WF, Collen D. Oxidized LDL and malondialdehyde-modified LDL in patients with acute coronary syndromes and stable coronary artery disease. *Circulation.* 1998;98:1487-94.

[5] Holvoet P, Mertens A, Verhamme P, Bogaerts K, Beyens G, Verhaeghe R et al. Circulating oxidized LDL is a useful marker for identifying patients with coronary artery disease. *Arterioscler Thromb Vasc Biol.* 2001;21:844-48.

[6] Wilson PW. Established risk factors and coronary artery disease: the Framingham Study. *Am J Hypertens.* 1994;7:7S-12S.

[7] Grundy SM, Pasternak R, Greenland P, Smith S Jr, Fuster V. Assessment of cardiovascular risk by use of multiple-risk-factor assessment equations: a statement for healthcare professionals from the American Heart Association and the American College of Cardiology. *Circulation.* 1999;100:1481-92.

[8] Ehara S, Ueda M, Naruko T, Haze K, Itoh A, Otsuka M et al. Elevated levels of oxidized low density lipoprotein show a positive relationship with the severity of acute coronary syndromes. *Circulation.* 2001;103:1955-60.

[9] Toshima S, Hasegawa A, Kurabayashi M, Itabe H, Takano T, Sugano J et al. Circulating oxidized low density lipoprotein levels. A biochemical risk marker for coronary heart disease. *Arterioscler Thromb Vasc Biol.* 2000;20:2243-47.

[10] Tsimikas S, Bergmark C, Beyer RW, Patel R, Pattison J, Miller E et al. Temporal increases in plasma markers of oxidized low-density lipoprotein strongly reflect the presence of acute coronary syndromes. *J Am Coll Cardiol.* 2003;41:360-370.

[11] Hulthe J, Fagerberg B. Circulating oxidized LDL is associated with increased levels of cell-adhesion molecules in clinically healthy 58-year old men (AIR study). *Med Sci Monit.* 2002;8:CR148-CR152.

[12] Hulthe J, Fagerberg B. Circulating oxidized LDL is associated with subclinical atherosclerosis development and inflammatory cytokines (AIR Study). *Arterioscler Thromb Vasc Biol.* 2002;22:1162-67.

[13] Holvoet P, Harris TB, Tracy RP, Verhamme P, Newman AB, Rubin SM et al. Association of High Coronary Heart Disease Risk Status With Circulating Oxidized LDL in the Well-Functioning Elderly: Findings From the Health, Aging, and Body Composition Study. *Arterioscler Thromb Vasc Biol.* 2003;23:1444-48.

[14] National Institutes of Health. Third Report of the National Cholesterol Education Program Expert Panel on Detection, Evaluation, and Treatment of High Blood Cholesterol in Adults (Adult Treatment Panel III). NIH Publication 01-3670. 2002. *Bethesda, Md: National Institutes of Health.* Ref Type: Report

[15] Isomaa B, Almgren P, Tuomi T, Forsen B, Lahti K, Nissen M et al. Cardiovascular morbidity and mortality associated with the metabolic syndrome. *Diabetes Care.* 2001;24:683-89.

[16] Trevisan M, Liu J, Bahsas FB, Menotti A. Syndrome X and mortality: a population-based study. Risk Factor and Life Expectancy Research Group. *Am J Epidemiol.* 1998;148:958-66.

[17] Ford ES, Giles WH, Dietz WH. Prevalence of the metabolic syndrome among US adults: findings from the third National Health and Nutrition Examination Survey. *JAMA.* 2002;287:356-59.

[18] Holvoet P, Kritchevsky SB, Tracy RP, Mertens A, Rubin SM, Butler J et al. The metabolic syndrome, circulating oxidized LDL, and risk of myocardial infarction in well-functioning elderly people in the health, aging, and body composition cohort. *Diabetes.* 2004;53:1068-73.

[19] Lindblad U, Langer RD, Wingard DL, Thomas RG, Barrett-Connor EL. Metabolic syndrome and ischemic heart disease in elderly men and women. *Am J Epidemiol.* 2001;153:481-89.

[20] Shepherd J. Issues surrounding age: vascular disease in the elderly. *Curr Opin Lipidol.* 2001;12:601-9.

[21] Holvoet P, Van Cleemput J, Collen D, Vanhaecke J. Oxidized low density lipoprotein is a prognostic marker of transplant- associated coronary artery disease. *Arterioscler Thromb Vasc Biol.* 2000;20:698-702.

[22] Cominacini L, Garbin U, Pasini AF, Davoli A, Campagnola M, Contessi GB et al. Antioxidants inhibit the expression of intercellular cell adhesion molecule-1 and

vascular cell adhesion molecule-1 induced by oxidized LDL on human umbilical vein endothelial cells. *Free Radic Biol Med.* 1997;22:117-27.

[23] Subbanagounder G, Leitinger N, Shih PT, Faull KF, Berliner JA. Evidence that phospholipid oxidation products and/or platelet-activating factor play an important role in early atherogenesis: in vitro and In vivo inhibition by WEB 2086. *Circ Res.* 1999;85:311-18.

[24] Metzler B, Hu Y, Dietrich H, Xu Q. Increased expression and activation of stress-activated protein kinases/c-Jun NH(2)-terminal protein kinases in atherosclerotic lesions coincide with p53. *Am J Pathol.* 2000;156:1875-86.

[25] Napoli C, Quehenberger O, de Nigris F, Abete P, Glass CK, Palinski W. Mildly oxidized low density lipoprotein activates multiple apoptotic signaling pathways in human coronary cells. *FASEB J.* 2000;14:1996-2007.

[26] Mertens A, Verhamme P, Bielicki JK, Phillips MC, Quarck R, Verreth W et al. Increased low-density lipoprotein oxidation and impaired high-density lipoprotein antioxidant defense are associated with increased macrophage homing and atherosclerosis in dyslipidemic obese mice: LCAT gene transfer decreases atherosclerosis. *Circulation.* 2003;107:1640-1646.

[27] Quarck R, De Geest B, Stengel D, Mertens A, Lox M, Theilmeier G et al. Adenovirus-mediated gene transfer of human platelet-activating factor- acetylhydrolase prevents injury-induced neointima formation and reduces spontaneous atherosclerosis in apolipoprotein E-deficient mice. *Circulation.* 2001;103:2495-500.

[28] Theilmeier G, De Geest B, Van Veldhoven PP, Stengel D, Michiels C, Lox M et al. HDL-associated PAF-AH reduces endothelial adhesiveness in apoE-/- mice. *FASEB J.* 2000;14:2032-39.

[29] McLaughlin T, Abbasi F, Kim HS, Lamendola C, Schaaf P, Reaven G. Relationship between insulin resistance, weight loss, and coronary heart disease risk in healthy, obese women. *Metabolism.* 2001;50:795-800.

[30] Henkin L, Bergman RN, Bowden DW, Ellsworth DL, Haffner SM, Langefeld CD et al. Genetic epidemiology of insulin resistance and visceral adiposity. The IRAS Family Study design and methods. *Ann Epidemiol.* 2003;13:211-17.

In: Cholesterol in Atherosclerosis and Coronary Heart Disease ISBN 1-59454-302-X
Editor: Jean P. Kovala, pp.45-62 

*Chapter III*

# Effects of Therapy with LDL Apheresis in Patients with Familial Hypercholesterolemia: The Dresden Experience

*U. Julius*[*] *and C. Namokel*
Medizinische Klinik und Poliklinik III, Universitätsklinikum Dresden, Germany

## Abstract

We report about our experience with LDL apheresis over more than 13 years. A total of 32 patients (19 males, 13 females; mean age at starting apheresis 50 years) were treated with different procedures (HELP, DALI, immunoadsorption, lipid filtration) for in the mean 80 months (6 to 161 months). According to the official rules an elevated atherosclerotic risk is a prerequisite for the indication of LDL apheresis. The intervals between two procedures were determined individually on the basis of LDL-C levels before procedures. 21 patients had a positive family history for either lipid disorders or coronary heart disease. The majority of patients suffered from a heterozygous form of hypercholesterolemia, in two patients a familial defective apolipoprotein B was found, in 9 patients a concomitant elevation of lipoprotein(a) was observed. 21 patients had also elevated triglyceride levels, at least temporarily. Before starting treatment with LDL apheresis in 25 patients an angiographically documented coronary atherosclerosis was found. 10 patients had suffered from a myocardial infarction, in 3 patients a PTCA was performed, 11 patients underwent a cardiac bypass operation. 5 patients were after a heart transplantation. In 6 patients a peripheral arterial occlusive disease was known. Only 3 patients were obese (Body Mass Index >= 30 $kg/m^2$). In 24 patients an accompanying hypertension and in 11 patients a diabetes mellitus was present. All

[*] Address of correspondence: Prof. Ulrich Julius, Medizinische Klinik und Poliklinik III, Universitätsklinikum Carl Gustav Carus Dresden, Fetscherstr. 74, 01307 Dresden, Germany. Tel.: +49 351 458 2306; FAX: +49 351 458 5306; E-mail: julius@rcs.urz.tu-dresden.de

patients were treated with a statin (atorvastatin, pravastatin, simvastatin, fluvastatin), in some patients (n = 14) ezetimibe was added recently. All LDL apheresis methods induced a reduction of LDL-C of at least 60 %. Lipoprotein(a) was reduced in the same range. Comparing the different LDL apheresis methods, in our hands the immunoadsorption and the DALI methods appeared to be the most effective ones. In no patient who was treated with LDL apheresis at our department a new myocardial infarction had developed. 5 patients underwent a PTCA and 3 patients a cardiac bypass surgery. One patient had died. In conclusion, it appears that LDL apheresis presents an effective tool in improving the prognosis in these high-risk patients.

## Introduction

In Dresden, we started in November 1990 with LDL apheresis. The reunification of Germany opened for us new possibilities. This paper gives an overview about our experience for up to more than 13 years. We started with 2 patients only and gradually added more patients. 4 patients stopped being treated at our center, one of them died. 2 of them went to another center, one female refused to be treated further on. We are going to report about the effectiveness of four methods of LDL apheresis and about the clinical results obtained. The generally accepted indication for the treatment by LDL apheresis is a disturbance of lipid metabolism that is refractory to diet and lipid-lowering drugs plus a documented atherosclerotic disease.

## Material and Methods

A total of 32 patients (19 males, 13 females; mean age at starting LDL apheresis 50 years; the youngest patient was 30 years old) were treated with different procedures (HELP, DALI, immunoadsorption, lipid filtration) for in the mean 80 months (6 to 161 months). 21 patients had a positive family history for either lipid disorders or coronary heart disease. The majority of patients suffered from a heterozygous form of hypercholesterolemia (genetic mutations of the LDL receptor gene that are responsible for a reduced function of the receptor have been found in 7 patients), in two patients a familial defective apolipoprotein B was found (mutation in apolipoprotein B at site of amino acid 3500 – arginine is replaced by glutamine), in 9 patients a concomitant elevation of lipoprotein(a) was observed. 21 patients had also elevated triglyceride levels, at least temporarily. Before starting treatment with LDL apheresis in 25 patients an angiographically documented coronary atherosclerosis was found. In 3 patients no coronary atherosclerosis had been seen. In 4 patients no angiography had been performed. 10 patients had suffered from a myocardial infarction, in 3 patients a PTCA was performed, 11 patients underwent a cardiac bypass operation. 5 patients were after a heart transplantation. In 6 patients a peripheral arterial occlusive disease was known. Only 3 patients were obese (Body Mass Index >= 30 kg/m$^2$). In 24 patients an accompanying hypertension and in 11 patients a diabetes mellitus was present. All patients were treated with a statin (atorvastatin, pravastatin, simvastatin, fluvastatin), in some patients (n = 14) ezetimibe was added recently. Only 1 patient had been treated with cerivastatin before starting the apheresis treatment. This drug was discontinued due to side effects. This is the only patient who was not treated with a statin during LDL apheresis procedures. Her highest LDL cholesterol level was 3.09 mmol/L, which is why she was not started with a statin again. But she had clearly elevated lipoprotein(a) concentrations.

4 methods of LDL apheresis have been used at our center. The first one to be introduced was the HELP method (heparin-induced extracorporeal lipoprotein precipitation; B. Braun Melsungen) [97, 13, 110, 94, 3, 27, 90, 91, 95, 60, 4, 89, 61, 92, 43, 100, 45, 38, 88, 8]. With this method also fibrinogen is being reduced. The second method was the immunoadsorption (immunoadsorbent consisting of sheep anti-LDL antibodies which had been coupled to Sepharose; previously produced by Baxter and Plasmaselect, now by Miltenyi Biotech Bergisch Gladbach) [83, 79, 37, 80, 87, 42b, 74, 84]. The next method was the DALI system (direct adsorption of lipoproteins by adsorption onto polyacrylate-coated polyacrylamide beads in an adsorber; Fresenius Bad Homburg) [26, 16, 40, 17b, 43, 111, 17a, 12, 17d, 98, 17c, 18, 14, 112]. In contrast to the other procedures no separation of plasma from the blood cells is needed here. The treatment time is the shortest one for all the methods we have used. The last method is the lipid filtration (using two filters: one in order to separate plasma and one in order to eliminate LDL particles; DIAMED Köln) [25, 99, 35, 29, 101, 7, 62, 20, 31, 109, 67, 45, 51, 52]. The latter method also reduces fibrinogen. All 4 methods also eliminate lipoprotein(a) from the blood [3, 85, 106, 79, 86, 4, 5, 62, 11, 63, 26, 16]. The intervals between two procedures were determined individually on the basis of LDL-C levels before procedures. Usually we started with weekly intervals and after at least 3 months we continued with biweekly intervals. Though those patients whose LDL cholesterol remained clearly elevated (> 4 mmol/L) were treated in weekly intervals over years.

For all patients the official German rules for the indication of LDL apheresis [21] had been checked and we got an agreement for each patient from his or her health insurance company for reimbursement.

Only standardized chemical methods were used to assess lipid concentrations.

The statistical analysis was done with the help of SPSS 10.0. We used an analysis of variance to compare different mean values.

## Results

The initial LDL cholesterol values before starting the first apheresis procedure were in the mean 5.95 mmol/L (range 2.86 to 15.21 mmol/L). 9 patients had already been treated at another center before they were referred to us. Their mean LDL cholesterol amounted to 2.48 mmol/L (range 0.34 to 4.6 mmol/L). Triglyceride values in those patients who started apheresis treatment at our center were 1.74 mmol/L (range 0.81 to 4.46 mmol/L), their HDL cholesterol concentrations were 1.15 mmol/L (range 0.66 to 1.54 mmol/L). The corresponding values for those patients who were treated at another center before were 4.46 mmol/L (range 0.69 to 20.5 mmol/L), their HDL cholesterol values were 1.29 mmol/L (range 0.23 to 2.43 mmol/L). Initial mean lipoprotein(a) levels in those 9 patients who had elevated levels were in the mean 1770.67 mg/L (range 400 to 7750 mg/L).

In total this paper analyzes 6472 procedures.

The different LDL apheresis methods had a different impact on the major lipid fractions (see Table 1).

**Table 1. Acute Reductions of Lipid Concentrations by Different LDL Apheresis Procedures (Mean Plus Range in %)**

| Method | LDL cholesterol | Triglycerides | HDL cholesterol |
|---|---|---|---|
| HELP | -62.83[a,b,c,] (+47.35 to -96.83) | -43.35[b,c] (+103.7 to –87.85) | -8.37[c] (+258.98 to –71.03) |
| Immunoadsorption | - 72.42[a,e] (+161.01 to – 100) | -41.24[d,e] (+286.21 to –84.75) | -8.91[e] (+258.82 to –91.48) |
| DALI | - 72.35[b,f] (-16.44 to -100) | -32.49[b,d,f] (+141.48 to –92.4) | -8.27[f] (+20.71 to –89.81) |
| Lipid filtration | - 65.03[c,e,f] (-42.83 to –97.83 | -47.69[c,e,f] (+113.2 to –78.57) | -15.55[c,e,f] (+6.25 to –31.34) |

Level of significance: $p < 0.05$.
[a] HELP vs immunoadsorption.
[b] HELP vs DALI.
[c] HELP vs lipid filtration.
[d] Immunoadsorption vs DALI.
[e] Immunoadsorption vs lipid filtration.
[f] DALI vs lipid filtration.

Elevations of LDL cholesterol and of triglyceride concentrations after a LDL apheresis (as indicated by the range) were only seen as a very unusual situation. This only happened when the values before the LDL apheresis were very low.

In those 9 patients with elevated lipoprotein(a) concentrations the absolute reductions of this parameter were as follows: -1196.22 mg/L (range + 320 to -7020 mg/L). This corresponds to a mean reduction by about 60 %.

Throughout the observation period referred to in this review 9 patients have been treated with the HELP procedure only, 4 patients with the DALI procedure only, and 2 patients with the immunoadsorption only. In all other patients at least two of the LDL apheresis methods have been used consecutively. There were different reasons for switching the method: low effectiveness with respect to LDL cholesterol lowering or lipoprotein(a) lowering with one method, the wish also to reduce fibrinogen, general recommendations (in Germany after heart transplantation there is only experience with the HELP procedure), the introduction of a new method at our center.

With the HELP method 2880.2 ml plasma (range 100 to 5000 ml) have been treated at each procedure. With the immunoadsorption 4667.98 ml (range 200 to 6090 ml) plasma have been processed. With the DALI system in the mean a blood volume of 8489.59 ml (range 860 to 10550 ml) have been treated. With the lipid filtration 3513.09 ml (range 2300 to 5000 ml) plasma have been processed.

The mean LDL cholesterol values before and after LDL apheresis are given in Figure 1.

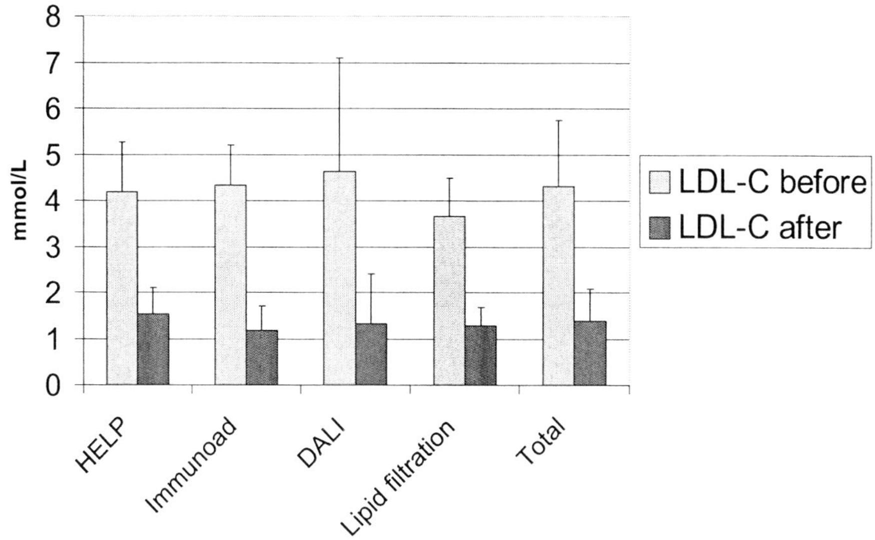


Figure 1. Mean LDL cholesterol values before and after LDL apheresis (mmol/L)

These mean values mask the fact that generally the LDL cholesterol concentrations were lowered the longer a patient was treated with LDL apheresis.

The corresponding triglyceride values before and after LDL apheresis are given in Figure 2.

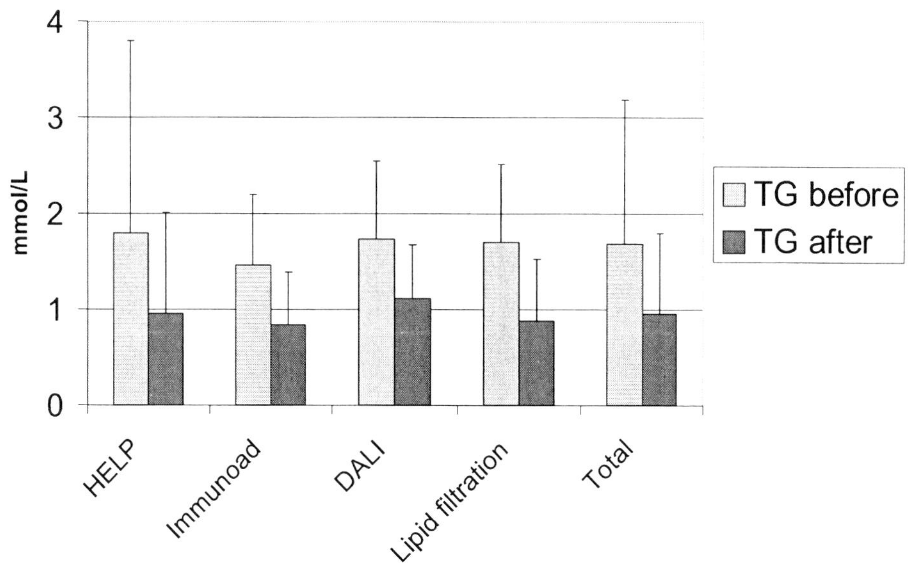


Figure 2. Mean triglyceride values before and after LDL apheresis (mmol/L)

The HDL cholesterol concentrations before and after LDL apheresis are depicted in Figure 3.

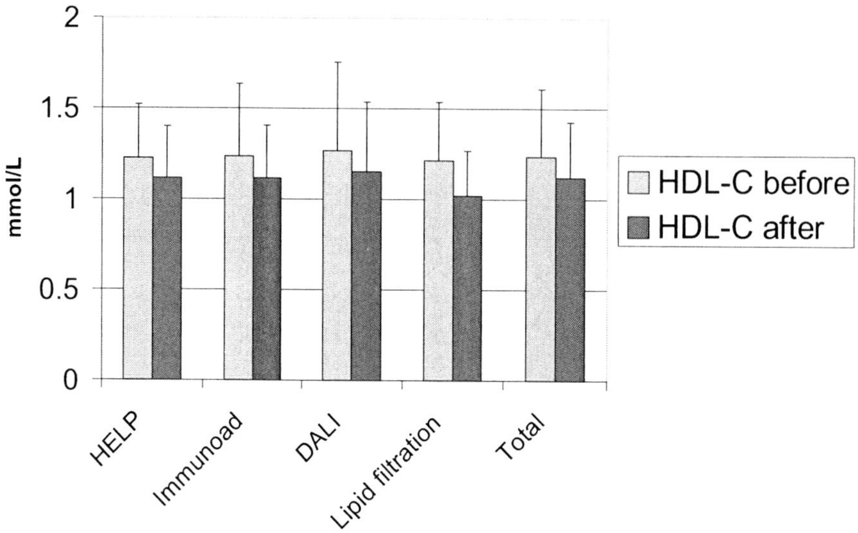


Figure 3. HDL cholesterol levels before and after LDL apheresis (mmol/L).

Lipoprotein(a) concentrations before and after all 4 apheresis methods used are depicted in Figure 4.

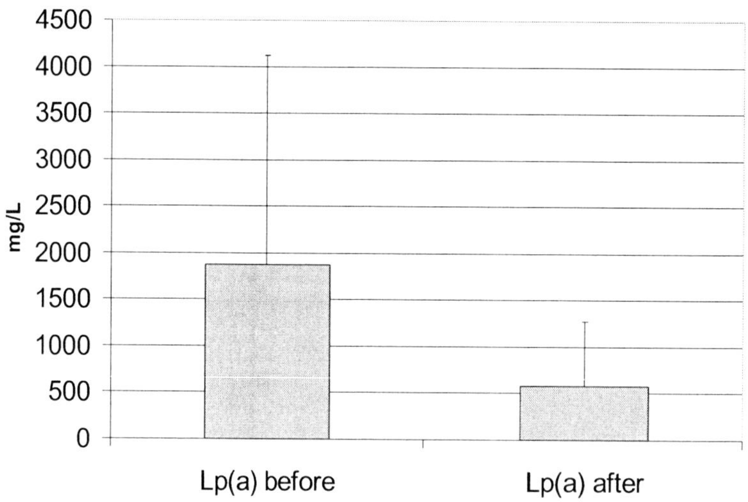


Figure 4. Lipoprotein(a) concentrations before and after all 4 apheresis methods (mg/L)

Side effects of apheresis procedures were very rare: mainly reductions of blood pressure, prolonged bleeding time after a procedure, paraesthesias when calcium levels were low. No life-threatening complications were seen. Sometimes we had difficulties with the venous access. In six patients an arterio-venous shunt had been implemented. 24 patients needed an iron therapy due to the development of an anemia, at least temporarily.

In several of our patients we had measured elevated homocysteine levels which were rather effectively reduced by a therapy including folic acid, vitamin B12 and vitamin B 6 [44].

In no patient who was treated with LDL apheresis at our department a new myocardial infarction had developed. 5 patients underwent a PTCA and 3 patients a cardiac bypass surgery. One patient had died due to an acute heart attack.

## Discussion

Elevated LDL cholesterol concentrations not adequately responding to diet and drug therapy represent an indication for extracorporeal LDL apheresis, which has become an highly effective and approved therapy for those patients in several countries [108]. All our patients were clearly at increased cardiovascular risk. Many of them showed initial LDL cholesterol concentrations that clearly exceeded those which are internationally recommended [28]. These elevated levels persisted despite the fact that the patients were on a statin therapy. All of them had been previously advised with respect to a lipid-modifying nutrition. In some patients a gene mutation of the LDL receptor gene had been detected [9]. 6 patients were smokers when they started the LDL apheresis therapy. At the end of the observation period reported here, only two patients remained smokers.

When considering the indication for a LDL apheresis therapy, the global risk has to be taken into consideration. Neither diet nor drugs are able to effectively reduce the atherogenic lipoprotein(a) levels. The only means is to use LDL apheresis ([107, 2, 33]. Some of our patients had been referred to our center because of this indication (and having a severe coronary atherosclerotic disease) though it is not officially recognized in the German rules [21].

In 24 patients a concomitant hypertension was present and in 11 patients a diabetes mellitus was diagnosed and treated. These factors clearly add to the cardiovascular risk. With the power of the 15 years of prospective evaluation, a study shows that increased smoking, hypertension and LDL cholesterol levels eight times more than HDL cholesterol predicts an adverse coronary heart disease event in patients with familial hypercholesterolemia [75]. In other studies the influence of a diabetes on the occurrence of a myocardial infarction could be shown [22, 72, 32].

The recently registered drug ezetimibe leads in our experience to a further reduction of LDL cholesterol values and has been given to all those patients whose LDL cholesterol concentrations still exceeded 4 mmol/L inspite of the combined treatment with a statin and LDL apheresis. Though in the patients after heart transplantation who are being treated with immunosuppressive agents it is not possible to use ezetimibe.

In the vast majority of our patients a coronary atherosclerosis has been documented by coronary angiography. 4 patients who did not underwent coronary angiography had a severe atherosclerosis at other sites (carotid arteries).

During all the years we did already LDL apheresis we never saw an acute myocardial infarction in our patients. We feel that this is an important step forward since the usual recurrence rate is at least 20 % in patients without hypercholesterolemia [32]. In those 5 patients who underwent a PTCA and in those 3 patients who had to be operated upon a progression of their coronary situation was to be suspected. Usually these interventions were done when the patients suffered from angina pectoris or had a pathological exercise testing. Not in all patients a reangiography has been performed. This means we do not have any prospective data with respect to the course of coronary atherosclerosis. Yet our longitudinal data point to a clear reduction in coronary events when comparing the preapheresis period with the period during apheresis in the same patients. Though we investigated our patients systematically by ultrasound to look at atherosclerotic plaques at the carotids. Only in 1 patient a carotid operation had to be performed. In the others a stable situation has been described. This is in accordance with data in the literature [57]. The one patient who died due to an acute heart attack had previously undergone a coronary bypass operation with 5 bypasses in 1988.

In the literature the positive effect on the course of coronary heart disease could be documented as well [81, 65, 15, 88, 93, 104, 34, 78, 36, 55, 68, 54, 71, 10, 46, 82, 73, 53, 23, 56, 64, 77, 81, 59, 89, 105]. In the studies with a clinical endpoint, approximately 50% reduction in incidence of major coronary events was achieved by LDL apheresis [104]. There also seems to be an effect on the prevention of restenosis after PTCA [30, 48, 70, 1, 24, 50, 113, 47, 114, 69] or after coronary bypass operation [102, 30, 49, 103, 114, 19] though not in all studies a positive result has been observed [115].

The main indication for performing LDL apheresis after a heart transplantation is post-transplant donor vessel disease which can be shown by angiography [39]. Almost all the patients who are treated at our center after heart transplantation have such a disease. One woman with a heart transplantation had been included due to refractory elevations of LDL cholesterol concentrations.

Comparing the different methods of LDL apheresis at our center, we state that based on the percent reductions of LDL cholesterol both the immunoadsorption and the DALI method appeared to be the most effective. In the papers of other groups the immunoadsorption also appeared the most effective method [76, 42a, 80]. The reason is that the plasma volume that can be proceeded is rather unlimited. In other papers similar reductions of LDL cholesterol for different methods have been described [51, 108, 45, 82, 81]. Following a single apheresis procedure LDL cholesterol concentrations increase. In this way, the concentrations before each therapy represent the highest LDL cholesterol values in a given patient. As could be demonstrated in Figure 1, mean LDL cholesterol concentrations before apheresis were about 4 mmol/L and were not found to be different between the different apheresis methods. After the procedures, mean LDL cholesterol concentrations amounted to about 1.5 mmol/L. One can calculate the mean LDL cholesterol concentrations between two treatments. These mean LDL cholesterol concentrations were: HELP 2.864 mmol/L, immunoadsorption 2.762 mmol/L, DALI 2.979 mmol/L, lipid filtration 2.476 mmol/L. They were all significantly different between each other. Most values exceed the internationally accepted target value of 2.6 mmol/L [28, 58]. Thus a certain atherosclerotic risk was still present in the majority of patients.

In those two patients with a familial defective apolipoprotein B the effectiveness of the LDL apheresis was comparable to the other patients. This is in good agreement with the literature [66].

The effectiveness of statins with respect to LDL cholesterol lowering is clearly different [41, 96]. In our hands, atorvastatin is the most effective one and is used in the majority of our patients.

Triglyceride levels were slightly elevated before apheresis and were reduced by all four apheresis methods in a comparable way. Only by the DALI method this reduction appeared to be less. Only the lipid filtration decreased the HDL cholesterol concentrations more strongly. But the values before the LDL apheresis procedures were rather comparable.

According to data in the literature during a single apheresis serum lipoprotein (a) levels fell by 45% and 58% [85], we saw a mean reduction of about 60 %. Other authors describe similar reductions [18, 111, 17b, 40, 16, 26, 6, 4, 79]. The clinical significance of this decrease is still open.

In conclusion, in more than 6000 procedures with LDL apheresis we could show that this method appears to be an effective one with regard to reducing LDL cholesterol concentrations. Clearly our patients suffered from less coronary heart disease than before this treatment. Side effects were rather seldom and no severe case occurred. Though we found small differences between the methods compared we conclude that all 4 methods used can be recommended in hypercholesterolemic patients who are refractory to diet and lipid-lowering drugs.

## Acknowledgments

The authors wish to thank the nurses of the Dresden Apheresis Center (Kerstin Johne, Franziska Meister, Christiane Wagner, Elke Neubert) for their hard work for the patients and their high degree of cooperation.

## References

[1] Adachi H, Niwa A, Shinoda T. Prevention of restenosis after coronary angioplasty with low-density lipoprotein apheresis. *Artif Organs* 1995; 19: 1243-7.

[2] Angelin B. Therapy for lowering lipoprotein (a) levels. *Curr Opin Lipidol* 1997; 8: 337-41.

[3] Armstrong V W, Schleef J, Thiery J, Muche R, Schuff-Werner P, Eisenhauer T, Seidel D. Effect of HELP-LDL-apheresis on serum concentrations of human lipoprotein(a): kinetic analysis of the post-treatment return to baseline levels. *Eur J Clin Invest* 1989; 19: 235-40.

[4] Armstrong V W, Schuff-Werner P, Eisenhauer T, Helmhold M, Stix M, Seidel D. Heparin extracorporeal LDL precipitation (HELP): an effective apheresis procedure for lowering Lp(a) levels. *Chem Phys Lipids* 1994; 67-68: 315-21.

[5] Bambauer R, Schiel R, Keller H E, Latza R. LDL-apheresis in two patients with extremely elevated lipoprotein (a) levels. *Int J Artif Organs* 1995; 18: 286-90.

[6] Banyai S, Streicher J, Strobl W, Gabriel H, Gottsauner-Wolf M, Rohac M, Weidinger F, Horl W H, Derfler K. Therapeutic efficiency of lipoprotein(a) reduction by low-density lipoprotein immunoapheresis. *Metabolism* 1998; 47: 1058-64.

[7] Barbagallo C M, Averna M R, DiMarco T, Spano L, Scafidi V, Marino G, Camemi A R, Notarbartolo A. Effectiveness of cascade filtration plasmapheresis in two patients affected by familial hypercholesterolemia. *J Clin Apheresis* 1995; 10: 96-100.
[8] Blessing F, Wang Y, Nagel D, Seidel D. The efficacy and safety of the new heparin-induced extracorporeal low-density lipoprotein precipitation system (Plasmat Futura) in comparison with the currently used system (Plasmat Secura). *Therap Apher Dial* 2004; 8: 33-8.
[9] Bochmann H, Geisel J, Herrmann W, Purcz T, Reuter W, Julius U, Metzler W, Bergmann S, Jaross W, Gehrisch S. Eight novel LDL receptor gene mutations among patients under LDL apheresis in Dresden and Leipzig. *Hum Mutat* 2001; 17: 76-7.
[10] Borberg H. Results of an open, longitudinal multicenter LDL-apheresis trial. *Transfus Sci* 1999; 20: 83-94.
[11] Bosch T. Low-density lipoprotein hemoperfusion using a modified polyacrylate adsorber: in vitro, ex vivo, and first clinical results. *Artif Organs* 1996; 20: 344-5.
[12] Bosch T. Direct adsorption of lipoproteins from whole blood by DALI apheresis: technique and effects. *Ther Apher* 2001; 5: 239-43.
[13] Bosch T. Recent advances in therapeutic apheresis. J Artif Organs 2003; 6: 1-8.
[14] Bosch T, Keller C. Clinical effects of direct adsorption of lipoprotein apheresis: beyond cholesterol reduction. *Therap Apher Dial* 2003; 7: 341-4.
[15] Bosch T, Wendler T. State of the Art of Low-density Lipoprotein Apheresis in the Year 2003. *Ther Apher* 2004; 8: 76-9.
[16] Bosch T, Lennertz A, Kordes B, Samtleben W. Low density lipoprotein hemoperfusion by direct adsorption of lipoproteins from whole blood (DALI apheresis): clinical experience from a single center. *Ther Apher* 1999; 3: 209-13.
[17] [17a] Bosch T, Heinemann O, Duhr C, Wendler T, Keller C, Fink E, Kirschner T, Klebert S, Samtleben W. Effect of low-dose citrate anticoagulation on the clinical safety and efficacy of direct adsorption of lipoproteins (DALI apheresis) in hypercholesterolemic patients: a prospective controlled clinical trial. *Artif Organs* 2000; 24: 790-6.
[18] [17b] Bosch T, Lennertz A, Schmidt B, Fink E, Keller C, Toepfer M, Drager J, Samtleben W. DALI apheresis in hyperlipidemic patients: biocompatibility, efficacy, and selectivity of direct adsorption of lipoproteins from whole blood. *Artif Organs* 2000; 24: 81-90.
[19] [17c] Bosch T, Wendler T, Jaeger B R, Samtleben W. Improvement of hemorheology by DALI apheresis: acute effects on plasma viscosity and erythrocyte aggregation in hypercholesterolemic patients. *Ther Apher* 2001; 5: 372-6.
[20] [17d] Bosch T, Lennertz A, Samtleben W. High-efficiency DALI apheresis using 1,250 ml adsorbers in a hypercholesterolemic obese patient: a case report. *Ther Apher* 2001; 5: 358-63.
[21] Bosch T, Lennertz A, Schenzle D, Drager J. Direct adsorption of low-density lipoprotein and lipoprotein(a) from whole blood: results of the first clinical long-term multicenter study using DALI apheresis. *J Clin Apheresis* 2002; 17: 161-9.

[22] Brown W V. Benefits of statin therapy in patients with special risks: coronary bypass surgery, stable coronary disease, and acute coronary syndromes. *Clin Cardiol* 2003; 26: III13-8.

[23] Brunner R, Widder R A, Walter P, Borberg H, Oette K. Change in hemorrheological and biochemical parameters following membrane differential filtration. *Int J Artif Organs* 1995; 18: 794-8.

[24] Bundesausschuss der Ärzte und Krankenkassen. Beschluss des Bundesausschusses der Ärzte und Krankenkassen über eine Änderung der Anlage A "Anerkannte Unteruchungs- und Behandlungsmethoden" der Richtlinien über die Bewertung ärztlicher Untersuchungs- und Behandlungsmethoden gemäß § 135 Abs. 1 des Fünften Buches Sozialgesetzbuch (BUB-Richtlinien). *Deutsches Ärzteblatt* 2003; 100: 1595-1596.

[25] Cho E, Rimm E B, Stampfer M J, Willett W C, Hu F B. The impact of diabetes mellitus and prior myocardial infarction on mortality from all causes and from coronary heart disease in men. *J Am Coll Cardiol* 2002; 40: 954-60.

[26] Daida H, Yamaguchi H. Clinical application and effectiveness of low-density lipoprotein apheresis in the treatment of coronary artery disease. *Ther Apher* 1997; 1: 253-4.

[27] Daida H, Lee Y J, Yokoi H, Kanoh T, Ishiwata S, Kato K, Nishikawa H, Takatsu F, Kato H, Kutsumi Y, et a l. Prevention of restenosis after percutaneous transluminal coronary angioplasty by reducing lipoprotein (a) levels with low-density lipoprotein apheresis. Low-Density Lipoprotein Apheresis Angioplasty Restenosis Trial (L-ART) Group. *Am J Cardiol* 1994; 73: 1037-40.

[28] Demetriou K, H'Maltezou E, Pierides A M. Familial homozygous hypercholesterolemia: effective long-term treatment with cascade double filtration plasmapheresis. *Blood Purif* 2001; 19: 308-13.

[29] Drager L J, Julius U, Kraenzle K, Schaper J, Toepfer M, Zygan K, Otto V, Steinhagen-Thiessen E. DALI the first human whole blood low-density lipoprotein and lipoprotein (a) apheresis system in clinical use: procedure and clinical results. *Eur J Clin Invest* 1998; 28: 994-1002.

[30] Eisenhauer T, Armstrong V W, Schuff-Werner P, Schutz E, Thiery J, Scheler F, Seidel D. Long-term clinical experience with HELP-LDL-apheresis in combination with HMG-CoA-reductase inhibitors for maximum treatment of coronary heart disease associated with severe hypercholesterolemia. *ASAIO Trans* 1989; 35: 580-3.

[31] Expert Panel on Detection E a T o H B C i A (T P I E s U S D o H a H S P H S N I o H N H L a B I 2 M 2. Third report of the National Cholesterol Education Program (NCEP). *JAMA* 2001; 285: 2486-2497.

[32] Franceschini G, Busnach G, Vaccarino V, Calabresi L, Gianfranceschi G, Sirtori C R. Apheretic treatment of severe familial hypercholesterolemia: comparison of dextran sulfate cellulose and double membrane filtration methods for low density lipoprotein removal. *Atherosclerosis* 1988; 73: 197-202.

[33] Fukuzawa S, Ozawa S, Inagaki M, Morooka S, Inoue T. Secondary prevention with lipid lowering therapy in familial hypercholesterolemia: a correlation between new

evolution of stenotic lesion and achieved cholesterol levels after revascularization procedures. *Intern Med* 1999; 38: 330-5.

[34] Geiss H C, Parhofer K G, Donner M G, Schwandt P. Low density lipoprotein apheresis by membrane differential filtration (cascade filtration). *Ther Apher* 1999; 3: 199-202.

[35] Haffner S M, Lehto S, Ronnemaa T, Pyorala K, Laakso M. Mortality from coronary heart disease in subjects with type 2 diabetes and in nondiabetic subjects with and without prior myocardial infarction. *N Engl J Med* 1998; 339: 229-34.

[36] Hajjar K A, Nachman R L. The role of lipoprotein(a) in atherogenesis and thrombosis. *Annu Rev Med* 1996; 47: 423-42.

[37] Higashikata T, Mabuchi H. Long-term effect of low-density lipoprotein apheresis in patients with heterozygous familial hypercholesterolemia. *Therap Apher Dial* 2003; 7: 402-7.

[38] Homma Y, Mikami Y, Tamachi H, Nakaya N, Nakamura H, Goto Y. Comparison of selectivity of LDL removal by double filtration and dextran-sulfate cellulose column plasmapheresis, and changes of subfractionated plasma lipoproteins after plasmapheresis in heterozygous familial hypercholesterolemia. *Metabolism* 1987; 36: 419-25.

[39] Hudgins L C, Gordon B R, Parker T S, Saal S D, Levine D M, Rubin A L. LDL Apheresis: an effective and safe treatment for refractory hypercholesterolemia. *Cardiovasc Drug Rev* 2002; 20: 271-80.

[40] Jacob B G, Richter W O, Schwandt P. Therapy of severe familial heterozygous hypercholesterolemia by low-density lipoprotein apheresis with immunoadsorption: effects of the addition of 3-hydroxy-3-methylglutaryl coenzyme A reductase inhibitors to therapy. *Clin Investig* 1993; 71: 908-12.

[41] Jaeger B R. The HELP system for the treatment of atherothrombotic disorders: a review. *Therap Apher Dial* 2003; 7: 391-6.

[42] Jaeger B R, Meiser B, Nagel D, Uberfuhr P, Thiery J, Brandl U, Bruckner W, von Scheidt W, Kreuzer E, Steinbeck G, Reichart B, Seidel D. Aggressive lowering of fibrinogen and cholesterol in the prevention of graft vessel disease after heart transplantation. *Circulation* 1997; 96: II-154-8.

[43] Jansen M, Banyai S, Schmaldienst S, Goldammer A, Rohac M, Horl W H, Derfler K. Direct adsorption of lipoproteins (DALI) from whole blood: first long-term clinical experience with a new LDL-apheresis system for the treatment of familial hypercholesterolaemia. *Wien Klin Wochenschr* 2000; 112: 61-9.

[44] Jones P H, Davidson M H, Stein E A, Bays H E, McKenney J M, Miller E, Cain V A, Blasetto J W. Comparison of the efficacy and safety of rosuvastatin versus atorvastatin, simvastatin, and pravastatin across doses (STELLAR* Trial). *Am J Cardiol* 2003; 92: 152-60.

[45] [42a] Jovin I S, Taborski U, Stehr A, Muller-Berghaus G. Lipid reductions by low-density lipoprotein apheresis: a comparison of three systems. *Metabolism* 2000; 49: 1431-3.

[46] [42b] Jovin I S, Taborski U, Muller-Berghaus G. Analysis of the long-term efficacy and selectivity of immunoadsorption columns for low density lipoprotein apheresis. *ASAIO J* 2000; 46: 298-300.

[47] Julius U, Siegert G, Gromeier S. Intraindividual comparison of the impact of two selective apheresis methods (DALI and HELP) on the coagulation system. *Int J Artif Organs* 2000; 23: 199-206.

[48] Julius U, Pietzsch J, Gromeier S, Schorr H, Herrmann W. Homocysteine levels in patients treated with lipid apheresis: effect of a vitamin therapy. *Eur J Clin Invest* 2001; 31: 667-71.

[49] Julius U, Metzler W, Pietzsch J, Fassbender T, Klingel R. Intraindividual comparison of two extracorporeal LDL apheresis methods: lipidfiltration and HELP. *Int J Artif Organs* 2002; 25: 1180-8.

[50] Kajinami K, Mabuchi H. Therapeutic effects of LDL apheresis in the prevention of atherosclerosis. *Curr Opin Lipidol* 1999; 10: 401-6.

[51] Kanemitsu S, Tekekoshi N, Murakami E. Effects of LDL apheresis on restenosis after angioplasty. *Chem Phys Lipids* 1994; 67-68: 339-43.

[52] Kanemitsu S, Takekoshi N, Matsui S, Tsugawa H, Ohkubo S, Kitayama M, Matsuda T, Senma J, Masuyama K, Yamagata T, Murakami E. Short-term and long-term effects of low-density lipoprotein (LDL) apheresis on restenosis after percutaneous transluminal coronary angioplasty (PTCA): is lowering Lp(a) by LDL apheresis effective on restenosis after PTCA?. *Ther Apher* 1998; 2: 65-70.

[53] Kawasuji M, Sakakibara N, Takemura H, Matsumoto Y, Mabuchi H, Watanabe Y. Coronary artery bypass grafting in familial hypercholesterolemia. *J Thorac Cardiovasc Surg* 1995; 109: 364-9.

[54] Kitabatake A, Sato H, Hori M, Kamada T, Kubori S, Hoki N, Minamino T, Yamada M, Kato T. Coronary atherosclerosis reduced in patients with familial hypercholesterolemia after intensive cholesterol lowering with low-density lipoprotein apheresis: 1 year follow up study. The Osaka LDL Apheresis Multicenter Trial Group. *Clin Ther* 1994; 16: 416-28.

[55] Klingel R, Fassbender T, Fassbender C, Gohlen B. From membrane differential filtration to lipidfiltration: technological progress in low-density lipoprotein apheresis. *Therap Apher Dial* 2003; 7: 350-8.

[56] Klingel R, Mausfeld P, Fassbender C, Goehlen B. Lipidfiltration--safe and effective methodology to perform lipid-apheresis. *Transfus Apheresis Sci* 2004; 30: 245-54.

[57] Koga N. The retardation of progression, stabilization, and regression of coronary and carotid atherosclerosis by low-density lipoprotein apheresis in patients with familial hypercholesterolemia. *Ther Apher* 1997; 1: 260-70.

[58] Koga N. Effects of low-density lipoprotein apheresis on coronary and carotid atherosclerosis and diabetic scleredema in patients with severe hypercholesterolemia. *Ther Apher* 2001; 5: 244-51.

[59] Koga N. Meaning of low-density lipoprotein-apheresis for hypercholesterolemic patients at high risk for recurrence of coronary heart disease. *Ther Apher* 2002; 6: 372-80.

[60] Koga N, Iwata Y, Yamamoto A. Angiographic and pathological studies on regression of coronary atherosclerosis of FH patients who received LDL-apheresis treatment. *Artif Organs* 1992; 16: 171-6.

[61] Koga N, Watanabe K, Kurashige Y, Sato T, Hiroki T. Long-term effects of LDL apheresis on carotid arterial atherosclerosis in familial hypercholesterolaemic patients. *J Intern Med* 1999; 246: 35-43.

[62] Krebs A, Krebs K, Keller F. Retrospective comparison of 5 different methods for long-term LDL-apheresis in 20 patients between 1986 and 2001. *Int J Artif Organs* 2004; 27: 137-48.

[63] Kroon A A, Aengevaeren W R, van der Werf T, Uijen G J, Reiber J H, Bruschke A V, Stalenhoef A F. LDL-Apheresis Atherosclerosis Regression Study (LAARS). Effect of aggressive versus conventional lipid lowering treatment on coronary atherosclerosis. *Circulation* 1996; 93: 1826-35.

[64] Lane D M, McConathy W J, Laughlin L O, Comp P C, von Albertini B, Gibson S M, Bricker L A, Kozlovskis P, Dorrier C. Weekly treatment of diet/drug-resistant hypercholesterolemia with the heparin-induced extracorporeal low-density lipoprotein precipitation (HELP) system by selective plasma low-density lipoprotein removal. *Am J Cardiol* 1993; 71: 816-22.

[65] Lees R S, Holmes N N, Stadler R W, Ibrahim S F, Lees A M. Treatment of hypercholesterolemia with heparin-induced extracorporeal low-density lipoprotein precipitation (HELP). *J Clin Apheresis* 1996; 11: 132-7.

[66] Legallais C, Moriniere P, Wojcicki J M, Lalau J D, Fournier A, Jaffrin M Y. A high selectivity cascade filtration technique for LDL-cholesterol and Lp(a) removal. *Artif Organs* 1995; 19: 887-95.

[67] Legallais C, Moriniere P, Fournier A, Jaffrin M Y. Pulsed flow cascade filtration. Long-term experience in low density lipoprotein and lipoprotein a removal. *ASAIO J* 1996; 42: M463-7.

[68] Mabuchi H, Koizumi J, Shimizu M, Kajinami K, Miyamoto S, Ueda K, Takegoshi T. Long-term efficacy of low-density lipoprotein apheresis on coronary heart disease in familial hypercholesterolemia. Hokuriku-FH-LDL-Apheresis Study Group. *Am J Cardiol* 1998; 82: 1489-95.

[69] Mabuchi H, Higashikata T, Kawashiri M A. Clinical applications of long-term LDL-apheresis on and beyond refractory hypercholesterolemia. *Transfus Apheresis Sci* 2004; 30: 233-43.

[70] Maher V M, Kitano Y, Neuwirth C, Gallagher J J, Thompson G R, Myant N B. Effective reduction of plasma LDL levels by LDL apheresis in familial defective apolipoprotein B-100. *Atherosclerosis* 1992; 95: 231-4.

[71] Matic G, Kohlschein P, Wallstab U, Tiess M, Winkler R, Prophet H, Ramlow W, Schuff-Werner P. Comparison of two filter combinations for low-density lipoprotein apheresis by membrane differential filtration: a prospective crossover controlled clinical study. *Artif Organs* 2002; 26: 371-7.

[72] Matsuzaki M, Hiramori K, Imaizumi T, Kitabatake A, Hishida H, Nomura M, Fujii T, Sakuma I, Fukami K, Honda T, Ogawa H, Yamagishi M. Intravascular ultrasound evaluation of coronary plaque regression by low density lipoprotein-apheresis in

familial hypercholesterolemia: the Low Density Lipoprotein-Apheresis Coronary Morphology and Reserve Trial (LACMART). *J Am Coll Cardiol* 2002; 40: 220-7.

[73] Messerli A W, Aronow H D, Sprecher D L. The Lescol Intervention Prevention Study (LIPS): start all patients on statins early after PCI. *Cleve Clin J Med* 2003; 70: 561-6.

[74] Miyamoto T, Niwa A, Sinoda T. State of percutaneous transluminal coronary artery angioplasty and effectiveness of low-density lipoprotein apheresis. *Ther Apher* 2001; 5: 226-31.

[75] Moriarty P M, Gibson C A. Low-density lipoprotein apheresis in the treatment of atherosclerosis and other potential uses. Curr Atheroscler Rep 2001; 3: 156-62.

[76] Mukamal K J, Nesto R W, Cohen M C, Muller J E, Maclure M, Sherwood J B, Mittleman M A. Impact of diabetes on long-term survival after acute myocardial infarction: comparability of risk with prior myocardial infarction. *Diabetes Care* 2001; 24: 1422-7.

[77] Nishimura S, Sekiguchi M, Kano T, Ishiwata S, Nagasaki F, Nishide T, Okimoto T, Kutsumi Y, Kuwabara Y, Takatsu F, Nishikawa H, Daida H, Yamaguchi H. Effects of intensive lipid lowering by low-density lipoprotein apheresis on regression of coronary atherosclerosis in patients with familial hypercholesterolemia: Japan Low-density Lipoprotein Apheresis Coronary Atherosclerosis Prospective Study (L-CAPS). *Atherosclerosis* 1999; 144: 409-17.

[78] Otto C, Geiss H C, Donner M G, Parhofer K G, Schwandt P. Influence of atorvastatin versus simvastatin on fibrinogen and other hemorheological parameters in patients with severe hypercholesterolemia treated with regular low-density lipoprotein immunoadsorption apheresis. *Ther Apher* 2000; 4: 244-8.

[79] Panagiotakos D B, Pitsavos C, Skoumas J, Chrysohoou C, Toutouza M, Stefanadis C I, Toutouzas P K. Importance of LDL/HDL cholesterol ratio as a predictor for coronary heart disease events in patients with heterozygous familial hypercholesterolaemia: a 15-year follow-up (1987-2002). *Curr Med Res Opin* 2003; 19: 89-94.

[80] Parhofer K G, Geiss H C, Schwandt P. Efficacy of different low-density lipoprotein apheresis methods. *Ther Apher* 2000; 4: 382-5.

[81] Park J W, Merz M, Braun P. Effect of HELP-LDL-apheresis on outcomes in patients with advanced coronary atherosclerosis and severe hypercholesterolemia. *Atherosclerosis* 1998; 139: 401-9.

[82] Ramunni A, Morrone L F, Baldassarre G, Montagna E, Saracino A, Coratelli P. Effectiveness of long-term heparin-induced extracorporeal LDL precipitation (HELP) in improving coronary calcifications. *Int J Artif Organs* 2003; 26: 252-5.

[83] Richter W O, Jacob B G, Ritter M M, Suhler K, Vierneisel K, Schwandt P. Three-year treatment of familial heterozygous hypercholesterolemia by extracorporeal low-density lipoprotein immunoadsorption with polyclonal apolipoprotein B antibodies. *Metabolism* 1993; 42: 888-94.

[84] Richter W O, Donner M G, Schwandt P. Short- and long-term effects on serum lipoproteins by three different techniques of apheresis. *Artif Organs* 1996; 20: 311-7.

[85] Richter W O, Donner M G, Hofling B, Schwandt P. Long-term effect of low-density lipoprotein apheresis on plasma lipoproteins and coronary heart disease in native

vessels and coronary bypass in severe heterozygous familial hypercholesterolemia. *Metabolism* 1998; 47: 863-8.
[86] Richter W O, Donner M G, Schwandt P. Three low density lipoprotein apheresis techniques in treatment of patients with familial hypercholesterolemia: a long-term evaluation. *Ther Apher* 1999; 3: 203-8.
[87] Riesen W F, Jaross W, Descoeudres C, Mordasini R, Koban F, Thulin H, Fisher S, Bergmann S. Lipoprotein changes in familial hypercholesterolemia after extracorporeal immunoadsorption of low density lipoproteins. *Ann Biol Clin (Paris)* 1988; 46: 787-91.
[88] Ritter M M, Parhofer K G. Extracorporal low-density lipoprotein elimination by immunoadsorption. *Therap Apher Dial* 2003; 7: 370-2.
[89] Ritter M M, Suhler K, Richter W, Schwandt P. Short- and long-term effects of LDL-apheresis on lipoprotein (a) serum levels. *Clin Chim Acta* 1990; 195: 9-15.
[90] Ritter M M, Richter W O, Schwandt P. Elimination of lipoprotein(a) by apheresis using polyclonal apo-B 100 antibodies. *J Clin Apheresis* 1994; 9: 240.
[91] Schmaldienst S, Goldammer A, Spitzauer S, Derfler K, Horl W H, Knobl P. Local anticoagulation of the extracorporeal circuit with heparin and subsequent neutralization with protamine during immunoadsorption. *Am J Kidney Dis* 2000; 36: 490-7.
[92] Schuff-Werner P. [Clinical long-term results of H.E.L.P.-apheresis]. *Z Kardiol* 2003; 92: III28-9.
[93] Schuff-Werner P, Gohlke H, Bartmann U, Baggio G, Corti M C, Dinsenbacher A, Eisenhauer T, Grutzmacher P, Keller C, Kettner U, et a l. The HELP-LDL-apheresis multicentre study, an angiographically assessed trial on the role of LDL-apheresis in the secondary prevention of coronary heart disease. II. Final evaluation of the effect of regular treatment on LDL-cholesterol plasma concentrations and the course of coronary heart disease. The HELP-Study Group. Heparin-induced extra-corporeal LDL-precipitation. *Eur J Clin Invest* 1994; 24: 724-32.
[94] Seidel D. The HELP system: an efficient and safe method of plasma therapy in the treatment of severe hypercholesterolemia. *Ther Umsch* 1990; 47: 514-9.
[95] Seidel D. The HELP-system in the treatment of severe hypercholesterolaemia: acute and long-term experience. *Adv Exp Med Biol* 1991; 285: 155-9.
[96] Seidel D. H.E.L.P. apheresis therapy in the treatment of severe hypercholesterolemia: 10 years of clinical experience. *Artif Organs* 1996; 20: 303-10.
[97] Seidel D. [LDL-apheresis in the treatment of coronary heart disease. Rationale for a specific adjuvant therapy]. *Z Kardiol* 2003; 92: III6-27.
[98] Seidel D, Armstrong V W, Schuff-Werner P, Eisenhauer T. Removal of low-density lipoproteins (LDL) and fibrinogen by precipitation with heparin at low pH: clinical application and experience. *J Clin Apheresis* 1988; 4: 78-81.
[99] Seidel D, Armstrong V W, Schuff-Werner P. The HELP-LDL-apheresis multicentre study, an angiographically assessed trial on the role of LDL-apheresis in the secondary prevention of coronary heart disease. I. Evaluation of safety and cholesterol-lowering effects during the first 12 months. HELP Study Group. *Eur J Clin Invest* 1991; 21: 375-83.

[100] Shepherd J, Hunninghake D B, Barter P, McKenney J M, Hutchinson H G. Guidelines for lowering lipids to reduce coronary artery disease risk: a comparison of rosuvastatin with atorvastatin, pravastatin, and simvastatin for achieving lipid-lowering goals. *Am J Cardiol* 2003; 91: 11C-17C; discussion 17C-19C.

[101] Siami G A, Siami F S. The current status of therapeutic apheresis devices in the United States. *Int J Artif Organs* 2002; 25: 499-502.

[102] Stefanutti C, Di Giacomo S, Di Caro M, Vivenzio A, Musca A. DALI low-density lipoprotein apheresis in homozygous and heterozygous familial hypercholesterolemic patients using low-dose citrate anticoagulation. *Ther Apher* 2001; 5: 364-71.

[103] Straube R, Gackler D, Thiele A, Muselmann L, Kingreen H, Klingel R. Membrane differential filtration is safe and effective for the long-term treatment of Refsum syndrome--an update of treatment modalities and pathophysiological cognition. *Transfus Apheresis Sci* 2003; 29: 85-91.

[104] Susca M. Heparin-Induced extracorporeal low-density lipoprotein precipitation futura, a new modification of HELP apheresis: technique and first clinical results. *Ther Apher* 2001; 5: 387-93.

[105] Taborski U, Kohler T, Schupphaus S, Hofmann M R, Muller-Berghaus G. Application of an automated plasma filtration device and a blood monitoring system for LDL apheresis. *Infusionsther Transfusionsmed* 1992; 19: 187-9.

[106] Takahashi K, Kobayashi J, Bujo H, Takahashi M, Taira K, Kaneko K, Tashiro J, Shinomiya M, Miyazaki A, Saito Y. Long-term (14 years) effect of LDL apheresis on obstructive changes in aortocoronary saphenous-vein bypass grafts in a case of heterozygous familial hypercholesterolemia with the LDL receptor proline664 to leucine mutation. *Intern Med* 2000; 39: 804-9.

[107] Takahashi T, Nakano S, Shimazaki Y, Kaneko M, Hirata N, Nakamura T, Matsuzawa Y, Kitamura S, Matsuda H. Long-term appraisal of coronary bypass operations in familial hypercholesterolemia. *Ann Thorac Surg* 1993; 56: 499-505.

[108] Tasaki H. Low-density lipoprotein apheresis in the prevention of recurrent coronary heart disease: a review. *Therap Apher Dial* 2003; 7: 408-12.

[109] Tatami R, Inoue N, Itoh H, Kishino B, Koga N, Nakashima Y, Nishide T, Okamura K, Saito Y, Teramoto T, et a l. Regression of coronary atherosclerosis by combined LDL-apheresis and lipid-lowering drug therapy in patients with familial hypercholesterolemia: a multicenter study. The LARS Investigators. *Atherosclerosis* 1992; 95: 1-13.

[110] Thiery J, Seidel D. LDL-apheresis: clinical experience and indications in the treatment of severe hypercholesterolemia. *Transfus Sci* 1993; 14: 249-59.

[111] Thomas H P, Steinhagen-Thiessen E. [Lipoprotein(a): Aspects of pathophysiology, epidemiology and treatment]. *Z Kardiol* 2003; 92: III53-8.

[112] Thompson G R. LDL apheresis. *Atherosclerosis* 2003; 167: 1-13.

[113] von Baeyer H, Schartl M, Bimmermann A. Outcome of patients on long term low-density lipoprotein apheresis with membrane differential filtration: a case study in three patients 14 years on treatment. *Ther Apher* 2000; 4: 386-94.

[114] Wang Y, Blessing F, Walli A K, Uberfuhr P, Fraunberger P, Seidel D. Effects of heparin-mediated extracorporeal low-density lipoprotein precipitation beyond

lowering proatherogenic lipoproteins-reduction of circulating proinflammatory and procoagulatory markers. *Atherosclerosis* 2004; 175: 145-50.

[115] Wendler T, Lennertz A, Heinemann O, Duhr C, Samtleben W, Bosch T. Heparin-free DALI LDL-apheresis in hyperlipidemic patients: efficacy, safety and biocompatibility. *Int J Artif Organs* 2000; 23: 710-7.

[116] Wendler T, Schilling R, Lennertz A, Sodemann K, Kleophas W, Messner H, Riechers G, Wagner J, Keller C, Bosch T. Efficacy and safety of DALI LDL-apheresis at high blood flow rates: a prospective multicenter study. *J Clin Apheresis* 2003; 18: 157-66.

[117] Yamaguchi H, Lee Y J, Daida H, Yokoi H, Miyano H, Kanoh T, Ishiwata S, Kato K, Nishikawa H, Takatsu F, et a l. Effectiveness of LDL-apheresis in preventing restenosis after percutaneous transluminal coronary angioplasty (PTCA): LDL-apheresis angioplasty restenosis trial (L-ART). *Chem Phys Lipids* 1994; 67-68: 399-403.

[118] Yamamoto A, Harada-Shiba M, Kawaguchi A, Tsushima M. Apheresis technology for prevention and regression of atherosclerosis. *Ther Apher* 2001; 5: 221-5.

[119] Yamashita K, Tasaki H, Tsuda Y, Himeno E, Nakashima Y. Can aggressive lipid lowering using low-density lipoprotein apheresis prevent restenosis after percutaneous transluminal coronary angioplasty in patients with normocholesterolemia?. *Ther Apher* 1998; 2: 210-7.

In: Cholesterol in Atherosclerosis and Coronary Heart Disease ISBN 1-59454-302-X
Editor: Jean P. Kovala, pp. 63-78 

*Chapter IV*

# HDL Cholesterol and CETP Inhibitors

***Hisashi Shinkai***
Central Pharmaceutical Research Institute, JT Inc.

## Abstract

Both a high plasma low-density lipoprotein (LDL) cholesterol level and a low plasma high-density lipoprotein (HDL) cholesterol level are critical risk factors for atherosclerosis and coronary heart disease. Therefore, increasing the plasma HDL cholesterol level is the next target for the treatment of atherosclerosis and coronary heart disease. Although statins, fibrates, and niacin can be used to improve low plasma HDL cholesterol levels, the effect of such drugs is limited. Agents that achieve better elevation of plasma HDL cholesterol levels are therefore needed. Among the many methods that may be used to raise the plasma HDL cholesterol level, this chapter focuses on cholesteryl ester transfer protein (CETP) inhibitors, including JTT-705 and torcetrapib.

## Introduction

Low-density lipoprotein (LDL) cholesterol is well known to be a major risk factor for atherosclerosis and coronary heart disease [1], and has been the primary target of therapeutic approaches to prevent coronary heart disease over the past two decades. 3-Hydroxy-3-methylglutaryl co-enzyme A (HMG-CoA) reductase inhibitors, which are also known as statins, achieve a marked reduction of plasma LDL cholesterol levels that is associated with a 30% to 45% decrease of clinical events [2-6]. However, many patients still suffer from cardiac events despite a decrease in plasma LDL cholesterol levels, which indicates that other risk factors besides a high plasma LDL cholesterol are also associated with the development of cardiac events. A low plasma high-density lipoprotein (HDL) cholesterol level has been noted as another risk factor for atherosclerosis and coronary heart disease [7-9]. Plasma levels of HDL cholesterol and its major protein component, apolipoprotein A-I (apoA-I), show a consistent inverse association with the risk of coronary heart disease in observational studies [10-12]. A 1% decrease of the plasma HDL cholesterol level is associated with a 1% to 2% increase in the risk of coronary heart disease [13]. Moreover, 5 weekly infusions of recombinant apoA-I Milano/phospholipid complex have been shown to decrease the total atheroma volume (measured using intravascular ultrasound) by 4.2% in 36 patients with acute coronary syndrome [14]. This effect on the atherosclerotic disease burden of a short-term treatment was greater than expected. The rapid regression observed in that study may provide evidence of a dynamic process associated with HDL-mediated reverse cholesterol transport. Interestingly, persons who are carriers of apoA-I Milano are protected from vascular disease. The substitution of cysteine for arginine at position 173 in the apoA-I Milano variant allows dimerization and the formation of large HDL particles that may be particularly active in reverse cholesterol transport. Although apoA-I Milano is a mutant of native apoA-I, it seems to be more atheroprotective than the native form protein and this suggests that raising plasma HDL cholesterol levels may be a useful therapeutic objective.

Reverse cholesterol transport mediated by HDL is the best known atheroprotective mechanism of HDL (Figure 1) [15, 16]. The excess cholesterol in peripheral tissues, including arterial macrophages, is removed through the ATP-binding cassette transporter 1 (ABCA1) to be taken up by lipid-poor apoA-I, forming pre-ß-HDL [17-21]. Lecithin-cholesterol acyltransferase (LCAT) then esterifies free cholesterol to form cholesteryl esters, thus converting pre- ß-HDL to mature spherical α-HDL [22]. After accepting excess cellular cholesterol from peripheral tissues, such as arterial macrophages, HDL returns it to the liver by two pathways. HDL can directly transfers cholesterol to the liver through the scavenger receptor BI (SR-BI), after which excretion in the bile occurs [23]. As an indirect pathway, the cholesteryl esters in HDL can be transferred by cholesteryl ester transfer protein (CETP) to very-low-density lipoprotein (VLDL) and LDL, and then partially returned to the liver via the LDL receptor [24]. A second major atheroprotective mechanism of HDL is that it protects LDL from oxidation [25, 26]. Unlike normal LDL, oxidized LDL is readily taken up by the macrophage scavenger receptor SR-A or CD36, resulting in the development of foam cells. Oxidized lipids are transferred to HDL from LDL and are hydrolyzed by HDL paraoxonase and platelet-activating factor acetylhydrolase [27, 28].

HDL has been noted as a potential new therapeutic target for the treatment of cardiovascular disease based on the recognition that a low plasma HDL cholesterol level is an independent risk factor for coronary heart disease. However, current therapies for increasing a low plasma HDL cholesterol level are not wholly satisfactory. Fibrates and statins produce only modest elevation of plasma HDL cholesterol (5% to 15%) [29, 30]. Nicotinic acid (niacin) increases plasma HDL cholesterol by 26%, but its side effects limit compliance with therapy [31]. Therefore, safer and more effective drugs that can significantly increase the plasma HDL cholesterol level are needed. There are many possible approaches to the elevation of plasma HDL cholesterol, such as increasing LCAT activity [32] or lipoprotein lipase activity [33], as well as increasing the levels of phospholipid transfer protein (PLTP) [34], apoA-I [35], or ABCA1 [36], modulating the expression of the hepatic HDL scavenger receptor [37], and inhibiting hepatic triglyceride lipase activity [33] or CETP activity [38, 39]. Among these targets, this chapter focuses on small molecule CETP inhibitors, due to some recent advances in this field.

# CETP

CETP is a hydrophobic plasma glycoprotein that was synthesized in the liver and is mainly bound to HDL [40, 41]. CETP mediates the transfer of cholesteryl esters from HDL to VLDL and LDL and the transfer of triglycerides from VLDL to HDL (Figure 1) [42]. This process not only decreases the level of anti-atherogenic HDL cholesterol but also increases pro-atherogenic VLDL cholesterol and LDL cholesterol, so CETP is a potentially atherogenic protein. However, a possible anti-atherogenic role of CETP has also been suggested because of its participation in reverse cholesterol transport [43-46]. If the increase of cholesteryl ester in LDL mediated by CETP mainly results in its return to the liver via the LDL receptor, CETP could be anti-atherogenic, but if the cholesteryl ester in LDL is taken up by arterial macrophages, CETP would be pro-atherogenic. Although the role of CETP in the progression of atherosclerosis remains controversial, many studies have shown that it has a pro-atherogenic effect.

Mice and rats are naturally deficient in CETP. These animals are relatively resistant to the development of dietary atherosclerosis and perform reverse cholesterol transport without a CETP-mediated pathway. If CETP is pro-atherogenic, mice should show a reduced ability to resist the development of dietary atherosclerosis when bearing CETP. Introduction of the human *CETP* gene into mice results in a dose-related reduction of plasma HDL levels, as well as a slight increase of plasma VLDL, LDL cholesterol, and apolipoprotein B (apoB) levels [47, 48]. Bile salt- and cholesterol-fed C57-B16 mice expressing the simian *CETP* gene show enhanced formation of fatty streaks compared with nonexpressing controls [49]. It has been suggested that the enhancement of lesions by CETP is secondary to redistribution of cholesterol from HDL to the VLDL/LDL fraction. These findings support the view that CETP is pro-atherogenic.

Rabbits have a naturally high level of CETP and tend to develop dietary atherosclerosis. This raises the question of whether rabbits would show a lower tendency to develop dietary atherosclerosis if CETP was inhibited. The inhibition of CETP in cholesterol-fed rabbits by intravenous injection of antisense oligodeoxynucleotides for CETP targeted to the liver results in a reduction of hepatic CETP mRNA, an increase of hepatic LDL receptor mRNA, a decrease of CETP mass, an increase of plasma HDL cholesterol, a decrease of total plasma cholesterol, and a decrease of the aortic cholesterol content and aortic percent lesion to total surface area [50]. An immunotherapeutic approach to decreasing CETP activity in vivo by using a vaccine to produce antibodies that bind to and block the function of CETP has also been investigated. In fact, CETP activity can be reduced in vivo by vaccination with a peptide derived from this protein. In a cholesterol-fed rabbit model of atherosclerosis, the CETP-vaccinated group showed a 42% increase of plasma HDL cholesterol, a 24% decrease of plasma LDL cholesterol, and a 39.6% decrease of the aortic surface exhibiting atherosclerosis lesions [51]. The marked reduction of atherosclerosis observed in rabbits after inhibition of CETP provides support for the concept that inhibition of CETP in vivo can be antiatherogenic.

In humans with elevated HDL cholesterol levels, several mutations of the *CETP* gene have been identified as a cause of CETP deficiency. A G-to-A mutation at the +1 position of intron 14 is present in up to 2% of the Japanese population and in 27% of the inhabitants of the Omagari district of Japan [52-56]. These people are homozygous for this mutation and have no CETP mass or activity. Their plasma HDL cholesterol and phospholipid levels are elevated by 3- to 4-fold and the apoA-I level is also elevated by 1.7-fold [53]. A D-to-G substitution at position 442 of exon 15 is another common functional mutation of the *CETP* gene [55]. Up to 7% of the Japanese population has this mutation and it leads to increased plasma HDL levels. Individuals homozygous for this D442G mutation only have partial CETP deficiency and 1- to 2-fold elevation of plasma HDL [55]. Plasma HDL cholesterol, apoA-I, apolipoprotein A-II (apoA-II), and apolipoprotein E (apoE) levels are elevated in subjects with homozygous CETP deficiency. The HDL fraction is especially rich in larger, less dense, cholesteryl ester- and apoE-rich $HDL_2$ particles [57]. Although large, apoE-rich $HDL_2$ particles are poor acceptors of arterial macrophage cholesterol, the apoE-free $HDL_2$ and the $HDL_3$ particles from homozygous CETP-deficient subjects function normally as acceptors of arterial macrophage cholesterol. Furthermore, the protective effect of HDL has been most consistently observed with respect to the large HDL subfraction, and some evidence suggests that small HDL levels may be positively correlated wtih the severity of coronary artery disease [58-62]. A study on the relationship of HDL subclass to the severity and rate of progression of coronary atherosclerosis in 60 men who survived myocardial infarction found a significant inverse correlation between the plasma level of the largest HDL particles (the $HDL_{2b}$ subclass) and both disease severity and the progression of coronary lesions [62]. A new and convenient procedure for quantifying plasma levels of lipoprotein subclasses by proton nuclear magnetic resonance (NMR) spectroscopy can simultaneously and rapidly determine the concentrations of VLDL, LDL, and HDL subspecies without the need for physical fractionation of the plasma [63]. In a study on the relationship of NMR-derived data on lipoprotein subclasses with the severity of arteriographically documented coronary artery disease in 158 men, subjects with relatively high levels of either small HDL or large VLDL particles were three to four times more likely to have extensive coronary artery disease, and the 27 men with high levels of both large VLDL and small HDL were 15 times more likely to have extensive coronary artery disease than the men with low levels of these particles. In addition to the elevation of plasma HDL cholesterol, subjects with CETP deficiency show a substantial reduction of plasma LDL cholesterol and apoB levels. A study on the metabolic basis for the decrease of plasma LDL cholesterol and apoB levels in CETP deficiency has shown that the fractional catabolic rate of LDL apoB is significantly increased in CETP-deficient subjects, while the production of apoB in VLDL and intermediate density lipoprotein is decreased by 55% and 81%, respectively. Decreased plasma LDL cholesterol and apoB levels in CETP-deficient subjects are associated with both a decrease of apoB production and a substantial increase of LDL apoB catabolism. The LDL receptor pathway may be up-regulated in CETP deficiency. The lipoprotein profile of CETP-deficient subjects seems to be anti-atherogenic, but the relationship between mutations of the CETP gene and susceptibility to atherosclerosis is complex. The available human studies on the relationship between CETP polymorphisms and atherosclerosis or coronary heart disease generally support the hypothesis that CETP deficiency is anti-atherogenic when it associated with a high HDL level, but these studies also suggest that atherosclerosis is promoted in some individuals who are heterozygous for CETP deficiency [64]. These conflicting results may be due to a small sample size, the confounding effect of other risk factors, or biases inherent in the study design [64].

Although it remains controversial whether CETP is anti-atherogenic or pro-atherogenic, many studies support the pro-atherogenicity of CETP and anti-atherogenicity of its inhibition [49-67], so the concept that effective and safe CETP inhibitors have potential as novel anti-atherogenic drugs has led to the development of CETP inhibitors. In fact, two small molecule CETP inhibitors, JTT-705 and torcetrapib, are currently undergoing clinical trials. Many compounds, such as cholesterol derivatives, natural products, and synthetic compounds, have been reported as CETP inhibitors. However, most of these only show a modest in vitro potency and have no in vivo activity. Because CETP is not an enzyme but a transfer protein and because its three-dimensional structure has not been identified, it may be difficult to generate potent and active CETP inhibitors. Among the various compounds, only JTT-705 and torcetrapib have survived to reach clinical trials.

## JTT-705

A benzenethiol derivative, JTT-705, was first reported to show an anti-atherogenic effect as a small molecule CETP inhibitor [68, 69]. JTT-705 was derived from an initial lead compound, bis(2-(acetylamino)phenyl) disulfide, that showed 50% inhibition of CETP activity in human plasma at a concentration of 500μM (Figure 2). The partial structures (alkyl, amide, benzene and disulfide moieties) of the initial lead compound were systematically varied to clarify structure-activity relationships and to determine an optimum CETP inhibitor. The alkyl moiety caused a marked increase of potency when it had the appropriate lipophilicity, size, and steric shape, indicating that this moiety might promote specific binding to CETP. In particular, tertiary alkyl groups, such as 1-substituted cyclohexyl groups, were specific for a high potency. The amide moiety could not be displaced by other structures, indicating its necessity. Introduction of electron-withdrawing groups into the benzene moiety increased in the vitro potency [70], probably due to increased reactivity of the thiol group that forms disulfide bond. However, the in vitro potency did not always reflect the in vivo potency. Under in vivo conditions, increased reactivity may cause a decrease of specificity. It was found that the disulfide moiety could be displaced by a thiol or thioester, indicating that the thiol and thioester groups played the same role as the disulfide group and that the dimeric structure of the initial lead compound was not essential. Since the thioester was readily hydrolyzed to a thiol in serum, it was suspected to actally be the precursor of a thiol. If the disulfide group and the thiol group were functionally equivalent, the common ability to form a disulfide bond with another thiol group could be important. If so, formation of a disulfide bond with this series of CETP inhibitors and a cysteine residue of CETP could be related to the mechanism of inhibition. Because the disulfides were not orally bioavailable and the thiols were potentially unstable, the reasonably stable and orally bioavailable thoesters were selected for further studies. As a result, thioester JTT-705 was selected as the optimum compound. Investigations based on point mutations of recombinant human CETP revealed the inhibitory mechanism of JTT-705. Human CETP consists of 476 amino acids and contains seven cysteines. As CETP is a monomer, it must possess at least one unpaired cysteine that forms a disulfide bond with another thiol or disulfide [27]. Each cysteine in CETP was replaced by serine and seven CETP mutants were constructed. Among these mutants, three in which the cysteine at residue 1 (C1S), 13 (C13S), or 131 (C131S) was replaced by serine maintained transfer activity. JTT-705 could inhibit the C1S and C131S mutants, but could not inhibit the C13S mutant, suggesting that the inhibitory mechanism involves the formation of a disulfide bond between the thiol form of JTT-705 and the cysteine residue at position 13 of CETP.

JTT-705 inhibited CETP activity in human plasma ($IC_{50}$ = 6~9 μM), and also produced 95% inhibition of CETP activity at an oral dose of 30 mg/kg in normal rabbits. Moreover, administration of JTT-705 (225 mg/kg/day) for six months caused a 90% increase of the plasma HDL cholesterol and decreased the plasma non-HDL cholesterol by 40-50% compared with the baseline values. As a result, JTT-705 decreased atherosclerotic lesions by 70% in cholesterol-fed rabbits, providing the first evidence that a small molecule CETP inhibitor can retard the progression of atherosclerosis.

The results of a randomized phase II dose-finding study of JTT-705 in 198 healthy subjects with mild hyerlipidemia (daily doses of 300, 600, or 900 mg) have also been reported [71]. CETP activity was inhibited by 15.4%, 29.6%, and 37.2% at 300, 600, and 900 mg/day, respectively. A dose-dependent decrease of CETP activity was observed after 1 week of treatment, with a maximum decrease of 37.2% from baseline after 4 weeks in the high-dose group. During treatment, the CETP concentration increased dose-dependently and a 66.8% increase of CETP mass was observed after 4 weeks in the high-dose group.

A dose-dependent increase of plasma HDL cholesterol was observed, reaching a plateau after the first week. The effect of JTT-705 (900 mg daily) on plasma HDL cholesterol was apparent after 4 weeks of treatment and there was an increase of 33.9%. The overall rise of plasma HDL cholesterol was caused by a significant increase of both $HDL_2$ and $HDL_3$. The increase of $HDL_2$ was dose-dependent over the dose range tested, whereas the increment of $HDL_3$ was slight in this dose range. The rise of plasma HDL cholesterol in all tested groups was also accompanied by significant increases of both apoA-I and apoA-II. All of the treated groups showed a decrease of plasma LDL cholesterol, with a 7.4% reduction in the high-dose group. A reduction of plasma LDL cholesterol is not unexpected in the context of reduced cholesteryl ester flux from HDL to LDL. The same effect is observed in individuals with a high baseline LDL cholesterol level, such as patients suffering from familial hypercholesterolemia who also have CETP gene mutations [72]. The levels of apoB, apoE, total cholesterol, and triglycerides were not significantly changed by JTT-705 at doses of up to 900 mg daily. The atherogenicity index, represented by the total cholesterol/HDL cholesterol ratio, was significantly reduced in all 3 active treatment groups compared with the placebo group. In this study, treatment with JTT-705 at 900 mg daily for 4 weeks led to a 37% decrease of CETP activity, a 34% increase of HDL cholesterol, a 16% increase of apoA-I, and a 7% decrease of LDL cholesterol, whereas the levels of triglycerides, PLTP, and LCAT were unaffected. It is important to note that inhibition of CETP by JTT-705 was not accompanied by any changes of PLTP and LCAT activity, underlining the specificity of this drug. The rise in plasma HDL cholesterol was caused by a significant increase of large cholesterol-rich $HDL_2$, which was expected to increase due to CETP inhibition, and also an increase of the $HDL_3$ subfraction. Although the biological effects of HDL subfractions are unclear, most evidence indicates that large cholesterol-rich $HDL_2$ represent the anti-atherogenic fraction [63]. Therefore, JTT-705 may have a favorable effect on the HDL subfraction composition. It is of interest to compare human genetic CETP deficiency with pharmacological inhibition of CETP. Absence of plasma CETP in homozygous CETP deficiency has been shown to result in a very high plasma HDL cholesterol level (2.5 to 3.5 times normal) and a significant reduction of plasma LDL cholesterol [53]. However, heterozygosity for CETP gene mutations resulting in a 35% to 39% decrease of CETP, similar to that seen in the high-dose group of the present study, is associated with a variable increase of plasma HDL cholesterol (10% to 32%) and a variable reduction of plasma LDL cholesterol (1% to 12%) [53, 73]. Heterozygous CETP deficiency has largely the same influence on lipids and lipoproteins as observed in the high-dose group in the present study. An effect not seen in genetic CETP deficiency is the profound dose-dependent increase of plasma CETP with JTT-705 treatment. It can be speculated that the liver and/or adipose tissue is compensating for loss of the active protein by the secretion of more CETP. However, CETP inhibition by an antisense oligodeoxynucleotide resulted in a decrease of the CETP concentration in rabbits [50]. Thus, it seems more likely that the increase of CETP observed in the present study was due to delayed clearance of inactivated CETP protein by the liver.

## Torcetrapib

The other CETP inhibitor is torcetrapib, which has a dihydroquinoline structure and evolved from a series of inhibitors identified by high throughput screening for inhibition of cholesteryl ester transfer activity in an assay using native human plasma CETP (Figure 3). Although the structure-activity relationship data have not been reported, the structure of torcetrapib seems to be thoroughly optimized. Torcetrapib does not form a disulfide bond with a cystein residue of CETP, so its mechanism of inhibition may be different from that of JTT-705. The $IC_{50}$ for trocetrapib determined in whole human plasma with a CETP concentration of 37 nM was about 50 nM.

Clinical studies of torcetrapib have also been reported. In the initial phase I multidose study, five groups of 8 healthy young subjects each were randomized to placebo (n=2) or torcetrapib (n=6) at 10, 30, 60, and 120 mg daily and 120 mg twice daily for 14 days [74]. The mean inhibition of CETP activity was 12%, 35%, 53%, and 80% in the 30-, 60-, 120-mg daily, and 120-mg twice-daily groups, respectively. Dose escalation led to an increase in the extent and duration of CETP inhibition, with up to 100% inhibition by 4 to 8 hours after the initial dose. Treatment with 10, 30, 60, and 120 mg daily, or 120 mg twice daily, resulted in a 16%, 28%, 62%, 73%, and 91% increase of plasma HDL cholesterol, respectively, with no significant change in total plasma cholesterol. This lack of effect on total plasma cholesterol despite the large increase in HDL cholesterol was caused by a reciprocal decrease in non-HDL cholesterol, with LDL cholesterol decreasing 21% at 120 mg daily and 42% at 120 mg twice daily. A significant increase of the HDL free cholesterol content was observed after 14 days of treatment at the highest dose. Because free cholesterol increased to a greater extent than cholesteryl ester, the free cholesterol/choesteryl ester ratio also increased. The plasma phospholipid profile of the 120 mg twice daily group demonstrated a 54% increase in HDL phospholipid, and a 33% reduction in LDL phospholipid. At the highest dose, apoA-I and apoE were respectively increased by 27% and 66%, whereas apoB was decreased by 26%. Presumably, much of this increased apoE was associated with HDL, and the increased free cholesterol content of HDL during torcetrapib therapy may be related to an increase of apoE-containing HDL. A shift to larger HDL particles was also evident with treatment. Lipoprotein lipid and apoprotein levels responded to CETP inhibition, and HDL cholesterol increased significantly with treatment at all doses tested. In contrast, non-HDL cholesterol decreased, resulting in no significant change of the total plasma cholesterol levle. Accompanying these lipoprotein changes were corresponding changes in apolipoproteins. ApoA-I and apoE both increased, while apoB decreased with treatment. These effects are consistent with those seen in human CETP deficiency. Complete CETP deficiency is associated with a 3- to 4- fold elevation of HDL cholesterol, an up to 40% reduction of LDL cholesterol, and a 40% to 90% increase of total plasma cholesterol relative to unaffected family members or controls [53, 75-77]. Furthermore, apoA-I and apoE levels were increased by 70% to 150% and 2- to 6-fold, respectively, while apoB was reduced by 30% to 40%. Partial CETP deficiency, with 40% to 70% of normal CETP activity or mass, has more modest effects: HDL cholesterol increases by 25% to70%, apoA-I and apoE increase by 20% to 40%, and total plasma cholesterol, LDL cholesterol, and apoB show little or no change [53, 78, 79]. By creating a range of partial deficiencies by inhibiting CETP activity using torcetrapib, the expected phenotypes were reproduced. During treatment, the CETP mass increased dose- and time-dependently and continued to increase throughout the 2-week study, with the change becoming significant for all groups by 14 days. An increase of the plasma CETP concentration by up to 3.5-fold occurred. The increase in CETP mass occurs within the first day, and subsequent 8-week studies have shown that the CETP mass plateaus at a 3- to 4-fold increase from baseline. By 2 hours after administration, the apparent molecular weight of CETP shows a shift to a larger form. By 36 hours, it largely returns to its former state. This drug-induced change of plasma CETP appears to occur because of the inhibitor's mechanism of action and represents the shift from free CETP to an HDL-bound form.

A single-blind, placebo-controlled study was also conducted to examine the effects of torcetrapib, alone or in combination with the HMG-CoA reductase inhibitor atorvastatin (20 mg/day), on the phenotype in 19 subjects with a low HDL cholesterol level [80]. The 19 subjects received torcetrapib for 4 weeks at a daily dose of 120 mg, either alone or in combination with 20 mg of atorvastatin daily, and 6 subjects in the torcetrapib-alone group received 120 mg of torcetrapib twice daily for an additional four weeks. Treatment with 120 mg of torcetrapib daily and 120 mg of torcetrapib twice daily resulted in a 28% and 65% decrease of the trough CETP activity. At a dose of 120 mg daily, torcetrapib in combination with atorvastatin decreased CETP activity by 38%. Torcetrapib had a striking effect on the plasma HDL cholesterol level, and the effect remained intact when it was administered in combination with a statin. Treatment with 120 mg of torcetrapib daily and 120 mg of torcetrapib twice daily resulted in a 46% and 106% increase of the HDL cholesterol level, respectively. Torcetrapib (at a dose of 120 mg daily) in combination with atorvastatin increased the HDL cholesterol level by 61%. Plasma HDL apoA-I and A-II levels were also significantly increased by torcetrapib, and this effect was still seen when it was administered in combination with a statin. The apoA-I and A-II levels were increased by 13% and 10%, respectively, in the subjects who received 120 mg daily with atorvastatin, by 16% and 12% in those who received 120 mg daily without atorvastatin, and by 36% and 21% in those who received 120 mg twice daily. Torcetrapib had a minimal effect on the plasma levels of total cholesterol and phospholipids. Torcetrapib also reduced the plasma levels of LDL cholesterol and apoB, and this effect was independent of that of the statin on LDL cholesterol and apoB. Among the subjects who received atorvastatin, torcetrapib reduced LDL cholesterol levels by 17% relative to placebo and reduced apoB levels by 14%. The corresponding reductions in the subjects who did not receive atorvastatin were 8% and 10%, respectively. Torcetrapib (at a dose of 120 mg twice daily) also caused a nonsignificant reduction in the plasma levels of LDL cholesterol (17%) and apoB (17%). This finding is consistent with the fact that patients with homozygous defects of the *CETP* gene have reduced levels of LDL cholesterol [52, 53]. The metabolic basis for the low levels of LDL cholesterol in persons with CETP deficiency is increased clearance of LDL cholesterol from the plasma [81], suggesting that the LDL receptor pathway may be up-regulated in CETP deficiency. Torcetrapib had a marked effect on the lipoprotein subclasses, and its effects remained intact when the drug was administered in combination with a statin. Treatment with 120 mg of torcetrapib daily or 120 mg of torcetrapib twice daily resulted in a 46% and 106% increase of $HDL_2$ cholesterol, respectively. Torcetrapib (at a dose of 120 mg daily) in combination with atorvastatin increased $HDL_2$ cholesterol by 61%. $HDL_3$ cholesterol levels were also increased by torcetrapib, but to a far lesser extent than $HDL_2$ cholesterol levels. Treatment with 120 mg of torcetrapib daily or 120 mg of torcetrapib twice daily resulted in a 29% and 56% increase of $HDL_3$ cholesterol, respectively. Torcetrapib (at a dose of 120 mg daily) in combination with atorvastatin increased $HDL_3$ cholesterol by 36%. The cholesterol content of large HDL particles, as assessed by NMR spectroscopy, increased by 133% in the subjects who received both atorvastatin at 20 mg daily and torcetrapib at 120 mg daily, by 199% in those who only received torctrapib at 120 mg daily, and by 446% in those who received torcetrapib at 120 mg twice daily. Torcetrapib also influenced the LDL subclass distribution, although the changes of LDL subclasses were not significant when it was administered in combination with atorvastatin. Without atorvastatin, torcetrapib administration at a dose of 120 mg once daily or 120 mg twice daily increased large LDL particles by 257% and 294%, respectively. Conversely, small LDL cholesterol was decreased by 73% at a dose of 120 mg daily without atorvastatin and by 93% when 120 mg of torcetrapib alone was given twice daily.

Despite the small number of patients, these results suggest that torcetrapib can effectively increase the HDL cholesterol level and also decrease LDL cholesterol. Moreover, these effects of torcetrapib remained intact when it was administered in combination with atorvastatin. Because the majority of patients who are candidates for CETP inhibitor therapy are also likely to be candidates for statin therapy, the potential value of combination therapy with atorvastatin and torcetrapib is notable.

## Conclusions

HMG-CoA reductase inhibitors (statins) cause a marked reduction of the plasma cholesterol level and are obviously beneficial for atherosclerosis and coronary heart disease.

However, 58% of patients with coronary heart disease do not have an elevated LDL cholesterol level [82]. A low level of HDL cholesterol is noted to be another risk factor for atherosclerosis and coronary heart disease, and increasing the HDL cholesterol level is the next target for the treatment of these conditions.

Inhibition of CETP is a potential method of increasing the HDL cholesterol level, and the small molecule CETP inhibitor JTT-705 has been shown to increase plasma HDL cholesterol, decrease plasma LDL cholesterol, and reduce atherosclerotic lesions in rabbits. These findings suggest the atherogenicity of endogenous CETP and that inhibition of CETP activity can retard the progression of atherosclerosis. Recently, JTT-705 and another CETP inhibitor (torcetrapib) were shown to significantly increase HDL cholesterol, particularly large $HDL_2$ cholesterol, and decrease LDL cholesterol in humans. The same changes of lipids and lipoproteins are observed in heterozygous CETP deficiency. Although large, apoE-rich $HDL_2$ are poor acceptors of cholesterol from arterial macrophages, there is much evidence that large cholesterol-rich $HDL_2$ represent the anti-atherogenic fraction [63]. Furthermore, the possibility of combination therapy with a statin and torcetrapib has been demonstrated. Although these results suggest the possibility of a new class of anti-atherogenic drugs, further studies are needed to establish whether CETP inhibitors will actually provide protection against cardiovascular disease in humans.

## References

[1] Gotto, A.M., Larosa, J.C., Hunninghake, D., Bush, D., Criqui, M.H., Getz, G.S., Gotto, A.M. Jr., Grundy, S.M., Rakita, L., Robertson, R.M., Weisfeldt, M.L. The cholesterol facts. A summary of the evidence relating dietary fats, serum cholesterol and coronary heart disease. *Circulation 81,* 1721-1733 (1990).

[2] Knopp, R.H. Drug treatment of lipid disorders. *N. Engl. J. Med. 341,* 498-511 (1999).

[3] Scandinavian Simvastatin Survival Study Group. Randomized trial of cholesterol lowering in 4444 patients with coronary heart disease: the scandinavian simvastatin survival study (4S). *Lancet 344,* 383-1389 (1994).

[4] Shepherd, J., Cobbe, S.M., Ford, I., Isles, C.G., Lorimer, A.R., Macfarlane, P.W., McKillop, J.H., Packard, C.J. Prevention of coronary heart disease with pravastatin in men with hypercholesterolemia. *N. Engl. J. Med. 333,* 1350-1351 (1995).

[5] Sacks, F.M., Pfeffer, M.A., Moye, L.A., Rouldeau, J.L., Futherford, J.D., Cole, T.G., Brown, L., Warnica, J.W., Arnold, J.M.O., Wun, C-C., Davis, B.R., Braunwald, E. The effect of pravastatin on coronary events after myocardial infraction in patients with average cholesterol levels. *N. Engl. J. Med. 335,* 1001-1009 (1996).

[6] Heart protection study collaborative group. MRC/BHF heart protection study of cholesterol lowering with simvastatin in 20,536 high-risk individuals: a randomized placebo-controlled trial. *Lancet 360,* 7-22 (2002).

[7] Gordon, D.J., Rifkind, B.M. High-density lipoprotein: the clinical implications of recent studies. *N. Engl. J. Med. 321,* 1311-1316 (1989).

[8] Lusis, A.J. Atherosclerosis. *Nature 407,* 233-241 (2000).

[9] Gotto, A.M. Jr. Low high-density lipoprotein cholesterol as a risk factor in coronary heart disease: a working group report. *Circulation 103,* 2213-2218 (2001).

[10] Barter, P., Kastelein, J., Nunn, A., Hobbs, R. High density lipoproteins (HDLs) and atherosclerosis; the unanswered questions. *Atherosclerosis 168,* 195-211 (2003).

[11] Rhoads, G.G., Gulbrandsen, C.L., Kagan, A. Serum lipoproteins and coronary heart disease in a population study of Hawaii Japanese men. *N. Engl. J. Med. 294,* 293-298 (1976).

[12] Gordon, T., Probstfield, J.L., Garrison, R.J., Neaton, J.D., Castelli, W.P., Knoke, J.D. High density lipoprotein cholesterol and cardiovascular disease. The Framingham study. *Am. J. Med. 62,* 707-714 (1977).

[13] Gordon, D.J., Probstfield, J.L., Garrison, R.J., Neaton, J.D., Castelli, W.P., Knoke, J.D., Jacobs, D.R. Jr., Bangdiwala, S., Tyroler, H.A. High density lipoprotein cholesterol and cardiovascular disease. Four prospective Am studies. *Circulation* 79, 8-15 (1989).

[14] Nissen, S.E., Tsunoda, T., Tuzcu, E.M., Schoenhagen, P., Cooper, C.J., Yasin, M., Eaton, G.M., Lauer, M.A., Sheldon, W.S., Grines, C.L., Halpern, S., Crowe, T., Blankenship, J.C., Kerensky, R. Effect of recombinant apoA-I milano on coronary atherosclerosis in patients with acute coronary syndromes. A randomized controlled trial. *JAMA. 290,* 2292-2300 (2003).

[15] Fielding, C.J., Fielding, P.E. Molecular physiology of reverse cholesterol transport. *J. Lipid Res. 36,* 211-228 (1995).

[16] Barter, P.J., Rye, K.A. Molecular mechanisms of reverse cholesterol transport. *Curr. Opin. Lipidol. 7,* 82-87 (1996).

[17] Schmitz, G., Kaminski, W.E., Orso, E. ABC transporters in cellular lipid trafficking. *Curr. Opin. Lipidol. 11,* 493-501 (2000).

[18] Tkahashi, Y., Smith. J.D. Cholesterol efflux to apolipoprotein AI involves endocytosis and resecretion in a calcium-dependent pathway. *Proc. Natl. Acad. Sci. U.S.A. 96,* 11358-11363 (1999).

[19] Remaley, A.T., Stonik, J.A., Demosky, S.J., Neufeld, E.B., Bocharov, A.V., Vishnyakova, T.G., Eggerman, T.L., Patterson, A.P., Duverger, N.J., Satamarina-Fojo, S., Brewer, H.B. Jr. Apolipoprotein specificity for lipid efflux by the human ABCA1 transporter. *Biochem. Biophys. Res. Commun. 280,* 818-823 (2001).

[20] Oram, J.F., Lawn, R.M. ABCA1: the gatekeeper for eliminating excess tissue cholesterol. *J. Lipid Res. 42,* 1173-1179 (2001).

[21] Liu, L., Bortnick, A.E., Nickel, M., Dhanasekaran, P., Subbaiah, P.V., Lund-Katz, S., Rothblat, G.H., Phillips, M.C. Effects of apolipoprotein A-I on ATP-binding cassette transporter A1-mediated efflux of macrophage phospholipids and cholesterol: formation of nascent high density lipoprotein particles. *J. Biol. Chem. 278,* 42976-42984 (2003).

[22] Castro, G.R., Fielding, C.J. Early incorporation of cell-derived cholesterol into pre-beta-migrating high-density lipoprotein. *Biochem. 27,* 25-29 (1988).

[23] Trigatti, B.L., Krieger, M., Rigotti, A. Influence of the HDL receptor SR-BI on lipoprotein metabolism and atherosclerosis. *Arterioscler. Thromb. Vasc. Biol. 23,* 1732-1738 (2003).

[24] Goldstein, J.L., Brown, M.S. Regulation of low-density lipoprotein receptors: implications for pathogenesis and therapy of hypercholesterolemia and atherosclerosis. *Circulation 76,* 504-507 (1987).

[25] Hegele, R.A. Paraoxonase -- genes and disease. *Ann. Med. 31,* 217-224 (1999).

[26] Shih, D.M., Xia, Y.-R., Wang, X.-P., Miller, E., Castellani, L.W., Subbanagounder, G., Cheroutre, H., Faull, K.F., Berliner, J.A., Witztum, J.L., Lusis, A.J. Combined serum paraoxonase knockout / apolipoprotein E knockout mice exhibit increased lipoprotein oxidation and atherosclerosis. *J. Biol. Chem. 276,* 17527-17535 (2000).

[27] Mackness, M.I., Arrol, S., Abbott, C., Durrington, P.N. Protection of low-density lipoprotein against oxidative modification by high-density lipoprotein associated paraoxonase. *Atherosclerosis 104,* 129-135 (1993).

[28] Marathe, G.K., Zimmerman, G.A., McIntyre, T.M. Platelet-activating factor acetylhydrolase and not paraoxonase-1, is the oxidized phospholipids hydrolase of high density lipoprotein particles. *J. Biol. Chem. 278,* 3937-3947 (2002).

[29] Rader, D.A. Effects of nonstatin lipid drug therapy on high-density lipoprotein metabolism. *Am. J. Cardiol. 91,* 18-23 (2003).

[30] Rakley, C.E. Monotherapy with HMG-CoA reductase inhibitors and secondary prevention in coronary artery disease. *Clin. Cardiol. 19,* 683-689 (1996).

[31] Goldberg, A., Alagona, P. Jr., Capuzzi, D.M., Guyton, J., Morgan, J.M., Rodgers, J., Sachson, R., Samuel, P. Multiple-dose efficacy and safety of an extended-release form of niacin in the management of hyperlipidemia. *Am. J. Cardiol. 85,* 1100-1105 (2000).

[32] Hoeg, J.M., Vaisman, B.L., Demosky, Jr. S.J., Meyn, S.M., Talley, G.D., Hoyt, Jr. R.F., Feldman, S., Berard, A.M., Sakai, N., Wood, D., Brousseau, M.E., Marcovina, S., Brewer, Jr. H.B., Santamarina-Fojo, S. Lecithin: cholesterol acyltransferase overexpression generates hyperalphalipoproteinemia and a non-atherogenic lipoprotein pattern in transgenic rabbits. *J. Biol. Chem. 271,* 4396-4402 (1996).

[33] Murdoch, S.J., Breckenridge, W.C. Influence of lipoprotein lipase and hepatic lipase on the transformation of VLDL and HDL during lipolysis of VLDL. *Atherosclerosis 118,* 193-212 (1995).

[34] Haperen, R., Tol, A., Vermeulen, P., Jauhiainen, M., Gent, T., van den Berg, P., Ehnholm, S., Grosveld, F., van der Kamp, A., Crom, R. Human plasma phospholipid transfer protein increases the antiatherogenic potential of high density lipoproteins in transgenic mice. *Arterioscler. Thromb. Vasc. Biol. 20,* 1082-1088 (2000).

[35] Holvoet, P., de Geest, B., van Linthout, S., Lox, M., Danloy, S., Raes, K., Collen, D. The arg 123 - tyr 166 central domain of human apoAI is critical for lecithin: cholesterol acyl transferase-induced hyperalphalipoproteinemia and HDL remodeling in transgenic mice. *Arterioscler. Thromb. Vasc. Biol. 20,* 459-466 (2000).

[36] Schwartz, K., Lawn, R.M., Wade, D.P. ABC1 gene expression and ApoA-I-mediated cholesterol efflux are regulated by LXR. *Biochem. Biophys. Res. Commun. 274,* 794-802 (2000).

[37] Kozarsky, K.F., Donahee, M.H., Glick, J.M., Krieger, M., Rader, D.J. Gene transfer and hepatic overexpression of the HDL receptor SR-BI reduces atherosclerosis in the cholesterol-fed LDL receptor-deficient mouse. *Arterioscler. Thromb. Vasc. Biol. 20,* 721-727 (2000).

[38] Shinkai, H. Cholesteryl ester transfer protein inhibitor. *Exp. Opin. Ther. Patents* 11, 739-745 (2001).

[39] Shinkai, H. New approaches to raising the HDL cholesterol level. *Mini Rev. Med. Chem.* 2, 271-276 (2002).

[40] Tall, A.R. Plasma cholesterol ester transfer protein. *J. Lipid. Res. 34,* 1255-1274 (1993).

[41] Lagrost, L. Regulation of cholesteryl ester transfer protein (CETP) activity: review of in vitro and in vivo studies. *Biochem. Biophys. Acta. 1215,* 209-236 (1994).

[42] Barter, P.J., Hopkins, C.J., Calvert, G.D. Transfers and exchanges of esterified cholesterol between plasma lipoproteins. *Biochem. J. 208,* 1-7 (1982).

[43] Bruce, C., Chouinard, Jr. R.A., Tall, A. R. Plasma lipid transfer proteins, high-density lipoproteins, and reverse cholesterol transport. *Annu. Rev. Nutr. 18,* 297-330 (1998).

[44] Fielding, C.J., Havel, R.J. Cholesteryl ester transfer protein: friend or foe? *J. Clin. Invest. 97,* 2687-2688 (1996).

[45] Hayek, T., Masucci-Magoulas, L., Jiang, X. Decreased early atherosclerotic lesions in hypertriglyceridemic mice expressing cholesteryl ester transfer protein transgene. *J. Clin. Invest. 96,* 2071-2074 (1995).

[46] Zhong, S., Sharp, D.S., Grove, J.S., Bruce, C., Yano, K., Curb, J.D., Tall, A.R. Increased coronary heart disease in Japanese-American men with mutation in the cholesteryl ester transfer protein gene despite increased HDL levels. *J. Clin. Invest. 97,* 2917-2923 (1996).

[47] Agellon, L.B., Walsh, A., Hayek, T., Moulin, P., Jiang, X.C., Shelanski, S.A., Breslow, J.L., Tall, A.R. Reduced high density lipoprotein cholesterol in human cholesteryl ester transfer protein transgenic mice. *J. Biol. Chem. 266,* 10796-10801 (1991).

[48] Jiang, X.C., Masucci-Magoulas, L, Mar, J., Lin, M., Walsh, A., Breslow, J.L., Tall, A.R. Down-regulation of mRNA for the low density lipoprotein receptor in transgenic mice containing the gene for human cholesteryl ester transfer protein: mechanism to explain accumulation of lipoprotein B particles. *J. Biol. Chem. 268,* 27406-27412 (1993).

[49] Marotti, K.R., Castle, C.K., Boyle, T.P., Lin, A.H., Murray, R.W., Melchior, G.W. Severe atherosclerosis in transgenic mice expressing simian cholesteryl ester transfer protein. *Nature 364*: 73-75 (1993).

[50] Sugano, M., Makino, N., Sawada, S., Otsuka, S., Watanabe, M., Okamoto, H., Kamada, M., Mizushima, A. Effect of antisense oligonucleotides against cholesteryl ester transfer protein on the development of atherosclerosis in cholesterol-fed rabbits. *J. Biol. Chem. 273,* 5033-5036 (1998).

[51] Rittershaus, C.W., Miller, D.P., Thomas, L.J., Picard, M.D., Honan, C.M., Emmett, C.D., Pettey, C.L., Adari, H., Hammond, R.A., Beattie, D.T., Callow, A.D., Marsh, H.C., Ryan, U.S. Vaccine-induced antibodies inhibit CETP activity in vivo and reduce aortic lesions in a rabbit model of atherosclerosis. *Arterioscler. Thromb. Vasc. Biol. 20,* 2106-2112 (2000).

[52] Brown, M.L., Inazu, A., Hesler, C.B., Agellon, L.B., Mann, C., Whitlock, M.E., Marcel, Y.L., Milne, R.W., Koizumi, J., Mabuchi, H., Tall, A.R. Molecular basis of lipid transfer protein deficiency in a family with increased high-density lipoproteins. *Nature 342,* 448-451 (1989).

[53] Inazu, A., Brown, M.L., Hesler, C.B., Agellon, L.B., Koizumi, J., Takata, K., Maruhama, Y., Mabuchi, H., Tall, A.R. Increased high-density lipoprotein levels caused by a common cholesteryl-ester transfer protein gene mutation. *N. Engl. J. Med. 323,* 1234-1238 (1990).

[54] Akita, H., Chiba, H., Tsuchihashi, K., Tsuji, M., Kumagai, M., Matsuno, K., Kobayashi, K. Cholesteryl ester transfer protein gene: two common mutations and their effect on plasma high-density lipoprotein cholesterol content. *J. Clin. Endorinol. Metab. 79,* 1615-1618 (1994).

[55] Inazu, A., Jiang, X.C., Haraki, T., Yagi, K., Kamon, N., Koizumi, J., Mabuchi, H., Takeda, R., Takata, K., Moriyama, Y., Doi, M., Tall, A.R. Genetic cholesteryl ester transfer protein deficiency caused by two prevalent mutations as a major determinant of increased levels of high density lipoprotein cholesterol. *J. Clin. Invest. 94,* 1872-1882 (1994).

[56] Hirano, K., Yamashita, S., Nakajima, N., Arai, T., Maruyama, T., Yoshida, Y., Ishigami, M., Sakai, N., Kameda-Takemura, K., Matsuzawa, Y. Genetic cholesteryl ester transfer protein deficiency is extremely frequent in the Omagari area of Japan. *Arterioscler. Thromb. Vasc. Biol. 17,* 1053-1059 (1997).

[57] Yamashita, S., Sprecher, D.L., Sakai, N., Matsuzawa, Y., Tarui, S., Hui, D.Y. Accumulation of apolipoprotein E-rich high density lipoproteins in hyperalphalipoproteinemic human subjects with deficiency of cholesteryl ester transfer protein. *J. Clin. Invest.* 86, 688-695 (1990).

[58] Fievet, C., Fruchart, J.C. HDL heterogeneity and coronary heart disease. *Diabetes Metab. Rev. 7,* 155-162 (1991).

[59] Wilson, H.M., Patel, J.C., Skinner, E.R. The distribution of high-density lipoprotein subfractions of lipoproteins in coronary survivors. *Biochem. Soc. Trans. 18,* 1175-1176 (1990).

[60] Miller, N.E. Associations of high density lipoprotein subclasses and apolipoproteins with ischemic heart disease and coronary atherosclerosis. *Am. Heart J. 113,* 589-597 (1987).

[61] Cheung, M.C., Brown, B.G., Wolf, A.C., Albers, J.J. Altered particle size distribution of apolipoprotein A-I-containing lipoproteins in subjects with coronary artery disease. *J. Lipid Res. 32,* 383-394 (1991).

[62] Johansson, J., Carlson, L.A., Landou, C., Hamsten, A. High density lipoproteins and coronary atherosclerosis. A strong inverse relation with the largest particles is confined to normotriglyceridemic patients. *Arterioscler. Thromb.* 11, 174-182 (1991).

[63] Freedman, D.S., Otvos, J.D., Jeyarajah, E.J., Barboriak, J.J., Anderson, A.J. Walker, J.A. Relation of lipoprotein subclasses as measured by proton nuclear magnetic resonance spectroscopy to coronary artery disease. *Arterioscler. Thromb. Vasc. Biol. 18,* 1046-1053 (1998).

[64] Barter, P.J., Brewer, H.B. Jr., Chapman, M.J., Hennekens, C.H., Rader, D.J., Tall, A.R. Cholesteryl ester transfer protein. A novel target for raising HDL and inhibiting atherosclerosis. *Arterioscler. Thromb. Vasc. Biol. 23,* 160-167 (2003).

[65] Bhatnagar, D., Durrington, P.N., Chennon, K.M., Prais, H., Mackness, M.I. Increased transfer of cholesteryl esters from high-density lipoproteins to low-density and very

low-density lipoproteins in patients with angiographic evidence of coronary artery disease. *Atehrosclerosis 98,* 25-32 (1993).

[66] Foger, B., Luef, G., Ritsch, A. Relationship of high-density lipoprotein subfractions and cholesteryl ester transfer protein in plasma to carotid artery wall thickness. *J. Mol. Med. 73,* 369-372 (1995).

[67] Kuivenhoven, J.A., Jukema, J.W., Zwinderman, A.H., Knijff, P., McPherson, R., Bruschke, A.V.G.; Lie, K.I.; Kastelein, J.J.P. The role of a common variant of the cholesteryl ester transfer protein gene in the progression of coronary atherosclerosis. *N. Engl. J. Med. 338,* 86-93 (1998).

[68] Okamoto, H., Yonemori, F., Wakitani, K., Minowa, T., Maeda, K., Shinkai, H. A cholesteryl ester transfer protein inhibitor attenuates atherosclerosis in rabbits. *Nature 406,* 203-207 (2000).

[69] Shinkai, H., Maeda, K., Yamasaki, T., Okamoto, H., Uchida, I. Bis(2-(acylamino)phenyl) disulfides, 2-(acylamino)benzenethiols, and S-(2-(acylamino)phenyl) alkanethioates as novel inhibitors of cholesteryl ester transfer protein. *J. Med. Chem. 43,* 3566-3572 (2000).

[70] Maeda, K., Okamoto, H., Shinkai, H. S-(2-(Acylamino)phenyl) 2,2-dimethylpropanethioates as CETP inhibitors. *Bioorg. Med. Chem. Lett. 14,* 2589-2591 (2004).

[71] de Grooth, G.J., Kuivenhoven, J.A., Stalenhoef, A.F.H., de Graaf, J., Zwiderman, A.H., Posma, J.L., van Tol, A., Kastelein, J.J.P. Efficacy and safety of a novel cholesteryl ester transfer protein inhibitor, JTT-705, in humans a randomized phase II dose-response study. *Circulation* 105, 2159-2165 (2002).

[72] Haraki, T., Inazu, A., Yagi, K., Kajinami, K., Koizumi, J., Mabuchi, H. Clinical characteristics of double heterozygotes with familial hypercholesterolemia and cholesteryl ester transfer protein deficiency. *Atherosclerosis 132,* 229-236 (1997).

[73] Zhong, S., Sharp, D.S., Grove, J.S., Bruce, C., Yano, K., Curb, J.D., Tall, A.R. Increased coronary heart disease in Japanese-American men with mutation in the cholestery ester transfer protein gene despite increased HDL levels. *J. Clin. Invest.* 97, 2917-2923 (1996).

[74] Clark, R.W., Sutfin, T.A., Ruggeri, R.B., Wilauer, A.T., Sugarman, E.D., Magnus-Aryitey, G., Cosgrove, P.G., Sand, T.M., Wester, R.T., Williams, J.A., Perlman, M.E., Bamverger, M.J. Raising high-density lipoprotein in humans through inhibition of cholesteryl ester transfer protein: an initial multidose study of torcetrapib. *Arterioscler. Thromb. Vasc. Biol. 24,* 490-497 (2004).

[75] Duverger, N., Rader, D., Ikewaki, K., Nishiwaki, M., Sakamoto, T., Ishikawa, T., Nagano, M., Nakamura, H., Brewer, H.B. Characterization of high-density apolipoprotein particles A-I and A-II isolated from human with cholesteryl ester transfer protein deficiency. *Eur. J. Bilchem. 227,* 123-129 (1995).

[76] Ohta, T., Nakamura, R., Takata., K., Saito, Y., Yamashita, S., Seikoh, S., Matsuda, I. Structural and functional differences of subspecies of apoA-I containing lipoprotein in patients with plasma cholesteryl ester transfer protein deficiency. *J. Lipid. Res.* 36, 696-704 (1995).

[77] Koizumi, J., Inazu, I., Yagi, K., Koizumi, I., Uno, Y., Kajinami, K., Miyamoto, S., Moulin, P., Tall, A.R., Mabuchi, H., Takeda, R. Serum lipoprotein lipid concentration and composition in homozygous and heterozygous patients with cholesteryl ester transfer protein deficiency. *Atherosclerosis 90,* 189-196 (1991).
[78] Chiba, H., Akita, H., Tsuchihashi, K., Hui, S., Takahashi, Y., Fuda, H., Suzuki, H., Shibuya, H., Tsuji, M., Kobayashi, K. Quantitative and compositional changes in high density lipoprotein subclasses in patients with various genotypes of cholesteryl ester transfer protein deficiency. *J. Lipid. Res. 38,* 1204-1216 (1997).
[79] Yamashita, S., Hui, D.Y., Wetterau, J.R., Sprecher, D.L., Harmony, J.A.K., Sakai, N., Matsuzawa, Y., Tarui, S. Characterization of plasma lipoproteins in patients heterozygous for human plasma cholesteryl ester transfer protein (CETP) deficiency: plasma CETP regulates high density lipoprotein concentration and composition. *Metabolism 40,* 756-763 (1991).
[80] Brousseau, M.E., Schaefer, E.J., Wolfe, M.L., Bloedon, L.T., Digenio, A.G., Clark, R.W., Mancuso, J.P., Rader, D.J. Effects of an inhibitor of cholesteryl ester transfer protein on HDL cholesterol. *N. Engl. J. Med. 350,* 1505-1515 (2004).
[81] Ikewaki, K., Nishiwaki, M., Sakamoto, T., Ishikawa, T., Fairwell, T., Zech, L.A., Nagano, M., Nakamura, H., Brewer, H.B. Jr., Rader, D.J. Increased catabolic rate of low density lipoproteins in humans with cholesteryl ester transfer protein deficiency. *J. Clin. Invest.* 96, 1573-1581 (1995).
[82] Rubins, H.B., Robins, S.J., Collins, D., Iranmanesh, A., Wilt, T.J., Mann, D., Mayo-Smith, M., Faas, F.H., Elam, M.B., Rutan, G.H., Anderson, J.W., Kashyap, M.L., Schectman, G. Distribution of lipid in 8,500 men with coronary artery disease. *Am. J. Cardiol. 75,* 1196-1201 (1995).

In: Cholesterol in Atherosclerosis and Coronary Heart Disease ISBN 1-59454-302-X
Editor: Jean P. Kovala, pp. 79-101 

*Chapter V*

# Differential Response of High Density Lipoprotein Cholesterol to Hypolipidemic Treatment

***Genovefa D. Kolovou**, *Katherine K. Anagnostopoulou and Dennis V. Cokkinos***
Cardiology Department, Onassis Cardiac Surgery Center, Athens, Greece

## Abstract

In a number of epidemiological studies, the high density lipoprotein (HDL) cholesterol has been identified as a powerful independent negative risk factor for coronary artery disease. Therefore, the increase of serum HDL cholesterol recently became a therapeutic target, in addition to low density lipoprotein (LDL) cholesterol. It has already been reported that the recommended lipid lowering diet reduces not only total cholesterol but HDL cholesterol levels as well. However, we have reported in a previous study, that in patients with baseline HDL cholesterol < 39 mg/dl, the hypolipidemic diet decreased total cholesterol and triglyceride levels, and increased HDL cholesterol, while in patients with HDL cholesterol ≥ 39 mg/dl the decrease of LDL cholesterol and triglyceride levels was followed by a decrease of HDL cholesterol. As an extension of this study, in another study, including a double number of patients, the decrease of HDL cholesterol levels in patients with baseline HDL cholesterol ≥ 39 mg/dl, after hypolipidemic diet, was again documented. Moreover, dyslipidemic individuals do not show uniform HDL response to the hypolipidemic drug treatment. Fibrates, nicotinic acid or its analogue may result in the decrease of total cholesterol, LDL cholesterol and triglyceride levels without a parallel decrease in HDL cholesterol. On the other hand, statins may decrease total cholesterol, LDL cholesterol and triglyceride levels with a concomitant significant decrease of HDL cholesterol levels. It seems that when the baseline HDL cholesterol

* Address of correspondence: Genovefa D. Kolovou, Associate Director, Onassis Cardiac Surgery Center, 356 Sygrou Ave Athens, Greece. Tel: +30 210 9493520, Fax: +30 210 9493336; e-mail: genkolovou@mail.gr

level is taken into account, a better selection of the optimal therapy could be made. In this chapter, besides the HDL metabolism and its pleiotropic effects, the results of the studies regarding the response of HDL cholesterol to hypolipidemic treatment will be analyzed.

## Introduction

High serum low density lipoprotein (LDL) cholesterol is a classical risk factor for premature coronary artery disease (CAD) [1-8]. However, even the aggressive lowering of LDL cholesterol cannot decrease the CAD risk and morbidity more than 23 to 44% [3,9,10]. This means, that the coronary events still occur in more than half of treated patients [11,12]. Therefore, treatment affecting other lipid parameters, besides LDL cholesterol [13] is likely to be required for many patients [14-15]. The high density lipoprotein (HDL) cholesterol has been considered such a candidate due to its important role in the reverse cholesterol transport [18] and its pleiotropic antiatherogenic effects [19]. Bar et al [20], first proposed HDL as a risk factor for CAD. The first prospective study was published 15 years later [21]. It was forgotten until 1975, when Miller and Miller [22] published an article detailing how HDL might be involved in reverse cholesterol transport. Afterwards, in a number of epidemiological studies [23-27], it has been identified as a powerful independent negative risk factor for CAD. The Air Force/Texas Coronary Atherosclerosis Prevention Study [28] showed that the LDL cholesterol is not a strong predictor for first coronary events, while apolipoprotein (apo) A (the main protein of HDL) and the ratio of apo B (the main protein of LDL) to apo A were powerful predictors of such risk. Furthermore, in Cox regression model, LDL cholesterol was found to predict acute myocardial events only when HDL cholesterol was included [24]. The antiatherogenic effects of HDL were directly proved in animal studies with intravenous injection of human HDL [25]. The Scandinavian Simvastatin Survival Study revealed that even a modest increase in HDL cholesterol could reduce coronary risk [26, 27]. The Veterans Affairs High-Density Lipoprotein Cholesterol Intervention Trial [29] was the first to relate the rise of HDL cholesterol levels in CAD patients, who had LDL cholesterol < 140 mg/dl and HDL cholesterol < 40mg/dl, with a significant reduction in coronary events. It was reported that a 6% increase of HDL cholesterol resulted in a significant 24% reduction in the risk for nonfatal myocardial infarction, coronary death and stroke, independently of LDL cholesterol and triglyceride changes [30, 31]. The Helsinki Heart Study [32] and the Veterans Affairs High-Density Lipoprotein Cholesterol Intervention Trial [29] showed that 1% increase of HDL cholesterol resulted to a 2% to 3% reduction in cardiovascular risk [29,30,32,33]. Therefore, the increase of serum HDL cholesterol recently became a therapeutic target, in addition to LDL cholesterol [34,35].

All these facts led us to evaluate the effect of various hypolipidemic treatments on HDL cholesterol levels. Previous studies [17,36,37] have shown that patients with baseline HDL cholesterol ≥ 39 mg/dl had significantly decreased total cholesterol levels with parallel reduction of HDL cholesterol, while patients with baseline serum HDL cholesterol < 39 mg/dl, had a decrease in total cholesterol and an increase in HDL cholesterol after lipid lowering diet [17] or hypolipidemic drugs [36] In this chapter, besides the HDL metabolism and its pleiotropic effects, the results of the studies regarding the response of HDL cholesterol to hypolipidemic treatment will be analyzed.

## HDL Metabolism

HDLs are heterogenous lipoprotein particles secreted by hepatocytes and enterocytes. They constitute a fraction of serum lipoproteins characterized by similar molecular density ($1.063 < d < 1.21$ g/ml) and size (5 – 17 nm in diameter). As a result of qualitative and quantitative differences in lipid, protein and enzyme content, HDL particles are multi-shaped molecules with varying density, fluidity, charge and anti-genicity. Isopycnic ultracentrifugation yields two major HDL fractions, $HDL_2$ and $HDL_3$. Unesterified cholesterol distributes between the surface and the core of HDL particles. Charged lipids, phopholipids and proteins are located primarily in the outer parts of the lipoprotein. The proteins of HDL are apo A-I (most abundant), A-II, A-IV, C, E and J (in lower amounts). The proteins associated with HDL and having enzyme activity are the lecithin-cholesterol acyltransferase, cholesterol ester transfer protein, phospholipid transfer protein, acetyl-PAF hydrolase and paraoxonase. Nonpolar elements of HDL such as triglycerides and esterified cholesterol are found in the center of the lipoprotein molecule. $HDL_2$ and $HDL_3$ have a globular shape and migrate on agarose gel electrophoresis in a fraction with α-electrophoretic mobility [38,39]. Newly synthesized HDL molecules lack the central nonpolar core, exhibit a disc-like bilayer structure and are characterized by electrophoretic pre-β or pre-α mobility. They have been identified in plasma [40] and intestinal fluid [41]. It is not known what regulates their concentration in plasma. Pre-β-particles usually contain apo A-I either as a free molecule or in association with a few molecules of sphingomyelin and phosphatidylcholine [38].

All human cells synthesize cholesterol and import cholesterol from plasma lipoproteins and from uptake of senescent erythrocytes. To achieve neutral cholesterol balance and prevent cholesterol overload, cell must export excess cholesterol. Cholesterol accumulation within cells is toxic as too much free cholesterol in the endoplasmic reticulum may disrupt the peptide biosynthetic machinery [42]. Therefore cells have to employ a number of safety devices to export cellular cholesterol and thus to limit the concentration of free cholesterol. The only quantitatively significant sink for excess cholesterol is the liver, owing to its unique ability to synthesize bile acids and to transport cholesterol into bile. Virtually all HDL particles are able to accept cholesterol from cells [43]. However, the preferred initial acceptor of cell cholesterol is the minor subpopulation of small, pre-β-migrating, apo A-I containing particles [40]. This process is dependent on functional ATP-binding cassette transporter 1 (ABCA1). ABCA1 is a member of the ABC transporter superfamily [44,45]. This family of large transmembrane proteins transports a large variety of molecules such as proteins, ions, and lipids across plasma membrane [46]. ABCA1 is ubiquitously expressed in tissues and is transcriptionally regulated by nuclear receptors and cAMP [47-50]. ABCA1 either directly or indirectly mediates transport of cholesterol and phospholipids across cellular membranes, where they are removed from cells by apolipoproteins. The role of ABCA1 as an exporter of cellular lipids became evident when it was discovered that it was the gene product defective in Tangier disease, a severe HDL deficiency characterized by deposition of sterols in tissue macrophages [42,51,52]. This discovery took place in 1999 by three different laboratories (led by Bodzioch et al [53], Rust et al [54], and Brooks-Wilson et al [55]) providing a new molecular key to understanding the mechanisms and regulation of cellular cholesterol efflux and it have shed further light on the process of reverse cholesterol transport. Human genetic deficiency states affecting HDL levels have considerably enhanced understanding the role of HDL particles and its contribution to reverse cholesterol transport. The process of reverse cholesterol transport involves the ability of HDL to remove cholesterol from the periphery for delivery to the liver and excretion in the bile [56]. This process is impaired in patients with Tangier disease. Cells isolated from Tangier disease homozygotes were shown to have a severely impaired ability to transport cholesterol and phospholipids to purified apolipoproteins [57].

Normally, cholesterol and phospholipid efflux takes place to free apo A-I, but has only a minor effect on efflux to mature HDL [58]. ABCA1 appears to be saturated at very low concentrations of free apo A-I (less than 15 μg/ml, plasma apo A-I 1mg/dl). This free apo A-I may be secreted from the liver or small intestine or may be regenerated in the circulation as a result of remodelling of HDL by cholesteryl ester transfer protein, followed by the action of hepatic lipase. Reduced expression of ABCA1 results in reduced lipidation and hypercatabolism of apo A-I.

Apo A-I-mediated cholesterol efflux from Tangier disease fibroblasts is severely impaired, where as passive desorption of cholesterol from Tangier disease cell plasma membrane to lipoprotein acceptors is intact. Moreover the translocation of newly synthesized cholesterol to plasma membrane (aberrant in Tangier disease cells) is dependent on protein kinase C, implicating impaired signal transduction in the pathogenesis of Tangier disease [58]. This inability to properly translocate cellular lipids from intracellular stores to the plasma membrane provides a mechanistic explanation for the excess lipid deposition observed in Tangier disease cells. In patients with Tangier disease, cholesteryl ester accumulation is noticed, but not in all and not in the same tissues. This suggests that probably there are other ways of cholesterol efflux besides the ABCA1 pathway [59]. The removal of cellular cholesterol in Tangier disease cells may occur by alternative mechanisms by passing the ABCA1 [60]. Some of the known mechanisms for cholesterol efflux include 1) aqueous diffusion to a phospholipid-containing acceptor [61,62], 2) facilitated efflux mediated by cell surface receptors such as scavenger receptor type B1 [61], 3) other genes besides the ABCA1, such as ABCG1, ABCG5 and ABCG8, involved in HDL homeostasis. [63].

The ABCA1-mediated cholesterol efflux pathway, shown to be defective in Tangier disease can either be modulated or bypassed after stimulation by products of phosphatidylcholine hydrolysis, diacylglycerol, and phospholipases. This raises the possibility that ABCA1 may be a proximal mediator to apo A-I cell interaction in cholesterol efflux or that other pathways of cholesterol movements to the plasma membrane can bypass the ABCA1 pathway. Therefore, increasing of cholesterol efflux cellular pathways can be used for potential therapeutic purposes in ABCA1 defects (Tangier disease, apo A deficiency). The increased abundance of pre-β HDL in certain HDL deficiency states provides evidence that this particle reflects the first step in the life cycle of an HDL particle. The phospholipids on HDL particles are made available during lipolysis of triglyceride-rich lipoproteins (chylomicrons and very low density lipoproteins). Proper lipidation is essential for the stability of HDL particles. The second main step in reverse cholesterol transport is the esterification of cholesterol on the surface of HDLs in a reaction catalysed by lecithin cholesterol acyltransferase [64]. This reaction depletes the HDL surface of unesterified cholesterol and thus generates a concentration gradient that promotes the transfer of cholesterol from cell membranes to HDLs. It is known that the rate of lecithin cholesterol acyltransferase reaction in plasma correlates negatively rather than positively with the concentration of HDL cholesterol [65]. Thus, subjects with low concentration of HDL cholesterol, especially if they also have elevated triglyceride levels [66] tend to have high rather than low rates of plasma cholesterol esterification, and by inference, higher than lower rates of reverse cholesterol transport.

The concept of reverse cholesterol transport provides the theoretical framework for understanding body cholesterol homeostasis. Approximately 9 mg cholesterol per kg body weight synthesized by peripheral tissues each day have to be moved to the liver for effective catabolism [67]. HDLs remove cholesterol from the arterial intima, thus preventing from foam cell formation [68-70]. Distortion of the reverse cholesterol transport may favor deposition of cholesterol in the arterial wall and thereby contribute to the development of atherosclerosis. In addition to reverse cholesterol transport, several other potentially anti-atherogenic activities are exerted by HDL presented below.

# Pleiotropic Effects of HDL

## Antioxidant Properties of HDLs

In addition to its role in reverse cholesterol transport, HDL may modify atherogenesis by transporting antioxidants. The oxidation of LDL is widely considered to be a major event in the inhibition and development of atherosclerosis [71]. Oxidized LDL acts as a chemoattractant for monocytes, transforms macrophages into foam cells, exerts cytotoxic effects on endothelial cells, increases thrombocyte activation, stimulates migration and proliferation of smooth muscle cells and antagonises the vasolidative effect of nitrogen oxide [72,73]. HDL inhibits the oxidation of LDL by transition metal ions [74,75]. This inhibition is usually attributed to the high content of anti-oxidative properties of apo A-I, as well as to the presence of paraoxonase [39,76] which is transported by HDL into the arterial wall where it protects LDL particles from oxidation. Additionally, paraoxonase decreases the lipid peroxide content in human coronary and carotid lesions [77]. The human paraoxonase-1 is a 354 amino acid calcium-dependent phosphotriesterase. Its name stems from its ability to metabolize paraoxon, the microsome-activated form of the pesticide parathion. Despite the intensive work on the protein, the structure of the enzyme and its catalytic mechanism are still not completely elucidated [78]. This enzyme is mainly expressed in the liver and is secreted in serum where it is associated with HDL [79].

Paraoxonase-1 possesses both arylesterase and organophosphatase activities and belongs to the family of phase I xenobiotic-metabolizing enzymes. Several heterocyclic compounds (lactones and thiolactones) were found to be paraoxonase-1 substrates, which include statin drugs [80].

In addition to its detoxification function, paraoxonase-1 is involved in the metabolism of endogenous substrates. This enzyme metabolizes oxidized phospholipids in HDL and LDL [81], homocysteine thiolactone [82], and platelet-activating factor [83]. Oxidized HDL loses its ability to induce efflux of cholesterol and does not show anti-aggregatory activity toward platelets [84-87]. Concerning the LDL molecule, it catalyses the breakdown of oxidized phospholipids in LDL (compounds that stimulate cytokine production and induce adhesion of monocytes to the endothelial surface) [88,89]. There are three genes identified so far encoding enzymes with paraoxonase activity: PON-1, PON-2 and PON-3 [90]. It was shown that PON-1-deficient mice are more susceptible to atherosclerosis than wild-type littermates, and several clinical studies report that paraoxonase-1 plays a role in the physiological prevention of cardiovascular disease [91].

Some clinical data suggest that treatment with hypolipidemic drugs may modulate serum paraoxonase-1 activity [92,93]. This activity is HDL-dependent, and several factors may be involved in its regulation. Some fibrates are shown to induce PON-1 gene expression, whereas statins have the opposite effect. Another HDL- associated antioxidant enzyme that may play a protective role is platelet activating factor acetylhydrolase [75], which catabolizes oxidised lipoproteins.

## Anti-Inflammatory Properties of HDLs

One of the earliest events induced in atherogenesis [84] and in the progression of mature atherosclerotic plaques is the expression of adhesion molecules, such as vascular cell adhesion molecule-1 (VCAM-1), intracellular adhesion molecule-1 (ICAM-1) and P- or E-selectin, and chemokines, including monocyte chemotactic protein-1, which attract leukocytes into the arterial wall [95-97]. VCAM-1 and ICAM-1 mediate adhesion of mononuclear cells including monocytes and lymphocytes. E- and P- selectins enabling tethering and rolling of monocytes and lymphocytes on the surface of endothelial cells. All these adhesion molecules are abundantly expressed in the atherosclerotic plaque [98-101]. Induction of VCAM-1 is one of the initial phenomena encountered in animals on a high cholesterol diet and precedes the transmigration of monocytes into the arterial wall [102]. Expression of VCAM-1 is induced by lysophosphatidylcholine present on oxidized LDL and by products of lipolysis [103,104]. Additionally, all these molecules are rapidly synthesised in response to the inflammatory cytokines, tumour necrosis factor-α and interleukin-1 as well as to intracellular synthesis of free radicals which activate the nuclear transcription factor NF-κB [105]. HDLs have the capacity to inhibit tumour necrosis factor-α and interleukin-1 expression of VCAM-1, ICAM-1 and selectins in endothelial cells grown in tissue culture [39,106]. The mechanism by which HDLs inhibit endothelial cell adhesion molecule expression has been partially evaluated. HDLs inhibit the tumour necrosis factor-α-induced translocation of NF-κB, the transcription factor essential for the expression of VCAM-1, ICAM-1 and E-selectin [107].

In addition to VCAM-1, ICAM-1 and selectins, fibrinogen can also mediate the adhesion of leukocytes to the endothelium [39,108]. Specifically, it creates bridges between integrins present on the surface of interacting cells. HDL can inhibit the adhesion of neutrophils to endothelial cells mediated by the fibrinogen receptor [109]. HDL also inhibits the binding of fibrinogen stimulated by ADP to monocytes [110].

# Response of HDL to Hypolipidemic Treatment

## Diet

It has been already reported that the recommended lipid lowering diet by previous and last NCEP ATP expert panel [111,112] reduces not only total cholesterol but serum HDL cholesterol levels as well [113-115]. We have shown that the response of serum HDL cholesterol to the first step lipid lowering diet is depended on baseline HDL cholesterol levels [17]. In patients with baseline HDL cholesterol < 39 mg/dl, the hypolipidemic diet decreased total cholesterol and triglyceride levels, and increased HDL cholesterol, while in patients with HDL cholesterol ≥ 39 mg/dl the decrease of LDL cholesterol and triglyceride levels was not followed by increase of HDL cholesterol [17]. In another study, where twice the number of patients was involved, the decrease of HDL cholesterol levels in patients with baseline HDL cholesterol ≥ 39 mg/dl, after hypolipidemic diet, was again documented [37] (Table 1). Similar decrease of HDL cholesterol after hypolipidemic diet was shown by Maki et al [116], beFIT and DAS studies [117] and others [118-120] (Table 2).

**Table 1. Effect of Statins, Fibrates and Nicotinic Acid or Acipimox on HDL Values**

| | **≥39 mg/dl** | **<39 mg/dl** |
|---|---|---|
| **Diet** | n=149 | n=92 |
| HDL baseline | 52 | 32 |
| Change (%) | -12* | +19* |
| **Statins** | n=206 | n=106 |
| HDL baseline | 54 | 32 |
| Change (%) | -7* | +22* |
| **Fibrates** | n=86 | n=79 |
| HDL baseline | 51 | 31 |
| Change (%) | +2 | +19* |
| **Nicotinic Acid/Acipimox** | n=50 | n=33 |
| HDL baseline | 48 | 30 |
| Change (%) | +6 | +27* |

HDL: high density lipoprotein cholesterol
*p<0.001 comparison before and after treatment.

## Fibrates

Fibric acid derivatives (fibrates), have been introduced in the treatment of dyslipidemia [121], since many decades (Table 2). There have been used mostly in the treatment of hypertriglyceridemia [122].

The large studies with fibrates reported an increase in HDL cholesterol from 6% [123], to 10% [32] and 18% [124] with simultaneous decreases of 10% [32] or no change [123] in LDL cholesterol and with triglyceride decrease of 21% [124], 31% [123] or 43% [32]. The Veterans Affairs High-Density Lipoprotein Cholesterol Intervention Trial and the Bezafibrate Infarction Prevention studies showed that treatment with fibrates is beneficial for patients with low HDL cholesterol levels and hypertriglyceridemia [123,124]. Our findings demonstrated that fibrates have no negative influence on HDL cholesterol concentrations in any baseline HDL cholesterol [121] (Table 1). Furthermore, the raise in HDL cholesterol (+18%) is seen when baseline HDL cholesterol is low similar to the BIP study (+18%) [123].

## Nicotinic Acid and its Analogue

Nicotinic acid is a well-established agent in the treatment of dyslipidemia. It is known to lower plasma cholesterol and triglyceride levels, reducing very low density lipoprotein and LDL cholesterol levels [124-126]. Nicotinic acid is also effective in raising HDL cholesterol [124-126] (Table 2). Moreover, the treatment with nicotinic acid reduces the risk for coronary heart disease and the recurrence rate of myocardial infarction [127,128]. The mechanism of its action has not been fully elucidated. However, it is speculated that nicotinic acid reduces the production of free fatty acids by inhibition of lipolysis in adipose tissue, which results in a reduced availability of substrate for very low density lipoprotein synthesis in the liver. It has also been suggested that nicotinic acid directly inhibits the synthesis of apolipoprotein B-containing lipoproteins in the liver [124,125,129].

Nicotinic acid was reported to produce the greatest (17 to 31%) HDL cholesterol increase with concomitant significant reduction of both LDL cholesterol (12 to 20%) and triglyceride levels [130]. Our data were similar concerning the nicotinic acid and its analogue, acipimox. However the patients with initial HDL cholesterol ≥ 39 mg/dl demonstrated a higher proportional decrease in LDL cholesterol and triglyceride levels [37]. The patients from this group with baseline HDL cholesterol < 39 mg/dl showed a greater HDL cholesterol increase, compared to the patients with baseline HDL cholesterol ≥ 39 mg/dl and to all other groups as well [37] (Table 1).

## Statins

The introduction of inhibitors of 3-hydroxy-3-methylglutaryl coenzyme A (HMG-CoA) reductase (statins), the rate-limiting enzyme in cholesterol synthesis, have revolutionised the treatment of dyslipidemia [36,112,131,132]. Administration of statins results in the upregulation of hepatic LDL receptors as a principal mechanism of maintaining intracellular cholesterol concentration. They are the most commonly prescribed lipid-lowering agents

**Table 2. Changes of Baseline HDL Cholesterol Levels in Various Studies of Cholesterol-lowering Interventions**

| Studies (year) [ref] | Number of Patients | Baseline HDL (mg/dl) | Type of Intervention | Change (%) |
|---|---|---|---|---|
| Diet | | | | |
| Kolovou et al (1994) [17] | 129 | 44 | Step I | -2 |
| Azen et al (1996) [120] | 162 | 42 | Step I | +2 |
| De Lorgeril et al (1999) [148] | 219 | 45 | mediterranean | +10 |
| Knopp et al (2000) [117] | 792 | 41 | Step II | -2.5 |
| Knopp et al (2000) [117] | 792 | 58 | Step II | -8 |
| Obarzanek et al (2001) [119] | 436 | 49 | DASH diet | -3 |
| Maki et al (2001) [116] | 75 | 52 | Step I + low sterols | -4 |
| Maki et al (2001) [116] | 35 | 52 | Step I + high sterols | -7 |
| Kolovou et al (2003) [37] | 241 | 45 | Step I | -4 |
| Fibrates | | | | |
| Manttari et al (1987) [149] | 4081 | 50 | Gemfibrozil | +10 |
| Steiner (1996) [150] | 418 | 39 | Fenofibrate | +7.5 |
| Frick et al (1997) [32] | 372 | 32 | Gemfibrozil | +15 |
| Rubins et al (1999) [29] | 2531 | 32 | Gemfibrozil | +6 |
| BIP Study Group (2000) [40] | 2825 | 35 | Bezafibrate | +18 |
| Sakai et al (2001) [151] | 65 | 31 | Gemfibrozil | +13 |
| Kolovou et al (2003) [37] | 165 | 41 | Fibrates[a] | +10 |
| Nicotinic Acid | | | | |
| Sakai et al (2001) [151] | 69 | 31 | N-SL | +22 |
| Cheung et al (2001) [152] | 146 | 31 | N+Simvastatin | +26 |
| Kolovou et al (2003) [37] | 83 | 41 | N or Acipimox | +10 |
| Statins | | | | |
| Sacks et al (1991) [153] | 4159 | 38 | Pravastatin | +4 |
| Shepherd et al (1995) [7] | 6595 | 43 | Pravastatin | +5 |
| 4S Study Group (1995) [154] | 4444 | 46 | Simvastatin | +8 |
| Bruschke et al (1995) [155] | 450 | 36 | Pravastatin | +9 |
| Herd et al (1994) [156] | 339 | 34 | Fluvastatin | +9 |
| Herd et al (1994 [156]) | 339 | 48 | Fluvastatin | +4 |
| Downs et al (1997) [28] | 5742 | 38 | Lovastatin | +6 |
| LIPID Study Group (1998) [157] | 7684 | 36 | Pravastatin | +5 |
| Schwartz et al (2001) [158] | 3086 | 46 | Atorvastatin | NC |
| Shepherd et al (2002) [159] | 5804 | 50 | Pravastatin | +5 |
| Colhoun et al (2002) [160] | 1421 | 52 | Atorvastatin | +1 |
| Sever et al (2003) [161] | 19342 | 51 | Pravastatin | NC |
| Kolovou et al (2003) [37] | 312 | 47 | Statins[b] | -2 |
| McKenney et al (2003) [162] | 313 | 51 | Rosuvastatin | +10 |
| McKenney et al (2003) [162] | 323 | 50 | Atorvastatin | +2 |
| McKenney et al (2003) [162] | 328 | 51 | Simvastatin | +7 |
| McKenney et al (2003) [162] | 321 | 50 | Pravastatin | +6 |
| Prove-it (2004) [139] | 2099 | 39 | Atorvastatin | +6.5 |
| Prove-it (2004) [139] | 2063 | 39 | Pravastatin | +8 |

[a]Fibrates used include: Gemfibrozil, Bezafibrate and Fenofibrate
[b]Statins used include: Lovastatin, Simvastatin, Pravastatin and Atorvastatin
HDL: high density lipoprotein cholesterol, N-SL: slow release, N: nicotinic acid, NC: no change
Step I & II diets according to NCEP ATP II guidelines [111]

because of their efficacy in reducing serum LDL cholesterol levels as well as because of their excellent tolerability and safety [133]. Statins have the proven ability to reduce overall mortality, the risk of myocardial infarction, stroke and the need for revascularisation [5,134-139]. The relationship between baseline and post-treatment LDL cholesterol levels and cardiovascular end points was evaluated in several clinical trials [5,6,138,140]. In our studies, statins also decreased total cholesterol, LDL cholesterol and triglyceride levels but "paid" it with a significant decrease of HDL cholesterol levels (Table 1). It is difficult to predict whether such a HDL cholesterol decrease would reflect an unfavourable influence in the patients` cardiovascular risk since, no such data exist. However, the Air Force/Texas Coronary Atherosclerosis Prevention Study demonstrated that patients in the lower 2 tertiles of baseline HDL cholesterol and average total cholesterol and LDL cholesterol levels, showed the greatest risk reductions after statin treatment (45% and 44%) [15,24,28]. Also, the greatest angiographic improvement after statin therapy was reported by Ballantyne et al. in patients with baseline HDL cholesterol concentrations < 35 mg/dl [141]. The statins used until now showed benefits mostly in patients with high or moderate LDL cholesterol concentrations [18]. The statins' effect on HDL cholesterol concentration is not well elucidated. It is possible that they may provoke selective upregulation of the scavenger receptor type B1 (one of the mechanism of cholesterol efflux mention above) resulting in increased $HDL_2$ removal by the liver, and as a consequence HDL cholesterol can be reduced [16]. On the other hand, statins are able to increase HDL cholesterol via peroxisome proliferator-activated receptor α-dependent apolipoprotein A-I oversynthesis [16]. It is also possible that different statins can have different influence on HDL cholesterol levels [16] (Table 2). The previous study [17] demonstrated that statins had no influence on HDL cholesterol in patients with HDL cholesterol ≥ 39 mg/dl. In the same study, 11% of the patients from the statins group were treated with simvastatin and no one with atorvastatin while in our study 21% of the patients were treated with simvastatin and 18% with atorvastatin. It has been reported that simvastatin can increase HDL cholesterol levels in dose dependent response, while atorvastatin is associated with progressively decreasing rises in HDL cholesterol as the dose increases (negative dose response) [142]. We have not evaluated HDL cholesterol response separately for every statin because of the relatively small patient number per drug. Moreover, the study was not designed to reveal differences between statins concerning the HDL cholesterol levels. However, this study pointed out, that after statin treatment, patients with baseline HDL cholesterol concentration ≥ 39 mg/dl, in parallel with significant beneficial decrease of total cholesterol, LDL cholesterol and triglyceride levels, demonstrated undesirable reduction of HDL cholesterol [37].

## Mechanism of HDL Behaviour after Treatment

The underlying mechanism of HDL cholesterol behaviour after treatment interventions is unclear. Lipoprotein heterogeneity is now well recognized as an important factor that reflects differences in lipoprotein composition, such as size and density. In populations with low HDL cholesterol levels and hypertriglyceridemia an increased number of small, dense LDL particles are found. In hypertriglyceridemic states, an enhanced exchange of triglycerides and cholesteryl esters from very low density lipoproteins to HDL by cholesterol ester transfer protein occurs. This leads to the formation of HDL, enriched with triglycerides. Such triglyceride-rich HDL particles appear to be more readily removed from the circulation by the kidney, resulting in low plasma HDL cholesterol levels. It is likely that the hypolipidemic drugs may affect the above mechanisms, leading to a different post treatment HDL cholesterol response. These mechanisms seem to be genetically controlled. There are studies which demonstrate that patients with gene variations have different response to hypolipidemic drugs. It has been recently shown that the ABCA1 is involved in reverse cholesterol transport, and that the scavenger receptor type B1 is an HDL receptor [143], and that the polymorphisms of lipoprotein lipase, cholesteryl-ester transfer protein [144], lecithin cholesterol acyl transferase [145] and hepatic lipase affect HDL metabolism [146]. However, there are still many conflicting points concerning the effect of various drugs on HDL cholesterol levels. Understanding the metabolism of HDL is helpful in the strategy of rising HDL cholesterol. Recently, a new drug has been proposed to rise HDL cholesterol levels, an inhibitor of cholesteryl ester transfer protein [147].

## Conclusions

During the last decade, there was a great progress in understanding the underlying mechanisms for HDL metabolism, which has been achieved by the findings of transgenic and knockout animals, the application of molecular biology, and the human genetics. The study of natural occurring mutations has considerably enhanced understanding the reverse cholesterol transport hypothesis and the role of HDL in atherosclerosis, though many aspects of the functions and characteristics of HDL remain to be elucidated. The aim of this chapter was to evaluate HDL cholesterol behaviour after the most common treatment regimens in clinical practice. Current therapeutic strategies include alteration of dietary habits, the use of fibrates which increase apo A-I production and lipoprotein lipase activity, nicotinic acid that increases HDL cholesterol and statins that reduce the cholesterol/HDL cholesterol ratio. Although statins have little effect on HDL, their favourable action is observed in low baseline HDL cholesterol levels. Potential therapeutic strategies include modulation of ABCA1 transporter and inhibition of cholesteryl ester transfer protein. The main message lies on the fact that if the baseline HDL cholesterol level is taken into account, a better selection of the optimal therapy can be made. This may permit a finer "tuning" of lipid lowering therapy.

## References

[1] Stamler, J; Daviglus, ML; Garside, DB; Dyer, AR; Greenland, P; Neaton, JD. Relationship of baseline serum cholesterol levels in 3 large cohorts of younger men to long-term coronary, cardiovascular, and all-cause mortality and to longevity. *JAMA,* 2000 284, 311-318.

[2] Stamler, J; Wentworth, D; Neaton, JD; for the MRFIT Research group. Is relationship between serum cholesterol and risk of premature death from coronary heart disease

continuous and graded? Findings in 352222 primary screeners of the Multiple Risk Factor Intervention Trial (MRFIT). *JAMA* 1986 256, 2823-2828.

[3] LaRosa J. Cholesterol lowering, low cholesterol, and mortality. *Am J Cardiol,* 1993 72, 776-786.

[4] Small, DM; Bond, MG; Waugh, D; Prack, M; Sawyer, JK. Physicochemical and histological changes in the arterial wall of non-human primates during progression and regression of atherosclerosis. *J Clin Invest,* 1984 73, 1590-1605.

[5] The Scandinavian Simvastatin Survival Study Group. Randomised trial of cholesterol lowering in 4444 patients with coronary heart disease: the Scandinavian Simvastatin Survival Study (4S). *Lancet,* 1994 344, 1383-1389.

[6] Cholesterol and Recurrent Events (CARE) Trial Investigators. The effect of pravastatin on coronary events after myocardial infarction in patients with average cholesterol levels. *N Engl J Med,* 1996 335, 1001-1009.

[7] Shepherd, J; Cobbe, SM; Ford, I; Isles, CG; Lorimer, AR; MacFarlane, PW; McKillop, JH; Packard, CJ; for the West of Scotland Coronary Prevention Study Group. Prevention of coronary heart disease with pravastatin in men with hypercholesterolemia. *N Engl J Med,* 1995 333, 1301-1307.

[8] Carmena, R; Duriez, P; Fruchart, JC. Atherogenic lipoprotein particles in atherosclerosis. *Circulation,* 2004 109, III2-7.

[9] Arntzenius, AC. Regression of atherosclerosis. Benefit can be expected from low LDL-C and high HDL-C levels. *Acta Cardiol,* 1991 46, 431-434.

[10] Gresser, U; Gathof, BS. Atorvastatin: gold standard for prophylaxis of myocardial ischemia and stroke - comparison of the clinical benefit of statins on the basis of randomized controlled endpoint studies. *Eur J Med Res,* 2004 9, 1-17.

[11] LaRosa, JC; He, J; Vupputuri, S. Effect of statins on risk of coronary disease: a meta-analysis of randomized controlled trials. *JAMA,* 1999 282, 2340-2346.

[12] Gotto; AM. High-density lipoprotein cholesterol and triglycerides as therapeutic targets for preventing and treating coronary artery disease. *Am Heart J,* 2002 144, S3-S42.

[13] Assmann, G; Schulte, H. Results and Conclusions of the Prospective Cardiovascular Munster (PROCAM) Study. In: Assmann G, editor. *Lipid Metabolism Disorders and Coronary Heart Disease.* Munchen: MMV Medizin-Verlag; 1993; 19-67.

[14] Superko, HR. Beyond LDL cholesterol reduction. *Circulation,* 1996 94, 2351-2354.

[15] Boden, WE; Pearson, TA. Raising low levels of high-density lipoprotein cholesterol is an omportent target of therapy. *Am J Cardiol,* 2000 85, 645-650.

[16] Assmann, G. Pro and con: high-density lipoprotein, triglycerides, and other lipid subfractions are the future of lipid management. *Am J Cardiol,* 2001 87, 2B-7B.

[17] Kolovou, G; Fostinis, Y; Athanassopoulos, G; Manolis, A; Cokkinos, DV. Differential response of high-density lipoproteins to first-step lipid-lowering diet according to their initial level. *Coronary Arter Dis,* 1994 5, 359-364.

[18] Gotto, A. Low High-density lipoprotein cholesterol as a risk factor in coronary heart disease. A Working Group Report. *Circulation,* 2001 103, 2213-2218.

[19] Kolovou, G; Cokkinos, DV. Low serum levels of high-density lipoprotein cholesterol and hypolipidemic treatment. *Curr Med Res Opin,* 2002 18, 265-268.

[20] Barr, DP; Russ, EM; Eder, HA. Protein-lipid relationships in human plasma. II. In atherosclerosis and related conditions. *Am J Med,* 1951 11, 480-493.

[21] Gofman, JW; Young, W; Tandy, R. Ischemic heart disease, atherosclerosis, and longevity. *Circulation,* 1966 34, 679-697.

[22] Miller, GJ; Miller, NE. Plasma-high-density-lipoprotein concentration and development of ischaemic heart-disease. *Lancet,* 1975 1, 16-19.

[23] Gordon, DJ; Rifkind, BM. High-density lipoprotein – the clinical implications of recent studies. *N Engl J Med,* 1989 321, 1311-1316.

[24] Gotto, AM Jr; Whitney, E; Stein, EA; Shapiro, DR; Clearfield, M; Weis, S; Jou, JY; Langendorfer, A; Beere, PA; Watson, DJ; Downs, JR; de Canis, JS. Relations between baseline and on-treatment lipid parameters and first acute major coronary events in the Air Force/Texas Coronary Atherosclerosis Prevention Study (AFCAPS/TexCAPS). *Circulation,* 2000 101, 477-484.

[25] Badimon, JJ; Badimon, L; Fuster, V. Regression of atherosclerotic lesions by high density lipoprotein plasma fraction in the cholesterol-fed rabbit. *J Clin Invest,* 1990 85, 1234-1243.

[26] Pedersen, TR; Olsson, AG; Faergeman, O; Kjekshus, J; Webel, H; Berg, K; Wilhelmsen, L; Haghfelt, T; Thorgeirsson, G; Pyorala, K; Miettinen, T; Christophersen, B; Tobert, JA; Musliner, TA; Cook, TJ. Lipoprotein changes and reduction in the incidence of major coronary heart disease events in the Scandinavian Simvastatin Survival Study (4S). *Circulation,* 1998 97, 1453-1460.

[27] Ronnemaa, T; Laakso, M; Kallio, V; Pyorala, K; Marniery, J; Puukka. Serum lipids, lipoproteins, and apolipoproteins and the excessive occurrence of coronary heart disease in non-insulin-dependent diabetic patients. *Am J Epidemiol,* 1989 130, 632-645.

[28] Downs, JR; Beere, PA; Whitney, E; Clearfield, M; Weis, S; Rochen, J; Stein, EA; Shapiro, DR; Langendorfer, A; Gotto, AM Jr. Design & rationale of the Air Force/Texas Coronary Atherosclerosis Prevention Study (AFCAPS/TexCAPS). *Am J Cardiol,* 1997 80, 287-293.

[29] Rubins, HB; Robins, SJ; Collins, D; Fye, CL; Anderson, JW; Elam, MB; Faas, FH; Linares, E; Schaefer, EJ; Schectman, G; Wilt, TJ; Wittes, J. Gemfibrozil for the secondary prevention of coronary heart disease in men with low levels of high-density lipoprotein cholesterol. Veterans Affairs High-Density Lipoprotein Cholesterol Intervention Trial Study Group. *N Engl J Med,* 1999 341, 410-418.

[30] Robins, SJ; Collins, D; Wittes, JT; Papademetriou, V; Deedwania, PC; Schaefer, EJ; McNamara, JR; Kashyap, ML; Hershman, JM; Wexler, LF; Rubins, HB; VA-HIT study group. Relation of gemfibrozil treatment and lipid levels with major coronary events. VA-HIT: a randomized controlled trial. *JAMA,* 2001 285, 1585-1591.

[31] Boden, WE. High-density lipoprotein cholesterol as an independent risk factor in cardiovascular disease: assessing the data from Framingham to the Veterans Affairs High-Density Lipoprotein Intervention Trial. *Am J Cardiol,* 2000 86, 19L-22L.

[32] Frick, MH; Elo, O; Haapa, K; Heinonen, OP; Heinsalmi, P; Helo, P; Huttunen, JK; Kaitaniemi, P; Koskinen, P; Manninen, V. Helsinki Heart Study: primary prevention

trial with gemfibrozil in middle-aged men with dyslipidemia. *N Engl J Med,* 1987 317, 1237-1245.

[33] Manninen, V; Elo, MO; Frick, MH; Haapa, K; Heinonen, OP; Heinsalmi, P; Helo, P; Huttunen, JK; Kaitaniemi, P; Koskinen, P. Lipid alterations and decline in the incidence of coronary heart disease in the Helsinki Heart Study. *JAMA,* 1988 260, 641-651.

[34] Sacks, FM. The role of high-density lipoprotein (HDL) cholesterol in the prevention and treatment of coronary artery disease: Expert group recommendations. *Am J Cardiol,* 2002 90, 139-143.

[35] Lamarche, B; Lewis, GF. Atherosclerosis prevention for the next decade: risk assessment beyond low density lipoprotein cholesterol. *Can J Cardiol,* 1998 14, 841-851.

[36] Kolovou, G; Fostinis, Y; Bilianou, H; Cokkinos, DV. Response of High-density lipoproteins to hypolipidemic drugs according to their initial level. *Am J Cardiol,* 1995 75, 293-295.

[37] Kolovou, G; Daskalova, D; Petropoulos, I; Anagnostopoulou, K; Bilianou, H; Pilatis, N; Pavlidis, A; and Cokkinos, DV. Effect of Baseline Levels on Response of High Density Lipoprotein Cholesterol to Hypolipidemic Treatment. *Am J Cardiol,* 2003 92, 1339-1342.

[38] von Eckardstein, A; Huang, Y; Assmann, G. Physiological role and clinical relevance of high-density lipoprotein subclasses. *Curr Opin Lipidol,* 1994 5, 404-416.

[39] Nofer, JR; Kehrel, B; Fobker, M; Levkau, B; Assmann, G; von Eckardstein, A. HDL and arteriosclerosis: Beyond reverse cholesterol transport. *Atherosclerosis,* 2002 161, 1-16.

[40] Castro, GR; Fielding, CJ. Early incorporation of cell-derived cholesterol into pre-beta-migrating high-density lipoprotein. *Biochemistry,* 1988 27, 25-29.

[41] Asztalos, BF; Sloop, CH; Wong, L; Roheim, PS. Comparison of apo A-I-containing subpopulations of dog plasma and prenodal peripheral lymph: evidence for alteration in subpopulations in the interstitial space. *Biochim Biophys Acta,* 1993 1169, 301-304.

[42] Oram, JF. HDL apolipoproteins and ABCA1. Partners in the removal of excess cellular cholesterol. *Arteriocler Thromb Vasc Biol,* 2003 23, 720-727.

[43] Barter, PJ. High-density lipoproteins and reverse cholesterol transport. *Curr Opin Lipid,* 1993 4, 210-217.

[44] Langmann, T; Klucken, J; Reil, M; Liebisch, G; Luciani, MF; Chimini, G; Kaminski, WE; Schmitz, G. Molecular cloning of the human ATP-binding cassette transporter 1 (hABC1): evidence for sterol-dependent regulation in macrophages. *Biochem Biophys Res Commun,* 1999 257, 29-33.

[45] Hyde, SC; Emsley, P; Hartshorn, MJ; Mimmack, MM; Gileadi, U; Pearce, SR; Gallagher, MP; Gill, DR; Hubbard, RE; Higgins, CF. Structural model of ATP-binding proteins associated with cystic fibrosis, multidrug resistance and bacterial transport. *Nature,* 1990 346, 362-365.

[46] Dean, M; Hamon, Y; Chimini, G. The human ATP-binding cassette (ABC) transporter superfamily. *J Lipid Res,* 2001 42, 1007-1017.

[47] Takahashi, Y; Miyata, M; Zheng, P; Imazato, T; Horwitz, A; Smith, JD. Identification of cAMP analogue inducible genes in RAW264 macrophages. *Biochim Biophys Acta,* 2000 1492, 385-394.

[48] Abe-Dohmae, S; Suzuki, S; Wada, Y; Aburatani, H; Vance, DE; Yokoyama, S. Characterization of apolipoprotein-mediated HDL generation induced by cAMP in a murine macrophage cell line. *Biochemistry,* 2000 39, 11092-11099.

[49] Sakr, SW; Williams, DL; Stoudt, GW; Phillips, MC; Rothblat, GH. Induction of cellular cholesterol efflux to lipid-free apolipoprotein A-I by cAMP. *Biochim Biophys Acta*, 1999 1438, 85-98.

[50] Marcil, M; Brooks-Wilson, A; Clee, SM; Roomp, K; Zhang, LH; Yu, L; Collins, JA; van Dam, M; Molhuizen, HO; Loubster, O; Ouellette, BF; Sensen, CW; Fichter, K; Mott, S; Denis, M; Boucher, B; Pimstone, S; Genest, J Jr; Kastelein, JJ; Hayden, MR. Mutations in the ABC1 gene in familial HDL deficiency with defective cholesterol efflux. *Lancet,* 1999 354, 1341-1346.

[51] Kolovou, G; Anagnostopoulou, K; Cokkinos, DV. A new ABCA1 mutation associated with low HDL cholesterol but without coronary artery disease. *Atherosclerosis,* 2003 169, 345-346.

[52] Kolovou, G; Daskalova, D; Anagnostopoulou, K; Hoursalas, I; Voudris, V; Mikhailidis, DP; Cokkinos, DV. Postprandial hypertriglyceridaemia in patients with Tangier disease. *J Clin Pathol,* 2003 56, 937-941.

[53] Bodzioch, M; Orso, E; Klucken, J; Langmann, T; Bottcher, A; Diederich, W; Drobnik, W; Barlage, S; Buchler, C; Porsch-Ozcurumez, M; Kaminski, WE; Hahmann, HW; Oette, K; Rothe, G; Aslanidis, C; Lackner, KJ; Schmitz, G. The gene encoding ATP-binding cassette transporter 1 is mutated in Tangier disease. *Nat Genet,* 1999 22, 347-351.

[54] Rust, S; Rosier, M, Funke, H; Real, J; Amoura, Z; Piette, JC; Deleuze, JF; Brewer, HB; Duverger, N; Denefle, P; Assmann, G. Tangier disease is caused by mutations in the gene encoding ATP-binding cassette transporter 1. *Nat Genet,* 1999 22, 352-355.

[55] Brooks-Wilson, A, Marcil, M; Clee, SM; Zhang, LH; Roomp, K; van Dam, M; Yu, L; Brewer, C; Collins, JA; Molhuizen, HO; Loubser, O; Ouelette, BF; Fichter, K; Ashbourne-Excoffon, KJ; Sensen, CW; Scherer, S; Mott, S; Denis, M; Martindale, D; Frohlich, J; Morgan, K; Koop, B; Pimstone, S; Kastelein, JJ; Hayden, MR. Mutations in ABC1 in Tangier disease and familial high-density lipoprotein deficiency. *Nat Genet,* 1999 22, 336-345.

[56] Tall, A. An overview of reverse cholesterol transport. *Europ Heart J,* 1998 19, A31-35.

[57] Francis, GA; Knopp, RH; Oram, JF. Defective removal of cellular cholesterol and phospholipids by apolipoprotein A-I in Tangier disease. *J Clin Invest,* 1995 96, 78-87.

[58] Mendez, AJ; Oram, JF; Bierman, EL. Protein kinase C as a mediator of high density lipoprotein receptor-dependent efflux of intracellular cholesterol. *J Biol Chem,* 1991 266, 10104-10111.

[59] Genest, J Jr; Bard, JM; Fruchart, JC; Ordovas, JM; Schaefer, EJ. Familial hypoalphalipoproteinemia in premature coronary artery disease. *Arterioscler Thromb,* 1993 13, 1728-1737.

[60] Rothblat, GH; de la Llera-Moya, M; Atger, V; Kellner-Weibel, G; Williams, DL; Phillips, MC. Cell cholesterol efflux: integration of old and new observations provides new insights. *J Lipid Res*, 1999 40, 781-796.

[61] Yancey, PG; Bortnick, AE; Kellner-Weibel, G; de le Llera-Moya, M; Phillips, MC; Rothblat, GH. Importance of different pathways of cellular cholesterol efflux. *Arterioscler Thromb Vasc Biol,* 2003 23, 712-719.

[62] Marcil, M; Yu, L; Krimbou, L; Boucher, B; Oram, JF; Cohn, JS; Genest, J Jr. Cellular cholesterol transport and efflux in fibroblasts are abnormal in subjects with familial HDL deficiency. *Arterioscler Thromb Vasc Biol,* 1999 19, 159-169.

[63] Wang, M; Briggs, MR. HDL: the metabolism, function, and therapeutic importance. *Chem Rev,* 2004 104, 119-137.

[64] Glomset, JA. The plasma lecithins:cholesterol acyltransferase reaction. *J Lipid Res,* 1968 9, 155-167.

[65] Wallentin, L; Vikrot, O. Lecithin:cholesterol acyl transfer in plasma of normal persons in relation to lipid and lipoprotein concentration. *Scand J Clin Lab Invest,* 1975 35, 669-676.

[66] Nestel, PJ; Monger, EA. Turnover of plasma esterified cholesterol in normocholesterolemic and hypercholesterolemic subjects and its relation to body build. *J Clin Invest,* 1967 46, 967-974.

[67] Dietschy, JM; Turley, SO; Spady, DK. Role of liver in the maintenance of cholesterol and low density lipoprotein homeostasis in different animal species. *J Lipid Res,* 1993 34, 1637-1639.

[68] Rader, DJ. Regulation of reverse cholesterol transport and clinical implications. *Am J Cardiol,* 2003 92, 42J-49J.

[69] Assmann, G; Gotto, AM Jr. HDL cholesterol and protective factors in atherosclerosis. *Circulation,* 2004 109, III8-14.

[70] Asztalos, BF. High-density lipoprotein metabolism and progression of atherosclerosis: new insights from the HDL Atherosclerosis Treatment Study. *Curr Opin Cardiol,* 2004 19, 385-391.

[71] Diaz, MN; Frei, B; Vita, J; Keaney, JF Jr. Antioxidants and atherosclerotic heart disease. *N Engl J Med,* 1997 337, 408-416.

[72] Holvoet, P; Collen, D. Oxidation of low density lipoproteins in the pathogenesis of atherosclerosis. *Atherosclerosis,* 1998 137 Suppl, S33-38.

[73] Yla-Herttuala, S. Oxidized LDL and atherogenesis. *Ann N Y Acad Sci,* 1999 874, 134-137.

[74] Hessler, JR; Robertson, AL Jr; Chisolm, GM 3rd. LDL-induced cytotoxicity and its inhibition by HDL in human vascular smooth muscle and endothelial cells in culture. *Atherosclerosis,* 1979 32, 213-229.

[75] Parthasarathy, S; Barnett, J; Fong, LG. High-density lipoprotein inhibits the oxidative modification of low-density lipoprotein. *Biochim Biophys Acta,* 1990 1044, 275-283.

[76] Mackness, MI; Mackness, B; Durrington, PN; Fogelman, AM; Berliner, J; Lusis, AJ; Navab, M; Shih, D; Fonarow, GC. Paraoxonase and coronary heart disease. *Curr Opin Lipidol,* 1998 9, 319-324.

[77] Aviram, M; Hardak, E; Vaya, J; Mahmood, S; Milo, S; Hoffman, A; Billicke, S; Draganov, D; Rosenblat, M. Human serum paraoxonases (PON1) Q and R selectively decrease lipid peroxides in human coronary and carotid atherosclerotic lesions: PON1 esterase and peroxidase-like activities. *Circulation,* 2000 101, 2510-2517.

[78] Josse, D; Xie, W; Renault, F; Rochu, D; Schopfer, LM; Masson, P; Lockridge, O. Identification of residues essential for human paraoxonase (PON1) arylesterase/organophosphatase activities. *Biochemistry,* 1999 38, 2816-2825.

[79] Kelso, GJ; Stuart, WD; Richter, RJ; Furlong, CE; Jordan-Starck, TC; Harmony, JA. Apolipoprotein J is associated with paraoxonase in human plasma. *Biochemistry,* 1994 33, 832-839.

[80] Billecke, S; Draganov, D; Counsell, R; Stetson, P; Watson, C; Hsu, C; La Du, BN. Human serum paraoxonase (PON1) isozymes Q and R hydrolyze lactones and cyclic carbonate esters. *Drug Metab Dispos,* 2000 28, 1335-1342.

[81] Aviram, M; Rosenblat, M; Bisgaier, CL; Newton, RS; Primo-Parmo, SL; La Du, BN. Paraoxonase inhibits high-density lipoprotein oxidation and preserves its functions. A possible peroxidative role for paraoxonase. *J Clin Investig,* 1998 101, 1581-1590.

[82] Jakubowski, H. Calcium-dependent human serum homocysteine thiolactone hydrolase. A protective mechanism against protein N-homocysteinylation. *J Biol Chem,* 2000 275, 3957-3962.

[83] Rodrigo, L; Mackness, B; Durrington, PN; Hernandez, A; Mackness, MI. Hydrolysis of platelet-activating factor by human serum paraoxonase. *Biochem J,* 2001 354, 1-7.

[84] Nagano, Y; Arai, H; Kita, T. High density lipoprotein loses its effect to stimulate efflux of cholesterol from foam cells after oxidative modification. *Proc Natl Acad Sci U S A,* 1991 88, 6457-6461.

[85] Morel, DW. Reduced cholesterol efflux to mildly oxidized high density lipoprotein. *Biochem Biophys Res Commun,* 1994 200, 408-416.

[86] Rifici, VA; Khachadurian, AK. Oxidation of high density lipoproteins: characterization and effects on cholesterol efflux from J774 macrophages. *Biochim Biophys Acta,* 1996 1299, 87-94.

[87] Takahashi, Y; Chiba, H; Matsuno, K; Akita, H; Hui, SP; Nagasaka, H; Nakamura, H; Kobayashi, K; Tandon, NN; Jamieson, GA. Native lipoproteins inhibit platelet activation induced by oxidized lipoproteins. *Biochem Biophys Res Commun,* 1996 222, 453-459.

[88] Navab, M; Berliner, JA; Watson, AD; Hama, SY; Territo, MC; Lusis, AJ; Shih, DM; Van Lenten, BJ; Frank, JS; Demer, LL; Edwards, PA; Fogelman, AM. The Yin and Yang of oxidation in the development of the fatty streak. A review based on the 1994 George Lyman Duff Memorial Lecture. *Arterioscler Thromb Vasc Biol,* 1996 16, 831-842.

[89] Watson, AD; Berliner, JA; Hama, SY; La Du, BN; Faull, KF; Fogelman, AM; Navab, M. Protective effect of high density lipoprotein associated paraoxonase. Inhibition of the biological activity of minimally oxidized low density lipoprotein. *J Clin Invest,* 1995 96, 2882-2891.

[90] Humbert, R; Adler, DA; Disteche, CM; Hassett, C; Omiecinski, CJ; Furlong, CE. The molecular basis of the human serum paraoxonase activity polymorphism. *Nat Genet,* 1993 3, 73-76.

[91] Mackness, B; Davies, GK; Turkie, W; Lee, E; Roberts, DH; Hill, E; Roberts, C; Durrington, PN; Mackness, MI. Paraoxonase status in coronary heart disease: are activity and concentration more important than genotype? *Arterioscler Thromb Vasc Biol,* 2001 21, 1451-1457.

[92] Tomas, M; Senti, M; Garcia-Faria, F; Vila, J; Torrents, A; Covas, M; Marrugat, J. Effect of simvastatin therapy on paraoxonase activity and related lipoproteins in familial hypercholesterolemic patients. *Arterioscler Thromb Vasc Biol,* 2000 20, 2113-2119.

[93] Balogh, Z; Seres, I; Harangi, M; Kovacs, P; Kakuk, G; Paragh, G. Gemfibrozil increases paraoxonase activity in type 2 diabetic patients. A new hypothesis of the beneficial action of fibrates? *Diabetes Metab,* 2001 27, 604-610.

[94] Cybulsky, MI; Gimbrone, MA Jr. Endothelial expression of a mononuclear leukocyte adhesion molecule during atherogenesis. *Science,* 1991 251, 788-791.

[95] Cockerill, GW; Reed, S. High-density lipoprotein: multipotent effects on cells of the vasculature. *Int Rev Cytol,* 1999 188, 257-297.

[96] Cockerill, GW; Huehns, TY; Weerasinghe, A; Stocker, C; Lerch, PG; Miller, NE; Haskard, DO. Elevation of plasma high-density lipoprotein concentration reduces interleukin-1-induced expression of E-selectin in an in vivo model of acute inflammation. *Circulation,* 2001 103, 108-112.

[97] Carter, AM; Anagnostopoulou, K; Mansfield, MW; Grant, PJ. Soluble P-selectin levels, P-selectin polymorphisms and cardiovascular disease. *J Thromb Haemost,* 2003 1, 1718-1723.

[98] Poston, RN; Haskard, DO; Coucher, JR; Gall, NP; Johnson-Tidey, RR. Expression of intercellular adhesion molecule-1 in atherosclerotic plaques. *Am J Pathol,* 1992 140, 665-673.

[99] van der Wal, AC; Das, PK; Tigges, AJ; Becker, AE. Adhesion molecules on the endothelium and mononuclear cells in human atherosclerotic lesions. *Am J Pathol,* 1992 141, 1427-1433.

[100] O'Brien, KD; Allen, MD; McDonald, TO; Chait, A; Harlan, JM; Fishbein, D; McCarty, J; Ferguson, M; Hudkins, K; Benjamin, CD; Lobb, R; Aplers, CE. Vascular cell adhesion molecule-1 is expressed in human coronary atherosclerotic plaques. Implications for the mode of progression of advanced coronary atherosclerosis. *J Clin Invest,* 1993 92, 945-951.

[101] Printseva, OYu; Peclo, MM; Gown, AM. Various cell types in human atherosclerotic lesions express ICAM-1. Further immunocytochemical and immunochemical studies employing monoclonal antibody 10F3. *Am J Pathol,* 1992 140, 889-896.

[102] Li, H; Cybulsky, MI; Gimbrone, MA Jr; Libby, P. An atherogenic diet rapidly induces VCAM-1, a cytokine-regulatable mononuclear leukocyte adhesion molecule, in rabbit aortic endothelium. *Arterioscler Thromb,* 1993 13, 197-204.

[103] Kume, N; Cybulsky, MI; Gimbrone, MA Jr. Lysophosphatidylcholine, a component of atherogenic lipoproteins, induces mononuclear leukocyte adhesion molecules in cultured human and rabbit arterial endothelial cells. *J Clin Invest,* 1992 90, 1138-1144.
[104] Saxena, U; Kulkarni, NM; Ferguson, E; Newton, RS. Lipoprotein lipase-mediated lipolysis of very low density lipoproteins increases monocyte adhesion to aortic endothelial cells. *Biochem Biophys Res Commun,* 1992 189, 1653-1658.
[105] Baeuerle, PA; Henkel, T. Function and activation of NF-kappa B in the immune system. *Annu Rev Immunol,* 1994 12, 141-179.
[106] Cockerill, GW; Rye, KA; Gamble, JR; Vadas, MA; Barter, PJ. High-density lipoproteins inhibit cytokine-induced expression of endothelial cell adhesion molecules. *Arterioscler Thromb Vasc Biol,* 1995 15, 1987-1994.
[107] Xia, P; Vadas, MA; Rye, KA; Barter, PJ; Gamble, JR. High density lipoproteins (HDL) interrupt the sphingosine kinase signaling pathway. A possible mechanism for protection against atherosclerosis by HDL. *J Biol Chem,* 1999 274, 33143-33147.
[108] Altieri, DC; Duperray, A; Plescia, J; Thornton, GB; Languino, LR. Structural recognition of a novel fibrinogen gamma chain sequence (117-133) by intercellular adhesion molecule-1 mediates leukocyte-endothelium interaction. *J Biol Chem,* 1995 270, 696-699.
[109] Moudry, R; Spycher, MO; Doran, JE. Reconstituted high density lipoprotein modulates adherence of polymorphonuclear leukocytes to human endothelial cells. *Shock,* 1997 7, 175-181.
[110] Neufeld, M; Nofer, JR; Becker, P; Langer, C; Assmann, G; Junker, R. High-density lipoproteins inhibit fibrinogen binding on adenosine diphosphate-activated monocytes. *Blood Coagul Fibrinolysis*, 2000 11, 505-509.
[111] Summary of the second report of the National Cholesterol Education Program (NCEP) Expert Panel on Detection, Evaluation, and Treatment of High Blood Cholesterol in Adults (Adult Treatment Panel II). *JAMA,* 1993 269, 3015-3023.
[112] Expert Panel on Detection, Evaluation, and Treatment of High Blood Cholesterol in Adults. Executive Summary of The Third Report of The National Cholesterol Education Program (NCEP) Expert Panel on Detection, Evaluation, And Treatment of High Blood Cholesterol In Adults (Adult Treatment Panel III). *JAMA,* 2001 285, 2486-2497.
[113] Ehnholm, C; Huttunen, JK; Pietinen, JK; Leino, U; Mutanen, M; Kostiainen, E; Pikkarainen, J; Dougherty, R; Iacono, J; Puska, P. Effect of diet on serum lipoproteins in a population with a high risk of coronary heart disease. *N Engl J Med,* 1982 307, 850-855.
[114] Arntzenius, AC; Kromhout, D; Barth, JD. Diet, lipoproteins, and the progression of coronary atherosclerosis: the Leiden Intervention Trial. *N Engl J Med,* 1985 312, 805-811.
[115] Ornish, D; Brown, SE; Scherwitz. Can lifestyle changes reverse coronary heart disease? The lifestyle heart trial. *Lancet,* 1990 336, 129-133.
[116] Maki, KC; Davidson, MH; Umporowicz, DM; Schaefer, EJ; Dicklin, MR; Ingram, KA; Chen, S; McNamara, JR; Gebhart, BW; Ribaya-Mercado, JD; Perrone, G; Robins, SJ; Franke, WC. Lipid responses to plant-sterol-enriched reduced-fat spreads incorporated

into a National Cholesterol Education Program Step I diet. *Am J Clin Nutr,* 2001 74, 33-43.

[117] Knopp, RH; Retzlaff, B; Walden, C; Fish, B; Buck, B; McCann, B. One-year effects of increasingly fat-restricted, carbohydrate-enriched diets on lipoprotein levels in free-living subjects. *Proc Soc Exp Biol Med,* 2000 225, 191-199.

[118] Watts, GF; Lewis, B; Brunt, JN; Lewis, ES; Coltart, DJ; Smith, LD; Mann, JI; Swan, AV. Effects on coronary artery disease of lipid-lowering diet, or diet plus cholestyramine, in the St Thomas' Atherosclerosis Regression Study (STARS). *Lancet,* 1992 339, 563-569.

[119] Obarzanek, E; Sacks, FM; Vollmer, WM; Bray, GA; Miller, ER 3rd; Lin, PH; Karanja, NM; Most-Windhauser, MM; Moore, TJ; Swain, JF; Bales, CW; Proschan,MA; DASH Research Group. Effects on blood lipids of a blood pressure-lowering diet: the Dietary Approaches to Stop Hypertension (DASH) Trial. *Am J Clin Nutr,* 2001 74, 80-89.

[120] Azen, SP; Mack, WJ; Cashin-Hemphill, L; LaBree, L; Shircore, AM; Selzer, RH; Blankenhorn, DH; Hodis, HN. Progression of coronary artery disease predicts clinical coronary events. Long-term follow-up from the Cholesterol Lowering Atherosclerosis Study. *Circulation,* 1996 93, 34-41.

[121] Diabetes Atherosclerosis Intervention Study Investigators. Effect of fenofibrate on progression of coronary artery disease in type 2 diabetes: the Diabetes Atherosclerosis Intervention Study, a randomised study. *Lancet,* 2001 357, 905-910.

[122] Todd, PA; Ward, A. Gemfibrozil. A review of its pharmacodynamic and pharmacokinetic properties, and therapeutic use in dyslipidaemia. *Drugs,* 1988 36, 314-39.

[123] The BIP Study Group. Secondary prevention by raising HDL cholesterol and reducing triglycerides in patients with coronary artery disease: the Bezafibrate Infarction Prevention (BIP) Study. *Circulation,* 2000 102, 21-27.

[124] Walldius G, Wahlberg G. Effects of nicotinic acid and its derivatives on lipid metabolism and other metabolic factors related to atherosclerosis. In: Kritchevsky D, Holmes WL, Paoletti R, editors. *Affecting Lipid Metabolism VIII Drugs.* New York: Plenum Publishing Corporation; 1985; 281-293.

[125] Carlson LA. Effects of nicotinic acid on serum lipids and lipoproteins. In: Carlson LA, Osslon AG, editors. *Treatment of Hyperlipoproteinemia.* Raven Press; 1984; 115.

[126] Blum, CB; Levy RI. Current therapy of Hypercholesterolemia. *JAMA,* 1989 261, 3582-3587.

[127] Canner, PL; Berge, KG; Wenger, NK; Stamler, J; Friedman, L; Prineas, RJ; et al. Fifteen year mortality in Coronary Drug Project patients: long term benefit with niacin. *J Am Coll Cardiol,* 1986 8, 1245-1255.

[128] The Coronary Drug Project Research Group. Clofibrate and niacin in coronary heart disease (the Coronary Drug Project). *J Am Med Assoc,* 1975 231, 360-381.

[129] Tatò, F; Vega, GL; Grundy, SM. Effects of crystalline nicotinic acid-induced hepatic dysfunction on serum low-density lipoprotein cholesterol and lecithin cholesteryl acyl transferase. *Am J Cardiol,* 1998 81, 805-808.

[130] Superko, HR; Krause, RM. Differential effects of nicotinic acid in subjects with different LDL subclass patterns. *Atherosclerosis,* 1992 95, 69-76.

[131] Smith, SC. Expanding the impact of statin therapy: would patients benefit from broader treatment and access? A Symposium: expanding the impact of statin therapy: would patients benefit from broader treatment and access? *Am J Cardiol,* 2000 85(12A), 1E-2E.

[132] Kolovou, G. The treatment of coronary heart disease. Statins beyond cholesterol lowering. *Curr Med Res Opin,* 2001 17, 34-37.

[133] Maron, DJ, Fazio, S; Linton, MF. Current perspectives on statins. *Circulation,* 2000 101, 207-213.

[134] Waters, D; Higginson, L; Gladstone, P; Kimball, B; Le May, M; Boccuzzi, SJ; Lesperance, J. Effects of monotherapy with an HMG-CoA reductase inhibitor on the progression of coronary atherosclerosis as assessed by serial quantitative arteriography. The Canadian Coronary Atherosclerosis Intervention Trial. *Circulation* 1994 89, 959-968.

[135] Sacks, FM; Pfeffer, MA; Moye, L; Rouleau, JL; Rutherford, JD; Cole, TG; Brown, L; Warnica, JW; Arnold, JM; Wun, CC; Davis, BR; Braunwald, E. The effect of pravastatin on coronary events after myocardial infarction in patients with average cholesterol levels. Cholesterol and Recurrent Events Trial investigators. *N Engl J Med,* 1996 335, 1001-1009.

[136] de Groot, E; Jukema, JW; Montauban van Swijndregt, AD; Zwinderman, AH; Ackerstaff, RG; van der Steen, AF; Bom, N; Lie, KI; Bruschke, AV. B-mode ultrasound assessment of pravastatin treatment effect on carotid and femoral artery walls and its correlations with coronary arteriographic findings: a report of the Regression Growth Evaluation Statin Study (REGRESS). *J Am Coll Cardiol,* 1998 31, 1561-1567.

[137] West of Scotland Coronary Prevention Study Group. Influence of pravastatin and plasma lipids on clinical events in the West of Scotland Coronary Prevention Study (WOSCOPS). *Circulation*, 1998 97, 1440-1445.

[138] Heart Protection Study Collaborative Group. MRC/BHF Heart Protection Study of cholesterol lowering with simvastatin in 20,536 high-risk individuals: a randomised placebo-controlled trial. *Lancet,* 2002 360, 7-22.

[139] Harrington, RA. Moderate versus aggressive lipid lowering with statins following an acute coronary syndrome: the pravastatin or atorvastatin evaluation and infection therapy trial. *Curr Cardiol Rep,* 2004 6, 272.

[140] Design features and baseline characteristics of the LIPID (Long-Term Intervention with Pravastatin in Ischemic Disease) Study: a randomized trial in patients with previous acute myocardial infarction and/or unstable angina pectoris. *Am J Cardiol,* 1995 76, 474-479.

[141] Ballantyne, CM; Herd, JA; Ferlic, LL; Dunn, JK; Farmer, JA; Jones, PH; Scheim, JR; Gotto, AM Jr. Influence of low HDL on progression of coronary artery disease and response to fluvastatin therapy. *Circulation*, 1999 99, 736-743.

[142] Mikhailidis, DP; Wierzbicki, AS. HDL-cholesterol and the treatment of coronary heart disease: contrasting effects of atorvastatin and simvastatin. *Curr Med Res Opin,* 2000 16, 139-146.

[143] Kzarsky, KF; Donahee, MH; Rigotti, A; Iqbal, S; Edelman, ER; Krieger, M. Overexpression of the HDL receptor SR-B1 alters plasma HDL and bile cholesterol levels. *Nature,* 1997 387, 414-417.

[144] Ritsch, A; Patsch, JR. Cholesteryl ester transfer protein: gathering momentum as a genetic marker and as drug target. *Curr Opin Lipidol,* 2003 14, 173-179.

[145] Lambert, G; Sakai, N; Vaisman, BL; Neufeld, EB; Marteyn, B; Chan, CC; Paigen, B; Lupia, E; Thomas, A; Striker, LJ; Blanchette-mackie, J. Analysis of glomarulosclerosis and atherosclerosis in lecithin cholesterolacyl transferase-deficient mice. *J Biol Chem,* 2001 276, 15090-15098.

[146] Ordovas, JM. HDL genetics: Candidate genes, genome wide scans and gene-environment interactions. *Cardiovasc Drugs Ther,* 2002 16, 273-281.

[147] Brousseau, ME; Schaefer, EJ; Wolfe, ML; Bloedon, LT; Digenio, AG; Clark, RW; Mancuso, JP; Rader, DJ. Effects of an inhibitor of cholesteryl ester transfer protein on HDL cholesterol. *N Engl J Med,* 2004 350, 1505-1515.

[148] de Lorgeril, M; Salen, P; Martin, JL; Monjaud, I; Delaye, J; Mamelle, N. Mediterranean diet, traditional risk factors, and the rate of cardiovascular complications after myocardial infarction: final report of the Lyon Diet Heart Study. *Circulation,* 1999 99, 779-785.

[149] Manttari, M; Elo, O; Frick, MH; Haapa, K; Heinonen, OP; Heinsalmi, P; Helo, P; Huttunen, JK; Kaitaniemi, P; Koskinen, P; et al The Helsinki Heart Study: basic design and randomization procedure. *Eur Heart J,* 1987 8, I1-I29.

[150] Steiner, G. The Diabetes Atherosclerosis Intervention Study (DAIS): a study conducted in cooperation with the World Health Organization. The DAIS Project Group. *Diabetologia,* 1996 39, 1655-1661.

[151] Sakai, T; Kamanna, V; Kashyap, M. Niacin, but Not Gemfibrozil, Selectively Increases LP-AI, a Cardioprotective Subfraction of HDL, in Patients with Low HDL Cholesterol. *Arteriosclerosis, Thrombosis, and Vascular Biology,* 2001 21, 1783-1789.

[152] Cheung, M; Zhao, X; Chait, A; Albers, J; Brown, BG. Antioxidant Supplements Block the Response of HDL to Simvastatin-Niacin Therapy in Patients with Coronary Artery Disease and Low HDL. *Arteriosclerosis, Thrombosis, and Vascular Biology,* 2001 21, 1320-1326.

[153] Sacks, FM; Pfeffer, MA; Moye,' L; Brown, LE; Hamm, P; Cole, TG; Hawkins, CM; Braunwald, E. Rationale and design of a secondary prevention trial of lowering normal plasma cholesterol levels after acute myocardial infarction: the Cholesterol and Recurrent Events trial (CARE). *Am J Cardiol,* 1991 68, 1436-1446.

[154] Baseline serum cholesterol and treatment effect in the Scandinavian Simvastatin Survival Study (4S). *Lancet,* 1995 345, 1274-1275.

[155] Bruschke, J: van Boven AV; Reiber, JH; Bal, ET; Zwinderman, AH; Jansen, H; Boerma, GJ; van Rappard, FM; Lie, KI; et al. Effects of lipid lowering by pravastatin on progression and regression of coronary artery disease in symptomatic men with normal to moderately elevated serum cholesterol levels. The Regression Growth Evaluation Statin Study (REGRESS). *Circulation,* 1995 91, 2528-2540.

[156] Herd, JA; West, MS; Ballantyne, C; Farmer, J; Gotto, AM Jr. Baseline characteristics of subjects in the Lipoprotein and Coronary Atherosclerosis Study (LCAS) with fluvastatin. *Am J Cardiol*, 1994 73, 42D-49D.

[157] Prevention of cardiovascular events and death with pravastatin in patients with coronary heart disease and a broad range of initial cholesterol levels. The Long-Term Intervention with Pravastatin in Ischaemic Disease (LIPID) Study Group. *N Engl J Med*, 1998 339, 1349-1357.

[158] Schwartz, GG; Olsson, AG; Ezekowitz, MD; Ganz, P; Oliver, MF; Waters, D; Zeiher, A; Chaitman, BR; Leslie, S; Stern, T; Myocardial Ischemia Reduction with Aggressive Cholesterol Lowering (MIRACL) Study Investigators. Effects of atorvastatin on early recurrent ischemic events in acute coronary syndromes: the MIRACL study: a randomized controlled trial. *JAMA,* 2001 285, 1711-1718.

[159] Shepherd, J; Blauw, GJ; Murphy, MB; Bollen, EL; Buckley, BM; Cobbe, SM; Ford, I; Gaw, A; Hyland, M; Jukema, JW; Kamper, AM; Macfarlane, PW; Meinders, AE; Norrie, J; Packard, CJ; Perry, IJ; Stott, DJ; Sweeney, BJ; Twomey, C; Westendorp, RG. PROSPER study group. PROspective Study of Pravastatin in the Elderly at Risk. Pravastatin in elderly individuals at risk of vascular disease (PROSPER): a randomised controlled trial. *Lancet,* 2002 360, 1623-1630.

[160] Colhoun, HM; Thomason, MJ; Mackness, MI; Maton, SM; Betteridge, DJ; Durrington, PN; Hitman, GA; Neil, HA; Fuller, JH; Collaborative AtoRvastatin Diabetes Study (CARDS). Design of the Collaborative AtoRvastatin Diabetes Study (CARDS) in patients with type 2 diabetes. *Diabet Med,* 2002 19, 201-211.

[161] Sever, PS; Dahlof, B; Poulter, NR; Wedel, H; Beevers, G; Caulfield, M; Collins, R; Kjeldsen, SE; Kristinsson, A; McInnes, GT; Mehlsen, J; Nieminen, M; O'Brien, E; Ostergren, J; ASCOT investigators. Prevention of coronary and stroke events with atorvastatin in hypertensive patients who have average or lower-than-average cholesterol concentrations, in the Anglo-Scandinavian Cardiac Outcomes Trial--Lipid Lowering Arm (ASCOT LLA): a multicentre randomised controlled trial. *Lancet,* 2003 61, 1149-1158.

[162] McKenney, JM; Jones, PH; Adamczyk, MA; Cain, VA; Bryzinski, BS; Blasetto, JW; STELLAR Study Group. Comparison of the efficacy of rosuvastatin versus atorvastatin, simvastatin, and pravastatin in achieving lipid goals: results from the STELLAR trial. *Curr Med Res Opin,* 2003 19, 689-698.

In: Cholesterol in Atherosclerosis and Coronary Heart Disease ISBN 1-59454-302-X
Editor: Jean P. Kovala, pp. 103-130 

*Chapter VI*

# Hyperlipidemia and Immunosuppressive Therapy: Pitfalls of Post Transplantation Management

*Marius Berman*
Tel Aviv University, Israel

## Abstract

Hyperlipidemia is a common and important risk factor after solid organ transplantation, mainly heart transplantation. Graft coronary vasculopathy is an accelerated form of atherosclerosis in transplanted hearts and has proven to be one of the most important late complications of heart transplantation and is the most limiting factor for long-term survival.

The most important factors favoring the development of hyperlipidemia after heart transplantation are inappropriate diet in combination with reduced physical activity, adverse effects of immunosuppressive therapy, such as steroids and cyclosporine, and polygenic hypercholesteremia in combination with ischemic cardiomyopathy.

Treatment of hyperlipidemia in heart transplant recipients results in a variety of complications and side effects. To note, interactions between lipid-lowering drugs and immunosuppressive therapy. The use of HMG-CoA reductase inhibitors (statins) achieved significant reduction in cholesterol levels. Use of these substances has resulted in significantly extended long-term survival times, significantly less graft coronary disease, and less severe graft rejection.

Blocking the cholesterol biosynthesis by statins resulted in lower levels of Coenzyme Q10, which plays an important role as a redox carrier in the mammalian respiratory transport chain, having a direct regulatory role on succinyl and reduced nicotinamide adenine dinucleotide (NADH) dehydrogenases. Enhancing the dietary uptake with Q10 may reduce the detrimental effect of statins therapy.

This chapter will review the common immunosuppressive drugs in clinical use, hyperlipidemia post transplantation and the current management therapies.

# Immunosuppressive Drugs

In the last few years, progress in the molecular understanding of the alloresponse has made new discoveries possible and allowed agents to be classified by mechanism of molecular action (Figure 1). (Reproducted with permission from Lawrence H. Cohn and L. Henry Edmunds, Cardiac Surgery in the Adult, 2$^{nd}$ edition, 2003, The McGraw-Hill Companies).

## Corticosteroids

Transplant physicians have recognized the benefits of corticosteroids from the very early days of clinical transplantation. These molecules have protean effects that are mediated through intracellular receptors that alter gene transcription. The predominant anti-inflammatory effects of glucocorticoids such as the blockade of NFKB-induced transcription of inflammatory cytokines and adhesion molecules derive from the inhibition of gene transcription. On the other hand, the metabolic side effects such as muscle wasting and diabetes derive from positive transcriptional effects [1]. This concept of differing mechanisms of action has prompted investigations to develop corticosteroid analogues that bind to intracellular receptors to promote the inflammatory effects without the metabolic effects. Glucocorticoids have been found to induce apoptosis in malignant T cells [2] and are therefore an especially appropriate choice of sole immunosuppression in the setting of posttransplant lymphoproliferative disorder. Outside of this subgroup, however, recent advances in the development of tolerance protocols have suggested that steroid use blocks certain immune signaling pathways necessary to induce donor-specific anergy or suppressor cells. In addition, steroid weaning reduces the tendency towards diabetes and dyslipidemia, which may decrease the incidence of AV [3].

### *Cytokine Synthesis Inhibitors*

*Cyclosporin* (CsA) inhibits the gene activation necessary for IL-2 production. To accomplish this, CsA inhibits the function of a $Ca^{2+}$ activated calcineurin phosphatase when bound to its cytoplasmic receptor [4]. This prevents the activation and nuclear translocation of the nuclear factor for activation of T cells (NFAT), precluding its engagement with the promoter sequence of the IL-2 gene. Blockade of the $Ca^{2+}$ calcineurin phosphatase complex also inhibits the production of nitric oxide synthetase, a potential mechanism by which CsA seems to promote AV in animal models [5].

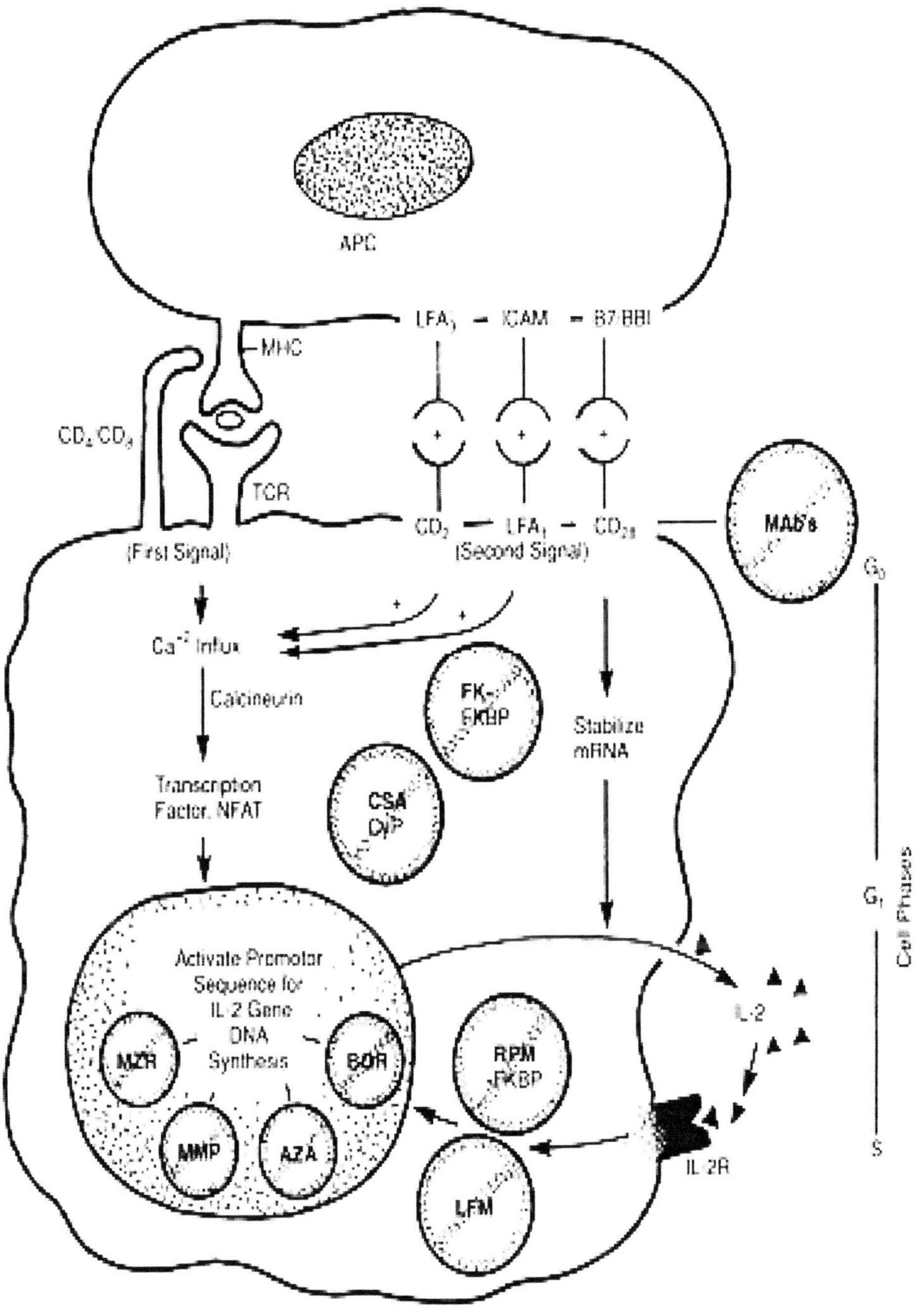


Figure 1. Immunosuppressants available to clinicians are directed toward inhibiting T-cell activation at various steps and by varied mechanisms, including interference with TCR complex (OKT3 Mab) and other surface ligands (anti–ICAM-1, anti-CD2, others); $Ca^{2+}$-dependent (CsA -ciclosporin, FK506 - tacrolimus) signal transduction; inhibition of cytokine IL-2 action in promoting cellular proliferation (RPM - rapamycin-, LFM); and inhibition of purine (AZA - azathioprine, MZR, MMP - Mycophenolate Mofetil) or pyrimidine synthesis BQR.

Originally oil-based, CsA has been replaced by a novel microemulsion formula, Neoral, which has significantly improved its bioavailability and reduced pharmacokinetic variability between patients. Approximately 30% of heart transplant recipients develop nephrotoxicity, the primary toxicity of CsA, which appears to be mediated by the inhibition of prostaglandin metabolites. In two recent series of heart transplant patients, calcineurin inhibition was the sole indication for metachronous kidney transplantation [6, 7]. CsA-induced alterations in cell phenotype explain other side effects such as hypertension and dyslipidemia [8, 9].

CsA was widely embraced as the central component for effective multidrug immunosuppression until FK506 (tacrolimus) was introduced to patients in Pittsburgh in 1988.

*Tacrolimus* combines with a different cytosolic protein than CsA (FK binding protein) but complexes with the same $Ca^{2+}$ activated calcineurin to prevent the activation of NFAT [10]. Tacrolimus has proven to be at least as effective in heart transplant patients [11] and possibly better in lung transplant patients [12]. It has found particular success following a switch from CsA-based immunosuppression when faced with a refractory acute rejection of the heart or lung [13] or bronchiolitis obliterans [14]. Given a mechanism of action similar to that of CsA, the reason for the improved effectiveness of tacrolimus in refractory rejection likely relates to more predictable pharmacokinetics [15]. Therefore, ongoing clinical trials comparing tacrolimus with Neoral are of great interest with regard to efficacy but are not likely to change the improved side effect profile already demonstrated with tacrolimus in multicenter trials [11]. Compared to recipients receiving CsA, tacrolimus was found to be associated with less facial disfigurement, hirsutism, hypertension, and hyperlipidemia but equal nephrotoxicity, and was perhaps associated with greater neurotoxic and diabetogenic effects.

### *Inhibitors of DNA Synthesis*

Antimetabolites are immunosuppressive because they inhibit the synthesis of nucleotides necessary for DNA's rapidly dividing cells. The classic antimetabolite has been azathioprine (AZA), which inhibits purine synthesis and therefore DNA and RNA synthesis throughout all dividing cells. Mycophenolate mofetil (MMF) appears to be more selective for T and B cells than AZA [16] based on its ability to block the activity of enzyme inosine monophosphate dehydrogenase, and therefore the synthesis of purines in the de novo pathway. Unlike other parenchymal and peripheral blood cells, T cells and B cells cannot use the salvage pathway and depend solely on the de novo pathway for purine synthesis. Compared to AZA, randomized clinical trials have shown a reduction in acute rejection events and antibody production with MMF in both heart [17] and lung [18] transplant patients. The reduction in chronic graft loss that has been demonstrated with the use of MMF versus AZA in renal transplantation has not yet been confirmed in cardiothoracic transplants. Neutropenia has not been a limiting factor as it has been with AZA.

### *IL-2 Signal Transduction Inhibitor*

*Rapamycin* (sirolimus; RPM) is structurally similar to tacrolimus and binds with FK binding protein (FKBP) but surprisingly does not inhibit the calcium-activated calcineurin [15]. Instead, RPM acts at a point downstream from the cytokine inhibitors and upstream from the antiproliferative agents. In alloreactive T cells, stimulation of the IL-2 receptor leads to clonal proliferation following initiation of the cell cycle and conversion from the resting ($G_0$] to proliferative ($G_1$/S) state. The RPM/FKBP complex binds the so-called "target of rapamycin," a lipid kinase [19], and prevents the signaling between IL-2 receptor activation and cell-cycle initiation. Because of theoretical concerns of competition for FK binding protein, sirolimus was combined initially with CsA [20] but recent clinical trials in renal transplantation have actually demonstrated greater success when combined with FK506 [21]. In vitro studies have demonstrated that RPM also induces cell cycle arrest in B cells and smooth muscle cells [22]. This smooth muscle cell antiproliferative effect is thought responsible for the arrest of AV in animal experimental models [23], and for the clinical prevention of restenosis after using RPM-coated intracoronary stents [24]. In preliminary randomized studies, the use of RPM instead of AZA following heart transplantation has resulted in reduced AV by IVUS evaluation at 6 months [25] and 1 year [26]. Sirolimus is not nephrotoxic but it may enhance the renal toxic effects of calcineurin inhibitors [20]; its main toxicity is hyperlipidemia. Combinations of these drugs that act at the level of cytokine production, the proliferative response to cytokines, and/or the signaling between the two have demonstrated additive immunosuppressive effects [27]. This will not only effectively reduce the alloresponse but also potentially do so with lower doses of each.

*Everolimus* (Certican) is a novel, orally active proliferation signal inhibitor with potent immunosuppressive activity. Everolimus blocks interleukin-2 and interleukin-15 pathways [28-30] to inhibit T-cell and non-hematopoietic cell proliferation, thus moderating the immune and non-immune response to the allograft and reducing the risk of acute rejection and coronary artery vasculopathy.

### *Receptor Antagonist and Monoclonal Antibodies*

Polyclonal anti–T-cell preparations (ATG) have been developed that recognize T-cell surface structures and kill these targets by inducing $F_C$-receptor–mediated cell lysis or by complement-dependent cell lysis. In the mid-1980s, the murine anti–human CD3 monoclonal antibody (OKT3) was developed that recognizes the epsilon protein of the CD3 complex on all T cells. When used as induction agents in thoracic transplantation, ATG and OKT3 have been found only to delay the onset of acute rejection at the expense of a profound, uncontrolled immunosuppression that increases the risk for opportunistic infections and malignancy [31]. Furthermore, their main toxicity, the cytokine release syndrome, is tolerated particularly poorly in heart and lung transplant recipients. As a result, their current use is limited in most centers for the treatment of refractory acute rejection and as a calcineurin-inhibitor sparing agent in those with prolonged postoperative renal dysfunction.

The development of a humanized monoclonal antibody (mAb) against the IL-2 receptor provided the opportunity for a more selective targeting of activated T cells, the only cells that express this receptor. In a small (55 heart transplant recipients), randomized, clinical trial, induction therapy using this mAb, dacluzimab, reduced the frequency and severity of acute rejection events over the study period. In addition, there were essentially no side effects and no increased risk of infections or malignancy [32]. Other monoclonal antibodies that are in various stages of clinical development may have a specific role in therapy, but hopes for a magic bullet likely will not be realized, as the immune response is far from simple and is based on redundancy by way of alternative pathways. A combination of various mAb would likely be the best protocol to address this redundancy. Unfortunately, no preclinical or clinical trials using a combination strategy have been performed in large part due to financial conflicts between the different pharmaceutical companies that own the rights to these agents.

# Hyperlipidemia after Solid Organ Transplantation

Hyperlipidemia is a major modifiable risk factor contributing to cardiovascular complication after solid organ transplantation [33]. Pathological changes in lipid parameters were found in about 60-80% of heart transplant recipients given standard triple immunosuppression consisting of cyclosporin, azathioprine and methylprednisolone [34-37]. Several studies, based on the transplanted population, found that plasma levels of total cholesterol, low-density lipoprotein (LDL), very low-density lipoprotein (VLDL), apolipoprotein B and triglycerides increase between 3 to 12 months post transplantation [38](Tables 1 and 2). The changes in apolipoproteins and lipid-related enzyme activity are shown in table 3. In the longer term, the elevated lipoprotein fractions show a gradual fall, although even then they remain above their respective normal range. Regarding high-density lipoprotein (HDL) cholesterol levels, the results are debatable; suggesting this lipoprotein fraction is not influenced b transplantation [39]. Similar confusion exists concerning lipoprotein (a) (Lp(a))levels which were found reduced after transplantation in 40% of patients [4], yet, other studies found elevated Lp(a) levels to be an independent risk factor for the development of graft coronary vasculopathy (GCV) [40, 41].

Three months after heart transplantation there is a marked increase in total cholesterol to a level about 40% higher than the pre transplant level [38], while LDL cholesterol increases by about 34% and triglycerides by up to 82%. The lipid levels rise most markedly in the first 3 months and then stabilize at abnormally high values even if systematic dietary measured are observed.

Hyperlipidemia develops after heart transplantation for a variety of reasons:

### *Genetics*

Some patients, in particular those in whom ischemic cardiomyopathy and hypercholesteremia are present even before transplantation, are genetically predisposed to the condition by polygenic dyslipidemia [42].

### *Dietary Factors*

Many patients have a low or ideal body-weight prior to transplantation. Following transplantation, 50% of patients put on weight as a result of a corticosteroid-induced increase in appetite [43]. A diet high in saturated fat, glucose and calories can contribute to excessive body-weight. Overweight, as in the general population, is associated to hypercholesteremia after heart transplantation.

**Table 1. Reproduced with Permission from Ichimaru et al: *Changes in Lipid Metabolism and Effect of Simvastatin in Renal transplant Recipients Induced by Cyclosporine or Tacrolimus***

Clinical characteristics of patients after renal transplantation[a]

| | | Cyclosporine ($n$ = 15) | Tacrolimus ($n$ = 17) |
|---|---|---|---|
| Total cholesterol (mg./dl.) | Before | 172 ± 43 | 176 ± 43 |
| | After | 223 ± 49** | 204 ± 37** |
| Triglycerides (mg./dl.) | Before | 120 ± 38 | 96 ± 35 |
| | After | 203 ± 115** | 138 ± 57* |
| LDL cholesterol (mg./dl.) | Before | 84 ± 28 | 90 ± 28 |
| | After | 105 ± 27** | 104 ± 26* |
| HDL cholesterol (mg./dl.) | Before | 43 ± 11 | 48 ± 11 |
| | After | 54 ± 8*** | 59 ± 17** |
| BUN (mg./dl.) | After | 21.8 ± 7.3 | 20.9 ± 6.2 |
| S-Cr (mg./dl.) | After | 1.5 ± 0.6 | 1.6 ± 0.6 |

[a] LDL, low density lipoprotein; HDL, high-density lipoprotein; BUN, blood urea nitrogen; S-Cr, serum creatinine. Data are expressed as mean ± S.D. * $P < 0.05$; **$P < 0.01$; ***$P < 0.001$ versus before transplantation as determined by paired $t$-test.

Source: Atherosclerosis 2001; 158: p. 417-423.

**Table 2. Reproduced with Permission from Ichimaru et al: *Changes in Lipid Metabolism and Effect of Simvastatin in Renal Transplant Recipients Induced by Cyclosporine or Tacrolimus***

Changes in cholesterol contents in the lipoprotein fractions after renal transplantation[a]

| | | Cyclosporine ($n$ = 15) | Tacrolimus ($n$ = 17) |
|---|---|---|---|
| VLDL (mg./dl.) | Before | 29.8 ± 8.9 | 26.2 ± 9.5 |
| | After | 47.9 ± 22.1* | 35.4 ± 15.0* |
| IDLs (mg./dl.) | Before | 15.1 ± 6.0 | 12.5 ± 5.1 |
| | After | 16.1 ± 11.4 | 9.0 ± 3.6* |
| LDL1 (mg./dl.) | Before | 72.9 ± 26.2 | 74.1 ± 25.3 |
| | After | 86.6 ± 25.4 | 85.0 ± 24.5 |
| LDL2 (mg./dl.) | Before | 10.9 ± 3.4 | 15.8 ± 6.1 |
| | After | 18.7 ± 5.2** | 18.6 ± 8.7 |
| HDL2 (mg./dl.) | Before | 28.9 ± 10.3 | 31.4 ± 11.0 |
| | After | 37.4 ± 8.4** | 40.0 ± 12.9* |
| HDL3 (mg./dl.) | Before | 14.1 ± 1.9 | 16.1 ± 2.2 |
| | After | 16.4 ± 2.9* | 18.7 ± 6.9 |

[a] VLDL, very-low density lipoprotein; IDL, intermediate high-density lipoprotein; LDL, low density lipoprotein HDL, high-density lipoprotein; BUN, blood urea nitrogen; S-Cr, serum creatinine. Data are expressed as mean ± S.D. * $P < 0.05$; **$P < 0.01$; ***$P < 0.001$ versus before transplantation as determined by paired $t$-test.

Source: Atherosclerosis 2001; 158: p.417-423.

**Table 3. Reproduced with Permission from Ichimaru et al:**
***Changes in Lipid Metabolism and Effect of Simvastatin in Renal Transplant Recipients Induced by Cyclosporine or Tacrolimus***

Changes in apolipoproteins and lipoprotein-related enzyme activity after renal transplantation[a]

| | | | Cyclosporine ($n$ = 15) | Tacrolimus ($n$ = 17) |
|---|---|---|---|---|
| Apolipoproteins | AI (mg./dl.) | Before | 121.3 ± 23.8 | 130.6 ± 24.1 |
| | | After | 142.1 ± 27.0* | 152.0 ± 26.9* |
| | AII (mg./dl.) | Before | 26.3 ± 3.8 | 28.0 ± 5.5 |
| | | After | 29.7 ± 7.8 | 27.8 ± 8.3 |
| | B (mg./dl.) | Before | 81.3 ± 20.9 | 78.1 ± 19.8 |
| | | After | 110.9 ± 30.0** | 90.2 ± 25.2* |
| | CII (mg./dl.) | Before | 3.6 ± 1.3 | 3.6 ± 1.2 |
| | | After | 5.3 ± 2.1** | 3.8 ± 1.3 |
| | CIII (mg./dl.) | Before | 15.4 ± 4.4 | 16.7 ± 5.6 |
| | | After | 22.6 ± 8.1** | 15.1 ± 4.5 |
| | E(mg./dl.) | Before | 4.1 ± 1.2 | 4.8 ± 2.5 |
| | | After | 6.9 ± 1.8*** | 5.7 ± 1.4 |
| Enzyme activity | LPL(μmol/ml./min.) | Before | 0.297 ± 0.086 | 0.321 ± 0.112 |
| | | After | 0.276 ± 0.078 | 0.372 ± 0.085 |
| | HTGL(μmol/ml./min.) | Before | 0.152 ± 0.072 | 0.190 ± 0.090 |
| | | After | 0.159 ± 0.057 | 0.241 ± 0.075* |
| | L-CAT(μmol/ml./h.) | Before | 338.0 ± 88.7 | 348.8 ± 102.4 |
| | | After | 410.9 ± 87.8** | 405.7 ± 87.3 |

[a] LDL, lipoprotein lipase; HTGL, hepatic triglyceride lipase; L-CAT, lecithin-cholesterol acyltransferase. Data are expressed as mean ± S.D.

* $P < 0.05$; **$P < 0.01$; ***$P < 0.001$ versus before transplantation as determined by paired $t$-test

Atherosclerosis 2001; 158: p.417-423.

## *Immunosuppressive Therapy*

*Corticosteroids* – act in various points in lipid metabolism, and, elevate a number of lipid parameters [43]. An increase in the activity of acetyl-coenzyme A (CoA) carboxylase and a consequent elevation of free fatty acid synthesis of long chain fatty acids. These processes lead to an increase in hepatic synthesis of VLDL. Hepatic LDL receptor activity is down regulated by corticosteroids. At the same time, activity of HMG-CoA reductase, the key enzyme in cholesterol biosynthesis, is markedly increased. In contrast, lipoprotein lipase activity is inhibited by corticosteroids. These various processes lead to markedly elevated plasma levels of VLDL, increased total cholesterol and triglycerides levels, and a marked reduction in HDL levels [43]. A high prevalence of severe glucose intolerance, hyperinsulinism, hypertriglyceridemia and hypercholesteremia has been reported in heart transplanted patients [44]. Insulin is crucial for the regulation of VLDL secretion and catabolism [45]. Insulin resistance enhances VLDL secretion and impedes the removal of triglycerides from VLDL in the circulation. This results in hypertriglyceridemia and high

VLDL levels. Furthermore, the expanded VLDL pool increases the transfer of cholesterol out of HDL and probably out of LDL to VLDL. This in turn leads to low levels of HDL cholesterol and the formation of small cholesterol depleted LDL. These small dense LDL particles are rich in triglycerides but contain relatively little cholesterol and are not readily cleared by the physiological LDL receptor. On the contrary, they readily undergo oxidative modification and become highly atherogenic. Thus, it has been suggested that the risk associated with hyperinsulinemia as a marker of insulin resistance is largely explained by lipid abnormalities [46].

*Cyclosporin* – also acts at various points in lipid metabolism. Cyclosporine inhibits the enzyme 26-hydrolase, which plays a crucial role in the biosynthesis of bile acids. Cyclosporin directly reduces conversion of cholesterol to bile acids and, thereby, reduces transport of cholesterol to the intestine [47]. Another mode of action of the cyclosporine is based upon the affinity of the cyclosporine molecule for the LDL receptors. Binding of cyclosporin to these receptors leads to an increased level of LDL cholesterol in peripheral blood [47]. Increased hepatic lipase activity and reduced lipoprotein lipase activity have also been observed in patients receiving cyclosporin. These changes lead to an imbalance between the LDL and VLDL lipoprotein fractions [48].

*Sirolimus* – Hyperlipidemia has been reported in up to 50% of kidney transplant recipients who received sirolimus as part of their immunosuppressive therapy [49]. The incidence of elevated lipid values in published reports of patients treated with sirolimus after liver transplantation ranges from 3.6-20% [50, 51]. The mechanism of sirolimus induced hyperlipidemia is not well understood, although effects on apoCIII and apo B100 have been proposed [52, 53].

*Tacrolimus* - Tacrolimus appears to have an advantage in controlling hyperlipidemia over CsA for the renal transplant patients with the risk factual disorders for CHD, however, tacrolimus also causes unfavorable effects on lipid metabolism. Post transplantation, both CsA and Tacrolimus showed significant increases in the serum lipid levels, with numerically higher increases in the CsA group [11, 54, 55]. A detailed examination of the effects of CsA and tacrolimus on the lipid metabolism showed cholesterol content in VLDL also increased significantly in both groups, but LDL2-C increased significantly CsA group. Therefore, hyperlipidemia induced by CsA or tacrolimus is associated with increased VLDL, suggesting that it may be not only secondary hypercholesteremia but also hypertriglyceridemia. An interaction was observed between pre transplant BMI and calcineurin inhibitors – among pre transplant normal weight patients (BMI<25 kg/m2), CsA produced a greater incidence of hyperlipidemia than tacrolimus (58% vs. 23%; p=.0001) while not among patients who were overweight (BMI > 25 kg/m2: pre transplant 58% vs. 42%; p=.341) [56].

*Receptor antagonists and monoclonal antibodies; ATG, OKT3* – to date, no relationship was found between these entities and dyslipidemia posttransplantation.

### *Miscellaneous*

Pre-existent hypercholesteremia prior to transplantation is an important predictor for the development of hypercholesteremia after kidney transplantation [57]. Same author suggested that there is significant regional variation in the severity and/or pattern of hyperlipidemia post transplantation, citing studies from Japan, Taiwan, Saudi Arabia, and Thailand.

# Graft Coronary Vasculopathy

The Framingham Study has shown that the prevalence of heart failure in the general population is about 1% in people in their 50s, rising progressively with age to affect 10% of people in their 80s [58]. In the transplanted population, the prevalence is much higher, greatly increasing morbidity and mortality. In a recent report from the Registry of the International Society for Heart and lung Transplantation, 45% of heart transplant recipients had a primary indication of coronary artery disease (CAD), and nearly 43% had a primary indication of cardiomyopathy [59]. Cardiac allograft vasculopathy (CAV), a type of cardiovascular disease that occurs uniquely in transplant recipients, is a rapidly progressive form of atherosclerosis characterized in its early stages by intimal proliferation, and in its later stages by luminal stenosis of epicardial branches, occlusion of smaller arteries and myocardial infarction [60]. CAV becomes clinically apparent in up to 50% of cardiac transplant recipients within the first 5 years after surgery. However, intimal thickening develops much earlier than that and is present in around 58% of transplant arteries by 1 year after transplantation.

Myocardial ischemia and infarction secondary to CAV in transplant patients are usually silent, due to a lack of cardial innervation. Instead of chest pain, more serious events, such as congestive heart failure, ventricular arrhythmias and sudden death, are commonly the first clinical manifestation [61]. Although CAV resembles atherosclerosis, there are few distinctive features such as; 1) intimal proliferation is concentric rather than eccentric and the lesions are diffuse, involving both distal and proximal coronary tree, 2) calcification is uncommon and the elastic lamina remains intact. This contrast with CAD, in which calcification is common and the internal elastic lamina is often severely disrupted. Occasionally, focal eccentric lesions associated with lipid depositions are found and may represent underlying, native (donor) atherosclerotic disease or late-stage degeneration [62]. A positive correlation has also been found between high donor age at the time of transplantation and postoperative development of CAV [63]. This association has been explained on the basis that the probability of pre-existing coronary disease increases with increasing donor age. The precise mechanism of CAV remains to be elucidated. It is likely that the initiating event is sub-clinical endothelial cell injury in the coronary graft mediated by cellular and humoral immune mechanisms in a milieu of additional non immunological risk factors [64]. These changes would produce inflammation and, ultimately, thrombosis, smooth muscle proliferation and vessel constriction.

Immunological risk factors for CAV:

1. A complete HLA-D-related mismatch is regarded as a risk factor for CAV, as is postoperative formation of anti-HLA antibodies [65],
2. Elevated levels of cytotoxic B-cell antibodies
3. Elevated levels of anti HLA antibodies
4. Increased incidence of acute cellular and humoral rejection
5. Cytomegalovirus infections
6. Sensitization to monoclonal antibodies
7. Early and persistent elevation of interleukin-2 receptor levels [7]

8. The occurrence of >= 2 major rejection episodes. Patients with evidence of cellular rejection, the rate of progression of CAV correlated significantly with the severity of rejection [66].

Non-immunologic risk factors for CAV:

1. Obesity
2. Smoking
3. Hypertension
4. Recipient age and sex
5. Overweight
6. Donor ischemia time

The liaison between hyperlipidemia and poorer outcome of transplanted patients remains unclear. Contradictory data shows no relation between hyperlipidemia and development of CAV [67] versus another study showing that low-density lipoprotein (LDL) cholesterol was significantly associated with intimal thickening (as measured by IVUS) [68]. Both triglyceride and high density lipoprotein (HDL) cholesterol predict cardiovascular disease after transplantation. The evidence linking hyperlipidemia and immunosuppressive therapy is conflicting; 2 studies found similar lipid profile 1-year post-transplant for patients receiving either cyclosporine or tacrolimus based- based immunosuppression [69, 70], while, other studies found that HDL cholesterol levels were significantly higher in cyclosporine-treated patients, as were all other lipid fractions [11, 23].

The medical treatment will be discussed in the next paragraph.

Once CAV has developed, the only definitive treatment is re-transplantation, which has risks for the patient and poses an ethical dilemma for the clinician in view of the scarcity of donor's organs. Other surgical approaches, such as stenting and angioplasty, may have a high re-stenosis rate and exposes the patient to the risk of another surgical procedure [71, 72]. Such procedures are inherently likely to be less effective than in non transplant patients because of the diffuse nature of CAV compared to CAD.

Because CAV has such an important influence on morbidity and mortality, it is evident that if further improvements in graft and patient survival are to be made, attention must focus on reducing the risk of CAV. As in the general population, modification of the classic (non-immunologic) risk factors may be used successfully to complement medical strategies. In transplant patients in particular, prevention is far better than cure.

# Treatment of Hyperlipidemia

## Dietary Measures

Systematic observance of a low cholesterol diet is the method of treating elevated LDL cholesterol levels in heart transplant recipients with the lowest incidence of adverse effects. All patients, together with their families, should receive extensive dietary counseling. The aim should be observance of an American Heart association (AHA) step I and II diet [73].

More ambitious dietary measures, although useful and desirable, are not satisfactorily tolerated by patients in the long term. Dietary measures alone are not sufficient of treating hypercholesteremia in heart transplant recipients, since most patients show persistent elevation of lipid levels despite following the diet [34]. In a study in which heart transplant recipients were followed up for 12 months postoperatively, a dietary program failed to bring about any striking change in lipoprotein profile, both LDL cholesterol and triglyceride remaining elevated [38]. Another first line therapy for dyslipidemia is weight reduction and physical activity. In ATP III (Adult Treatment Panel of National Cholesterol Education Program) [74], overweight and obesity are recognized as major, underlying risk factor for dyslipidemia. Weight reduction will enhance LDL lowering and reduce all the risk factors of the metabolic syndrome. Physical inactivity augments the lipid and nonlipid risk factors of the metabolic syndrome. Regular physical activity reduces VLDL levels, raises HDL and, in some persons lowers LDL levels. It was notable that despite good dietary observance, optimal drug therapy of hypertension and improved immunosuppressive therapy, the patients still showed elevated lipid levels. This indicates that drug therapy is required.

## Modification of Immunosuppressive Therapy

Immunosuppressive agents, in particular ciclosporin and prednisolone play a significant role in the development of post-transplant hyperlipidemia [38]. One way of treating hyperlipidemia is, therefore, to modify the patient's immunosuppressive agents. Many US transplant centers have attempted to reduce cholesterol levels in heart transplant recipients by dose reduction or discontinuation of corticosteroids [75-77]; however, the effectiveness of this measure has been highly variable. Reductions of 6% to 26% in total cholesterol level have been achieved, but not all patients benefited from this measure. Between 56% and 89% of the transplanted recipients investigated showed reductions in lipid levels after discontinuation or dose reduction of corticosteroids [76, 77]. However, the results of these studies indicate that elimination of corticosteroids from the immunosuppressive regimen does not necessarily lead to a reduction in cardiovascular risk profile. In another study, use of a steroid-free immunosuppressive regimen led to a 16% and 17% reduction in total and LDL cholesterol respectively [78]. However, HDL cholesterol decreased at the same time by 18%, with the result that the patients' cardiovascular risk profile was not significantly improved.

The calcineurin inhibitors are currently the mainstay of immunosuppressive therapy after transplantation and have greatly reduced the incidence of acute rejection, but they have little impact on the outcome of CAV. Even triple-drug therapy of cyclosporine, azathioprine and prednisone has not reduced the incidence of CAV [79]. Several mechanisms have been proposed for this lack of long-term effectiveness against CAV. First, neither calcineurin inhibitors nor purine synthesis inhibitors (azathioprine and MMF) prevent intimal thickening, as assessed by IVUS (intra vascular ultrasound), in the first year post-transplant [17, 69]. Second, calcineurin may be only partly inhibited by clinical doses of cyclosporine [80] and this partial inhibition may initiate the immune rejection process, leading to CAV [61]. In a number of clinical trials, tacrolimus not only achieved significantly better results in terms of reduced graft rejection but also caused significantly less elevation of cholesterol levels, as compared with ciclosporin [11]. Total cholesterol was found to be 13% and LDL cholesterol 12% less than in patients treated with ciclosporin. These findings were later reproduced in renal and liver transplant recipients [81, 82].

Sirolimus (Rapamycin) did not significantly increase cholesterol levels compared with ciclosporin [83-85]. In randomized studies, the use of sirolimus led to significantly reduced development of CAV compared with standard care (ciclosporin, prednisolone, azathioprine) [86, 87].

Everolimus is the only immunosuppressive agent that has been shown to significantly reduce the incidence and severity of CAV in heart transplant recipients in a large, well-controlled study. A 2-year international, multicenter, randomized study compared the efficacy and safety of everolimus with azathioprine in 634 de novo heart transplantation recipients receiving concomitant full dose cyclosporine and corticosteroids. At 24 months, both average intimal thickness and the incidence of CAV were significantly less in patients receiving everolimus than those receiving azathioprine [88].

## Drug Therapy

### *HMG-CoA Reductase Inhibitors (Statins)*

The introduction of statins constitutes a breakthrough in the treatment of hypercholesteremia in transplantation medicine. The primary objective of antihyperlipidemic therapy is to reduce total and LDL cholesterol to levels at which the risk for atherosclerosis is low. On the basis of these excellent results, lovastatin, pravastatin and simvastatin were introduced in transplantation medicine.

**Table 4. Reproduced with Permission from Ichimaru et al:**
***Changes in Lipid Metabolism and Effect of Simvastatin in Renal Transplant Recipients Induced by Cyclosporine or Tacrolimus***

The effects of simvastatin on serum lipid levels in post-transplant hyperlipidemia[a]

| Fractions | Simvastatin treatment | | | |
|---|---|---|---|---|
| | 0M | 1M | 3M | 6M |
| Total cholesterol | 240 ± 29 | 210 ± 21*** | 193 ± 24*** | 200 ± 22*** |
| Triglycerides | 217 ± 103 | 168 ± 106* | 158 ± 116* | 130 ± 38** |
| LDL cholesterol | 114 ± 20 | 99 ± 14* | 89 ± 19** | 99 ± 17* |
| HDL cholesterol | 57 ± 26 | 54 ± 14 | 54 ± 11 | 58 ± 13 |

[a] LDL, low density lipoprotein; HDL, high-density lipoprotein. Data are expressed as mean ± S.D.

* $P < 0.05$; **$P < 0.01$; ***$P < 0.001$ versus 0M as determined by paired *t*-test

Atherosclerosis 2001; 158: p.417-423.

By inhibiting HMG-CoA reductase, the key enzyme of cholesterol biosynthesis, substances of the statin class (lovastatin, pravastatin, simvastatin, atorvastatin), directly reduce the biosynthesis of cholesterol. This causes a marked reduction in cholesterol concentration in hepatocytes. This shortage of intracellular cholesterol leads to a compensatory increase in the number of newly formed LDL receptors in the liver. By increasing the uptake of LDL cholesterol, these newly formed LDL receptors bring about a marked reduction in the blood cholesterol levels [89] (Tables 4 and 5). Statins are metabolized in the liver via the cytochrome P450 (CYP) system. Simultaneous administration of ciclosporin, which is also metabolized via CYP, can lead to an increase in the plasma concentration of both drugs (Table 6). Statins have been shown in a number of prospective randomized long-term studies to significantly reduce total and LDL cholesterol levels. They also achieved a significant increase in patient survival times and a significant reduction in the number of late coronary events [90-92]. In secondary prevention studies on non-transplanted coronary patients, treatment with simvastatin led to an approximately 33% reduction in mortality and an approximately 42% reduction in myocardial infarction risk [91]. A number of authors reported 25-32% reductions in total cholesterol level within 6-96 months after transplantation, while LDL cholesterol was reduced by 40% from baseline levels [93-103]. To date, there are only two prospective randomized studies regarding the use of statins after heart transplantation [99, 103]. In the first study, 97 heart transplant recipients were treated in the early postoperative period with either pravastatin 40mg/day (n=47) or diet alone (n=50) as a control [99]. Total cholesterol levels over the first year were significantly lower in the active treatment group than in the control group, at 193 mg/dl versus 248 mg/dl ($p<0.0001$). In addition to the cholesterol lowering effect of pravastatin, other positive effects were observed. In particular, the incidence of clinically severe hemodynamically relevant graft rejection in the first year was significantly less with pravastatin than in the control group. Also, the 1-year survival rate was significantly greater in patients treated with pravastatin than in the control group, at 94% versus 78%, respectively ($p<0.02$). The incidence of CAV, as determined by IVUS, showed significantly less intimal thickening in the pravastatin group than in the control patients. Another positive effect of pravastatin therapy was a reduction in the cytotoxicity of natural killer cells. Pravastatin is a hydrophilic HMG-CoA reductase inhibitor. Therefore, it develops smaller intracellular concentrations in striated muscle than do lipophilic agents such as lovastatin and simvastatin [104] and may have fewer toxic effects on skeletal muscle. Moreover, pravastatin is not metabolized through the cytochrome P450 pathway (Phase I reaction), but is eliminated primarily through gastric degradation and metabolism to a 3alpha-hydroxy isomeric metabolite through Phase II reactions [105]. This seems to make pravastatin preferable in a setting of frequent P450 inhibitor use, such as therapy with cyclosporine, diltiazem, omeprazole, fluconazole, ketoconazole and others. Pravastatin may have an immunomodulatory benefit [99]. Seipelt [106] reported similar beneficial effect of pravastatin in pediatric heart transplant recipients. A second prospective, randomized study investigated simvastatin over a period of 8 years [103]. Thirty-five patients received simvastatin 5-20mg/day, while 37 patients in a control group were treated with diet alone. The survival rate was significantly higher in the active treatment group, at 88.6% versus 59.5% ($p<0.006$), and the incidence of angiographically and IVUS confirmed CAV was significantly lower in the active treatment than the control group.

In both studies the positive effects of statin therapy were not limited to cholesterol reduction. Simvastatin is known to inhibit proliferation of vascular smooth muscle cells (VSMC) [107]. In addition, statins exert a direct influence on the gene expression of growth factors that are required for proliferation of on the gene expression of VSMC [108]. Furthermore, simvastatin has been found to exert a direct influence on the gene expression of endothelin-1 in cultured endothelial cells, thereby markedly improving endothelial function and consequently providing protection against atherosclerosis [109]. Monocyte adhesion to endothelial cells is similarly inhibited by simvastatin [110]. Statins may have immunomodulatory effects. In both aforementioned studies, the survival rate was better in the patients treated with statins. This was mostly due to a lower rate of severe rejection reactions and associated graft failure. Statin themselves have no immunosuppressive actions [111], however, in the presence of cyclosporine, statins appear to develop such actions. Thus, they have reported to reduce the number of natural killer cells, inhibit T-cell proliferation and reduce T-cell toxicity, suppress T-cell response, reduce chemokine synthesis in peripheral blood mononuclear cells and inhibit expression of MHC-II genes [111-116]. In order to explain these effects of statins, it might be postulated that statin-induced LDL receptor activation also results in increased intracellular availability of LDL-bound ciclosporin and, thus, more inhibition of immunologically competent cells [34].

**Table 5. Reproduced with Permission from Ichimaru et al:**
***Changes in Lipid Metabolism and Effect of Simvastatin in Renal Transplant Recipients Induced by Cyclosporine or Tacrolimus***

| Fractions | Simvastatin treatment | | | |
|---|---|---|---|---|
| | 0M | 1M | 3M | 6M |
| VLDL (mg./dl.) | 52.5 ± 19.6 | 38.9 ± 24.5** | 35.6 ± 15.7*** | 29.3 ± 9.8*** |
| IDLs (mg./dl.) | 15.4 ± 10.8 | 14.1 ± 7.3 | 11.8 ± 4.9 | 9.9 ± 4.8* |
| LDL1 (mg./dl.) | 94.5 ± 20.1 | 78.9 ± 12.5* | 72.5 ± 16.2** | 78.5 ± 16.0* |
| LDL2 (mg./dl.) | 19.3 ± 8.4 | 15.3 ± 6.7* | 13.8 ± 6.0* | 17.7 ± 6.3 |
| HDL2 (mg./dl.) | 37.7 ± 12.8 | 37.1 ± 13.1 | 38.5 ± 9.6 | 42.2 ± 10.9 |
| HDL3 (mg./dl.) | 18.1 ± 6.5 | 18.2 ± 3.4 | 16.6 ± 2.5 | 17.4 ± 3.1 |

[a] VLDL, very-low density lipoprotein; IDL, intermediate-density lipoprotein; LDL, low-density lipoprotein HDL, high-density lipoprotein. Data are expressed as mean ± S.D. * $P < 0.05$; ** $P < 0.01$; *** $P < 0.001$ versus 0M as determined by paired *t*-test. M, months of treatment.
Atherosclerosis 2001; 158: p.417-423.

Excessive plasma statin concentrations can cause myopathy and rhabdomyolysis [89, 117]. These risks can be largely eliminated by regular monitoring of liver enzymes (transaminases), bilirubin and muscle enzyme levels (creatine kinase), and determining drug concentrations as well as adjusting dosages appropriately during the first months of statin therapy.

**Table 6. Reproduced with Permission from Ichimaru et al:**
***Changes in Lipid Metabolism and Effect of Simvastatin in Renal Transplant Recipients Induced by Cyclosporine or Tacrolimus***

Pharmakinetics of simvastatin administered with and without cyclosporine tacrolimus[a]

| | Tmax(h) | Cmax(ng ml) | AUC [b] (ng/h ml) | T1/2 (h) |
|---|---|---|---|---|
| With cyclosporine ($n$ = 6) | 2.9 ± 0.7 | 18.9 ± 11.3** | 78.1± 36.6** | 2.9 ± 0.8 |
| Simvastatin alone ($n$ = 6) | 2.0 ± 0.5 | 2.5 ± 1.5 | 9.8 ± 6.3 | 3.2 ± 1.1 |
| With tacrolimus ($n$ = 4) | 3.5 ± 1.5 | 3.6 ± 0.5 | 18.7 ± 3.8 | 4.7 ± 2.5 |
| Simvastatin alone ($n$ = 4) | 2.3 ± 0.4 | 2.8 ± 0.8 | 17.7 ± 7.0 | 4.8 ± 1.0 |

[a] Data are expressed as mean ± S.D. [b] AUCs of simvastatin were calculated over 0-12 h.
** $P < 0.01$ versus simvastatin alone as determined by unpaired $t$-test
Source: Atherosclerosis 2001; 158: p417-423.

### *Coenzyme Q10 (Ubiquinone)*

CoQ10 plays an important role as a redox carrier in the mammalian respiratory transport chain, having a direct regulatory role on succinyl and reduced nicotinamide adenine dinucleotide (NADH) dehydrogenases [118]. Lower-than-normal levels of CoQ10 have also been found in blood samples [119] from patients with cardiovascular diseases compared to levels in healthy human subjects and in myocardial biopsies assessing different cardiac pathologies [120-123]. Interestingly, it appears to be a relationship between HMG-CoA reductase treatment (statins), and CoQ10. HMG-CoA is enzymically converted to mevalonate by HMG-CoA reductase. Similar to cholesterol synthesis, the primary regulation of Coenzyme Q10 biosynthesis is the HMG-CoA reductase reaction, providing its isoprenyl side chain deriving from mevalonate. Therefore, inhibition of HMG-CoA reductase by statins will decrease not only intrinsic cholesterol production, but also CoQ10 [124]. Similar decreased CoQ10 blood levels were found in patients who were exposed for statin therapy. [125-127]. Phillips [128], found muscle weakness during statin therapy that reversed during placebo use. Muscle biopsies showed evidence of mitochondrial dysfunction, including abnormally increased lipid stores, fibers that did not stain for cytochrome oxidase activity, and ragged red fibers, suggesting that CoQ10 deficiency might be the cause of it [128, 129]. Furthermore, in one study [130], statin induced coenzyme Q10 reduction was prevented by exogenous coenzyme Q10 supplementation.

Several authors reported the correlation between acute rejection after heart transplantation and low CoQ10 levels of blood and endomyocardial biopsies [131, 132].

Treatment with Ultrasome (CoQ10) in patients with end stage heart failure awaiting heart transplantation improved the clinical capacity and daily functional independence [133], suggesting that myocardial mitochondrial CoQ10 depletion may have a role in patient clinical deterioration.

Further investigation is needed in order to determine whether the transplantation community should adopt these reports, at least after heart transplantation, and routinely use CoQ10 in order to diminish the notorious effects of well established statin treatment.

### *Cholesterol Absorption Inhibitors*

Ezetimibe [134] is the only available representative of this group. In non transplant recipients, ezetimibe significantly reduces total and LDL cholesterol, apolipoprotein B and triglycerides levels while increasing HDL levels. These effects are due to selective inhibition of intestinal absorption of cholesterol and related phytosterols, and are seen both with monotherapy and in combination with statins [135]. Caution is needed when initiating treatment in patients receiving ciclosporin, since increased plasma ezetimibe concentrations have been reported in this setup [135, 136].

### *Bile Acid Binding Agents*

Bile acid binding agents (colestipol, cholestyramine) bind to bile acids inhibiting their reabsorption and, thereby, interrupting their enterohepatic circulation. This results in increased intrahepatic synthesis of bile acids and increased hepatic LDL receptor activity, leading to increased clearance of circulating LDL cholesterol. This mechanism of action suggests that intestinal absorption of lipid soluble substances such as ciclosporin could be disturbed. In clinical trials in heart transplant recipients, treatment with cholestyramine led to a 14% reduction in total cholesterol levels [137]. However, in the same time, unusually wide fluctuations in blood ciclosporin concentrations were observed. Also, bile acid-binding drugs were found to increase serum triglyceride levels in heart transplant recipients [138]. Because of these undesirable effects, bile acid-binding drugs have limited use in post-transplantation medical therapy.

### *Fibric Acid Derivatives*

Fibric acid derivatives are gemfibrozil, clofibrate, bezafibrate and fenofibrate. This family of drugs is mostly used in patients with significant elevation of triglycerides levels. Reductions in levels of total cholesterol and its fractions are only moderate, at 15-20% [139]. Therefore, use of fibric acid derivatives is only rarely indicated in heart transplant recipients, since hypercholesteremia is generally the most prominent lipid abnormality in these patients. Only patients whose hypercholesteremia is accompanied by hypertriglyceridemia are candidates for adjuvant therapy with fibric acid derivatives [140]. Side effects are mainly elevation of blood urea and creatinine levels associated with reduction of renal function, particularly in heart transplant recipients [140]. Intestinal absorption of ciclosporin is impaired during treatment with fibric acid derivatives, sometimes resulting in large blood levels fluctuations [137].

### *Probucol*

Rarely used, mainly in patients who are intolerant of other antihyperlipidemic agents. Probucol lowers both total and LDL cholesterol levels by about 15%. It also delays oxidation of LDL cholesterol. A reduction of HDL cholesterol has also been observed. It has no effect on triglycerides [141]. In heart transplant recipients, it was found to be well tolerated but to reduce cyclosporine concentrations by up to 28% [141].

*Omega-3 fatty acids*

Epidemiological studies have shown an inverse correlation between consumption of fish or other source of omega-3 (n-3) fatty acids and cardiovascular events [142]. Large doses of n-3 fatty acids lower cholesterol levels [143]. Increased levels of HDL cholesterol in response to n-3 supplementation were observed in most, but not all, studies [142]. In heart transplant recipients, endothelium-dependent coronary vasodilatation, as assessed after acetylin infusion, was normal after 3 weeks of consuming 5g dietary n-3 fatty acids a day, whereas it was pathological in otherwise matched controls [143]. This could contribute to the inhibition of CAV and longer cardiac graft survival seen in animal models of cardiac transplantation [144]. The utility of n-3 fatty acid in heart transplant recipient is under investigation.

*Heparin-induced Extracorporeal Low-density Lipoprotein Precipitation (HELP)*

In a small proportion of heart transplant recipients with heterozygous familial hypercholesteremia, even maximal dietary and drug therapy fails to reduce LDL cholesterol levels. In this group of patients, drug therapy can be supplemented by extracorporeal treatment methods that can reduce the elevated LDL cholesterol levels to within target range (<100mg/dl) [145]. The HELP system is based on precipitations of LDL cholesterol from the plasma. This is induced by heparinization and acidification of the plasma (PH 5.12). The precipitated LDL cholesterol is eliminated by means of an extracorporeal filter system and the purified plasma is then returned to the patient's blood circulation. In 1991 the HELP system was first used in heart transplant recipients with familial hypercholesteremia. In a small group of patients, the mean LDL cholesterol blood levels were reduced from 172 mg/dl to 125 mg/dl, with the aid of the HELP system. The procedure had no influence on the blood ciclosporin levels, nor was any other negative effects observed. The heart transplant recipients treated in this way showed no increased incidence of infection and no impairment of organ function attributable to the procedure [146, 147]. Others authors have reported significant regression of existing CAV with the aid of the HELP system [148, 149]. In a controlled trial in 20 heart transplant recipients with severe hypercholesteremia, regular weekly use of the HELP technique in combination with simvastatin (n=10) led to a significant reduction in fibrinogen, LDL cholesterol and Lp(a) levels, and a lower incidence of CAV compared with patients treated with simvastatin alone [150].

The HELP system is costly, time consuming and of potential benefit only to a small and selected group of patients.

## Summary

More than 60% of heart transplant recipients develop elevated lipid levels, especially LDL cholesterol postoperatively. Dietary factors, overweight, physical inactivity, genetic predisposition and immunosuppressive therapy have been identified as dyslipidemia enhancing factors. Elevated cholesterol levels correlate in heart transplant recipients with an increased risk for CAV and other vascular disorders. To date, international accepted guidelines for drug therapy in heart transplant recipients are still lacking.

Guidelines for the treatment of hyperlipidemia in heart transplant recipients should be based on the NCEP guidelines [34, 74]. According to these, lipid-lowering therapy should be initiated in all patients with a total cholesterol >200mg/dl, LDL cholesterol >130mg/dl and triglycerides >200mg/dl, while LDL cholesterol >100mg/dl and triglycerides >150mg/dl constitute relative indications. Lipid lowering therapy should be initiated earlier and be more aggressive in heart transplant recipients than in non-transplant patients, as CAV develops soon after transplantation and can become clinically significant within one year.

The statins are the most intensively investigated of the drugs currently available for lowering cholesterol levels in solid organ transplant recipients [34, 54,151]. In addition to these cholesterol-lowering effects, these drugs have been shown to have immunomodulatory effects. Their clinical use has resulted in significantly better survival rates, a significantly lower incidence of CAV and fewer graft rejections. Statin therapy in combination with a systematic diet (AHA step I and II) should, therefore, be initiated in all solid organ transplant recipients as soon as possible after transplantation. Meticulous biochemical and clinical monitoring of these patients is needed in order to minimize the risk of myositis and rhabdomyolysis. Coenzyme Q10 addition should be considered due to the lowering effect of statin treatment and possible consequences of CoQ10 depletion. Treatment with fibric acid derivatives may be considered in heart transplant recipients with hypertriglyceridemia (>150-200 mg/dl) that cannot be controlled by diet alone. Strict renal function monitoring is required. HELP is required only in a small percentage of patients with familial hypercholesteremia refractory to diet and cholesterol-lowering drug treatment.

In conclusion, the current data, which the main ideas are expressed in this chapter, shows that solid organ transplant recipients and their care givers should closely monitor hyperlipidemia post transplantation and start treatment prophylactically in order to improve quality of life and survival.

## References


[1] Newton R: Molecular mechanisms of glucocorticoid action: what is important? *Thorax* 2000; 55:603.

[2] Ramdas J, Hasday JD: Glucocorticoid-induced apoptosis and regulation of NF-kappaB activity in human leukemic T cells. *Endocrinology* 1998; 139:3813.

[3] Baran DA, Segura L, Kushwaha S, et al: Tacrolimus monotherapy in adult cardiac transplant recipients: intermediate-term results. *J Heart Lung Transplant* 2001; 20:59.

[4] Clipstone NA, Crabtree GR: Calcineurin is a key signaling enzyme in T lymphocyte activation and the target of immunosuppressive drugs cyclosporin A and FK 506. *Ann NY Acad Sci* 1993; 696:20.

[5] Sudhir K, MacGregor JS, DeMarco T, et al: Cyclosporine impairs release of endothelium-derived relaxing factors in epicardial and resistance coronary arteries. *Circulation* 1994; 90:3018.

[6] Poston R, McCurry K, Griffith B: Kidney transplantation following heart transplantation: effects on cardiac outcome. *J Heart Lung Transplant* 2002; 21:102.

[7] Coopersmith CM, Brennan DC, Miller B, et al: Renal transplantation following previous heart, liver, and lung transplantation: an 8–year single-center experience. *Surgery* 2001; 130:457.

[8] Wu J, Zhu H, Patel SB: CsA-induced dyslipoproteinemia is associated with selective activation of SREBP-2. *Am Physiol Soc* 1999; 277:E1087.

[9] Ventura HO, Malik FS, Mehra MR, et al: Mechanisms of hypertension and the role of CsA. *Curr Opin Cardiol* 1997; 12:375.

[10] Mathew P, Bozeman P, Krance RA et al: Bronchiolitis obliterans organizing pneumonia in children after allogenic bone marrow transplantation. *Bone Marrow Transplant* 1994; 13: 221.

[11] Taylor DO, Barr ML, Radovancevic B, et al: A randomised, multicenter comparison of TAC and CsA immunosuppressive regimens in cardiac transplantation: decreased hyperlipidemia and hypertension with TAC. *J Heart Lung Transplant* 1999; 18:336.

[12] Treede H, Klepetko W, Reichenspurner H, et al: Tacrolimus versus cyclosporine after lung transplantation: a prospective, open, randomized two-center trial comparing two different immunosuppressive protocols. *J Heart Lung Transplant* 2001; 20:511.

[13] Onsager DR, Canver CC, Jahania MS, et al: Efficacy of tacrolimus in the treatment of refractory rejection in heart and lung transplant recipients. *J Heart Lung Transplant* 1999; 18:448.

[14] Ross DJ, Lewis MI, Kramer M, et al; FK506 ''rescue'' immunosuppression for obliterative bronchiolitis after lung transplantation. *Chest* 1997; 112: 1175.

[15] Fruman D, Burakoff SJ, Biarer BE: Molecular actions of cyclosporin A, FK 506 and rapamycin, in Thompson AW, Starzl TE (eds): *Immunosuppressive Drugs: Developments in Anti-Rejection Therapy*. London, Edward Arnold, 1994; p 15.

[16] Allison A, Eugui EM: Mycophenolate mofetil (RS-61443): mode of action and effects on graft rejection, in Thompson AW, Starzl TE (eds): *Immunosuppressive Drugs: Developments in Anti-Rejection Therapy*. London, Edward Arnold, 1994; p 144.

[17] Kobashigawa J, Miller L, Renlund D, et al: A randomized active-controlled trial of mycophenolate mofetil in heart transplant recipients. Mycophenolate Mofetil Investigators. *Transplantation* 1998; 66:507.

[18] Corris P, Glanville A, McNeil K, et al: One year analysis of an ongoing international randomized study of mycophenolate mofetil (MMF) vs azathioprine (AZA) in lung transplantation. *J Heart Lung Transplant* 2001; 20:149.

[19] Kuntz J, Henriquez R, Schneider U, et al: Target of rapamycin in yeast TOR2, as an essential phosphatidylinositol kinase homolog required for G1 progression. *Cell* 1993; 73:585.

[20] Halloran PF: Immunosuppressive agents in clinical trials in transplantation. *Am J Med Sci* 1997; 313:283.

[21] McAlister VC, Gao Z, Peltekian K, et al: Sirolimus-tacrolimus combination immunosuppression. *Lancet* 2000; 355:376.

[22] Gregory CR, Huang X, Pratt RE, et al: Treatment with rapamycin and mycophenolic acid reduces arterial intimal thickening after balloon catheter injury and allows endothelial replacement. *Transplantation* 1995; 59:655.

[23] Ikonen TS, Gummert JF, Hayase M, et al: Sirolimus (rapamycin) halts and reverses progression of allograft vascular disease in non-human primates. *Transplantation* 2000; 70:969.

[24] Morice M-C, Serruys PW, Sousa JE, et al: A randomized comparison of a sirolimus-eluting stent with a standard stent for coronary revascularization. *N Engl J Med* 2002; 346:1773.

[25] Keogh A: Progression of graft vessel disease in cardiac allograft recipients is significantly reduced by sirolimus immunotherapy: 6-month results from a phase 2, open-label study [abstract #431]. *Am J Transpl* 2002; 2(suppl 3):246.

[26] Tuzcu EM, Schoenhagen P, Starling RC, et al: Impact of everolimus on allograft vasculopathy: the SDZ RAD/heart intravascular ultrasound study. *J Heart Lung Transplant* 2002; 21:68.

[27] Hausen B, Gummert J, Berry GJ, et al: Prevention of acute allograft rejection in nonhuman primate lung transplant recipients: induction with chimeric anti-interleukin-2 receptor monoclonal antibody improves the tolerability and potentiates the immunosuppressive activity of a regimen using low doses of both microemulsion cyclosporine and 40–O-(2–hydroxyethyl)-rapamycin. *Transplantation* 2000; 69:488.

[28] Nashan B. The role of Certican (everolimus) in the many pathways of chronic rejection. *Transplant Proc* 2001; 33: 3215.

[29] Schuler W, Sedrani R, Cottens S, et al. SDZ RAD, a new rapamycin derivative: pharmacological properties in vitro and in vivo. *Transplantation* 1997; 64: 36-42.

[30] Schuurman HJ, Cottens S, Fuchs S et al. SDZ RAD, a new rapamycin derivative: synergism with cyclosporin. *Transplantation* 1997; 64: 32-5.

[31] Johnson MR, Mullen GM, O'Sullivan EJ, et al: Risk/benefit ratio of perioperative OKT3 in cardiac transplantation *Am J Cardiol* 1994; 74:261.

[32] Beniaminovitz A, Itescu S, Lietz K, et al: Prevention of rejection in cardiac transplantation by blockade of the interleukin-2 receptor with a monoclonal antibody. *N Engl J Med* 2000; 342:613.

[33] Kendrick E. Cardiovascular Disease and the renal transplant recipient (Review). *Am J Kidney Dis* 2001; 38(Suppl. 6): s36.

[34] Wenke K. Management of hyperlipidemia associated with heart transplantation. *Drugs* 2004; 64(10): 1053.

[35] Carrier M, Rivard M, Kostuk W et al. Tha Canadian study of cardiac transplantation atherosclerosis. *Can J Cardiol* 1999; 15: 1337.

[36] Farmer JA, Ballantyne CM, Frazier OH et al. Lipoprotein(a) and apolipoproteins changes after cardiac transplantation. *J Am Coll Cardiol* 1991; 18: 926.

[37] Gao SZ, Schrodeder JA, Alderman EL et al. Prevalence of accelerated coronary artery disease in heart transplant survivors: comparison of ciclosporin and azathioprine regiments. *Circulation* 1989; 80 suppl 3: III-100.

[38] Ballantyne CM, Radovancevic B, Farmer JA, et al. Hyperlipidemia after heart transplantation: report of a 6-year experience with treatment recommendations. *J Am Coll Cardiol* 1992; 19: 1315.

[39] Hosenpud JD, Shipley GD, Wagner CR. Cardiac allograft vasculopathy: current concepts, recent developments and future directions. *J Heart Lung Transplant* 1992; 11: 9

[40] Barbir M, Kushwaha S, Hunt B, et al. Lipoprotein (a) and accelerated coronary artery disease in cardiac transplant recipients. *Lancet* 1992; 340: 1500.

[41] Kobashigawa JA, Kasiske BL. Hyperlipidemia in solid organ transplantation. *Transplantation* 1997; 63: 331.

[42] McGriffin DC, Savumen T, Kirklin JK, et al. Cardiac transplant coronary disease: a multivariate analysis of pretransplant risk factors for disease development and morbid events. *J Thorac Cardiovasc Surg* 1995; 109: 1082.

[43] Becker DM, Chamberlain B, Swank R, et al. Relationship between corticosteroid exposure and plasma lipid levels in heart transplant recipients. *Am J Med* 1988; 85: 632.

[44] Kemna MS, Valentine HA, Hunt SA et al. Metabolic risk factors for atherosclerosis in heart transplant recipients. *Am Heart J* 1994; 128: 68.

[45] Bagdade JD, Lane JT, Subbaiah PV et al. Accelerated cholesteryl ester transfer in non-insulin dependent diabetes mellitus. *Atherosclerosis* 1993; 104: 69.

[46] Valentine HA, Schroeder JS. HMG-CoA reductase inhibitors reduce transplant coronary artery disease and mortality. *Circulation* 1997; 96: 1370.

[47] De Groen PC. Cyclosporine, low density lipoprotein, and cholesterol. *Mayo Clinic Proc* 1988; 63: 1012.

[48] Chan MK, Varghese Z, Moohead JF. Lipid abnormalities in uremia, dialysis and transplantation. *Kidney Int* 1981; 19: 625.

[49] MacDonald ASfor the Rapamune Global Study Group. A World-wide, phase III, randomized, controlled, safety and efficacy study of a sirolimus/cyclosporine regimen for prevention of acute rejection in recipients of primary mismatched renal allografts. *Transplantation* 2001; 71: 271.

[50] Trotter JF, Wachs ME, Trouillot TE, et al. Dyslipidemia during sirolimus therapy in liver transplant recipients occurs with concomitant cyclosporine but not tacrolimus. *Liver Transpl* 2001; 7: 401.

[51] Watson CJE, Friend PJ, Jamienson NV, et al. Sirolimus: a potent new immunosuppressant for liver transplantation. *Transplantation* 1999; 67: 505.

[52] Tur MD, Garrigue V, Vela C, et al. Apolipoprotein CIII is upregulated by anticalcineurins and rapamycin: implications in transplantation-induced dyslipidemia. *Tranplant Proc* 2000; 32: 278.

[53] Hoogeveen RC, Ballantyne CM, Pownall HJ, et al. Effect of sirolimus on the metabolism of ApoB100-containing lipoproteins in renal transplant patients. *Clin Transpl* 2001; 72: 1244.

[54] Ichimaru N, Takahara S, Kokado Y, et al. Changes in lipid metabolism and effect of simvastatin in renal transplant recipients induced by cyclosporine or tacrolimus. *Atherosclerosis* 2001; 158: 417.

[55] Berman M, Ben-Gal T, Stamler A, et al. Lipid metabolism and immunosuppressive therapy in heart transplant recipients. *Transpl Proc* 2003; 35(2): 677.

[56] Hernandez D, Alvarez A, Torres A et al. Cardiovascular Risk profile in nondiabetic renal transplant patients: cyclosporine versus tacrolimus. *Transpl Proc* 2003; 35(5): 1727.

[57] Tse KC, Lam MF, Yip PS et al. A long term study on hyperlipidemia in stable renal transplant recipients. *Clin Transplant* 2004; 18: 274.

[58] Kannel WB, Belanger AJ. Epidemiology of heart failure. *Am Heart J* 1991; 121: 951.

[59] Taylor DO, Edwards LB, Mohacsi PJ et al. The registry of the international society for heart and lung transplantation: twentieth official adult heart transplant report -2003. *J Heart Lung Transplant* 2003; 22: 616.

[60] Billingham ME. Histopathology of graft coronary disease. *J Heart Lung Transplant* 1992; 11(suppl): s38.

[61] Moien-Afshari F, McManus BM, Laher I. Immunosuppression and transplant vascular disease: benefits and adverse effects. *Pharmacol Ther* 2003; 100:141.

[62] Radio S, Wood S, Wilson j, et al. Allograft vascular disease: comparison of heart and other grafted organs. *Transplant Proc* 1996; 28: 496.

[63] Bieber CP, Hunt SA, Schwinn DA, et al. Complications in long term survivors of cardiac transplantation. *Transplant Proc* 1981; 13(1): 207.

[64] Paavonen T, Mennander A, Lautenschlager I, et al. Endothelialitis and accelerated arteriosclerosis in human heart transplant coronaries. *J Heart Lung Transplant* 1993; 12: 117.

[65] Libby P, Swanson SJ, Tanaka H, et al. Immunopathology of coronary arteriosclerosis in transplanted hearts. *J Heart Lung Transplant* 1992; 11: 5.

[66] Valantine H. Cardiac allograft vasculopathy after heart transplantation: risk factors and management. *J Heart Lung Transplant* 2004; 23: s187.

[67] Radovancevic B, Poindexter S, Birovljev S, et al. Risk factors for development of accelerated coronary artery disease in cardiac transplant recipients. *Eur J Cardiothorac Surg* 1990; 4: 309.

[68] Kapadia SR, Ziada KM, L'Allier PI et al. Intravascular ultrasound imaging after cardiac transplantation: advantages of multivessel imaging. *J Heart Lung Transplant* 2000; 19: 167.

[69] Klauss V, Konig A, Spes C, et al. Cyclosporine versus tacrolimus for prevention of cardiac allograft vasculopathy. *Am J Cardiol* 2000; 85: 266.

[70] Reichart B, Meiser B, Vigano M, et al. European multicenter tacrolimus heart pilot study- one year results- European Tacrolimus Multicenter Heart Study Group. *J Heart Lung Transplant* 1998; 17: 775.

[71] Halle AAI, DiSciascio G, Massin EK, et al. Coronary angioplasty, atherectomy, and bypass surgery in cardiac transplant recipients. *J Am Coll Cardiol* 1995; 26: 120.

[72] Radonnet M, Tron C, Koning R, et al. Coronary angioplasty and stenting in cardiac allograft vasculopathy following heart transplantation. *Transplant Proc* 2000; 32: 463.

[73] Adult Treatment Panel II. Summary of the second report of the National Cholesterol Education Program. *JAMA* 1993; 269: 3015.

[74] Executive Summary of the third report of the National Cholesterol Education Program expert Panel on detection, evaluation and treatment of high blood cholesterol in adults (Adult Treatment Panel III). *JAMA* 2001; 285: 2486.

[75] Renlund DG, Bristow MR, Crandall BG et al. Hypercholesterolemia after heart transplantation: amelioration by corticosteroids-free maintenance immunosuppression. *J Heart Lung Transplant* 1989; 8: 214.

[76] Keogh A, Macdonald P, Harvison A et al. Initial steroid-free versus steroid-based maintenance therapy and steroid withdrawal after heart transplantation: two views of the steroid question. *J Heart Lung Transplant* 1992; 11: 421.

[77] Kobashigawa JA, Stevenson LW, Brownfield EB et al. Corticosteroid weaning late after cardiac transplantation: relation to HLA-DR mismatching and long-term metabolic benefits. *J Heart Lung Transplant* 1995; 14: 963.

[78] Hricik DE, Bartucci MR, Mayes JT et al. The effects of steroid withdrawal on the lipoprotein profiles of cyclosporine-treated kidney and kidney-pancreas transplant recipients. *Transplantation* 1992; 54: 868.

[79] Olivari MT, Kubo SH, Braunlin EA et al. Five year experience with triple-drug immunosuppressive therapy in cardiac transplantation. *Circulation* 1990; 82(suppl IV): 276

[80] Batiuk TD, Pazderka F, Halloran PF. Calcineurin activity in only partially inhibited in leukocytes of cyclosporine-treated patients. *Transplantation* 1995; 59: 1400.

[81] McCune TR, Thacker LR, Peters TG et al. Effects of tacrolimus on hyperlipidemia after successful renal transplantation. *Transplantation* 1998; 65: 87.

[82] Cleasson K, Mayer AD, Squifflet JP et al. Lipoprotein patterns in renal transplant patients: a compairison between FK 506 and cyclosporine A patients. *Transplant Proc* 1998; 30: 1292.

[83] Groth C, Backmann L, Morales J, et al. Sirolimus based therapy in human renal transplantation. *Transplantation* 1999; 67: 1036.

[84] Kahan BD. Efficacy of sirolimus compared with azathioprine for reduction of acute renal allograft rejection: a randomized multicenter study. *Lancet* 2000; 356: 194.

[85] Edelman ER, Danenberg HD. Rapamycin for cardiac transplant rejection and vasculopathy: one stone, two birds. *Circulation* 2003; 108: 6.

[86] Mancini D, Pinney S, Burkhoff D et al. Use of rapamycin slows progression of cardiac transplantation vasculopathy. *Circulation* 2003; 108: 48.

[87] Dambrin C, Klupp J, Birsan T, et al. Sirolimus monotherapy prevents graft vascular disease in non human primate recipients of orthotopic aortic allografts. *Circulation* 2003; 107: 2369.

[88] Mancini D, Vigano M, Pulpon LA et al. 24-month results of a multicenter study of Certican for the prevention of allograft rejection and vasculopathy in de novo cardiac transplant recipients. *Am J Transpalnt* 2003; 3(suppl 5): 550.

[89] Plosker GL, McTavish D. Simvastatin: a reappraisal of its pharmacology and therapeutic efficacy in hypercholesterolemia. *Drugs* 1995; 50: 334.

[90] Shepard J, Cobbe SM, Ford I et al. prevention of coronary heart disease with pravastatin in men with hypercholesterolemia. *N Engl J Med* 1995; 333: 1301.

[91] The Scandinavian Simvastatin Survival Study Group. Randomized trial of cholesterol lowering in 4444 patients with coronary artery disease: the Scandinavian Simvastatin Survival Study. *Lancet* 1994; 344: 1383.

[92] Heart Protection Collaborative Group. MRC/BHF heart protection study of cholesterol with simvastatin in 20536 high-risk individuals: a placebo-controlled trial. *Lancet* 2002; 360: 7.

[93] Kobashigawa JA, Murphy FL, Stevenson LW et al. Low-dose lovastatin safely lowers cholesterol after cardiac transplantation. *Circulation* 1990; 82(5 suppl): 281.

[94] Babir M, Rose M, Kushwaha S et al. Low-dose simvastatin for treatment of hypercholesterolemia in recipients of cardiac transplantation. *Int J Cardiol* 1991; 33: 241.

[95] Kobashigawa JA, Brownfield ED, Stevenson LW et al. Effects of pravastatin for hypercholesterolemia in cardiac transplant recipients. *J Am Coll Cardiol* 1993; 21: 141.

[96] Vanhaecke J, van Cleemput J, van Lierde J et al. Safety and efficacy of low dose simvastatin in cardiac transplant recipients treated with cyclosporine. *Transplantation* 1994; 58: 42.

[97] Carrier M, Pelletier GB, Genest Jr J, et al. Cholesterol lowering intervention and coronary artery disease after cardiac transplantation. *Ann Thorac Surg* 1994; 57: 353.

[98] Campana C, Iacona I, Regazzi MB et al. Efficacy and pharmacokinetics of simvastatin in heart transplant recipients. *Ann Pharmacother* 1995; 29: 235.

[99] Kobashigawa JA, Katznelson W, Laks H et al. Effects of pravastatin on outcome after cardiac transplantation. *N Engl J Med* 1995; 333: 621.

[100] Wenke K, Thiery J, Meiser B et al. long-term simvastatin therapy for hypercholesterolemia in heart transplant recipients. *Z Kardiol* 1995; 84: 130.

[101] Pflugfelder PW, Huff M, Oskalns R et al. Cholesterol lowering therapy after heart transplantation: a 12-month randomized trial. *J Heart Lung Transplant* 1995; 14: 613.

[102] Mehra MR, Uber PA, Vivekananthan K et al. Comparative beneficial effects of simvastatin and pravastatin on cardiac allograft rejection and survival. *J Am Coll Cardiol* 2002; 40: 1609.

[103] Wenke K, Meiser B, Thiery J, et al. Simvastatin initiated early after heart transplantation: 8-year prospective experience. *Circulation* 2003; 107: 93.

[104] Gatbut A, Caruso A, Galper J. Differential sensitivity of C2-C12 stirated muscle cells to lovastatin and pravastatin. *J Mol Cell Cardiol* 1995; 27: 2397.

[105] Christians U, Jacobsen W, Floren LC. Metabolism and drug interactions of 3-hydroxy-3-methylglutaryl coenzyme A reductase inhibitors in transplant patients: are the statins mechanistically similar? *Pharmacol Ther* 1998; 80: 1.

[106] Seipelt IM, Crawford SE, Rodgers S et al. Hypercholesterolemia is common after pediatric heart transplantation: initial experience with pravastatin. *J Heart Lung Transplant* 2004; 23: 317.

[107] Corsini A, Raiteri M, Soma MR. et al. Simvastatin but not pravastatin has a direct inhibitory effect on rat and human myocyte proliferation. *Clin Biochem* 1992; 25: 399.

[108] Farmer JA. Pleiotropic effect of statins. *Curr Atheroscler Rep* 2000; 2: 208.

[109] Alfon J, Guasch JF, Berropze M et al. Nitric oxide synthetase II gene expression correlates with atherosclerotic intimal thickening: preventive effect of HMG-CoA reductase inhibitors. *Atherosclerosis* 1999; 145: 325.

[110] Hernandez-Perera O, Perea-Salea D, Navarro-Antolin J, et al. Effects of HMH-CoA reductase inhibitors, atorvastatin and simvastatin on the expression of endothelin nitric oxide synthetase in vascular endothelial cells. *J Clin Invest* 1998; 101: 2711.

[111] Muldoon MF, Flory JD, Marsland A et al. Effects of lovastatin on the immune system. *Am J Cardiol* 1997; 80: 1391.

[112] Katzenelson S, Huang XM, Chia D et al. The inhibitor effects of pravastatin on natural killer T cell activity in vivo in cytotoxic T lymphocyte activity in vitro. *J Heart Lung Transplant* 1998; 259: 414.

[113] McPherson R, Tsoukas C, Baines MG et al. Effects of lovastatin on natural killer cell function and other immunological papremeters in men. *J Clin Immunol* 1993; 13: 439.

[114] Kurakata S, Kada M, Shimada Y et al. Effect of different inhibitors of HMG-CoA reductase, pravastatin sodium and simvastatin on sterol synthesis and immunological functions in human lymphocyte in vitro. *Immunopharmacol* 1996; 34: 51.

[115] Kano H, Hayashi T, Sumi D et al. A HMG-CoA reductase inhibitor improved progression of atherosclerosis in rabbit aorta without affecting serum lipid levels: possible relevance of upregulating of endothelial nitric oxide synthetase mRNA. *Biochem Biophys Res Commun* 1999; 259: 414.

[116] Kwak B, Mulhaupt F, Myit S et al. Statins as a newly recognized typr of immunomodulator. *Nat Med* 2000; 80: 1095.

[117] East C, Alivizatos PA, Grundy SM et al. Rhabdomyolysis in patients receiving lovastatin after cardiac transplantation. *N Engl J Med* 1988; 318: 47.

[118] Crane FL, Hatefi Y, Lester RL, Widmer G. Isolation of a quinone from beef heart mitochondria. *Biochem Biophys Acta* 1957; 25:220-221.

[119] Folkers K, Baker L, Richardson PC, Shizukuishi S, Takamura K, Drzewoski J, Lewandowski J, Ellis JM. New progress on the biomedical and clinical research in coenzyme Q,. In: Folkers K, Yamamura Y eds. *Biomedical and clinical aspects of coenzyme* Q, Vol. 3, Elsevier/North Holland Biomedical press, Amsterdam: Elsevier/North-Holland, 1981: 399-412.

[120] Folkers K, Littaru GP, Ho L, Runge TM, Havanonda S, Cooley D. Evidence for a deficiency of coenzyme Q10 in human heart disease. *Int J Vitamin Res* 1970; 40, 380-390.

[121] Littaru GP, Ho L, Folkers K. Deficiency of coenzyme Q10 in human heart disease Part 1. *Int J Vitamin Res* 1972 ; 42: 291-305.

[122] Littaru GP, Ho L, Folkers K. Deficiency of coenzyme Q10 in human heart disease Part 2. *Int J Vitamin Res* 1972 ; 42: 413-434.

[123] Mortensen SA. Perspectives on therapy of cardiovascular diseases with coenzyme Q10 (Ubiquinone). *Clin Investig* 1993; 71S: 116-123.

[124] Folkers K, Langsjoen P, Willis R et al. Lovastatin decreases coenzyme Q levels in humans. *Proc Natl Acad Sci* 1990; 87: 8931-4.

[125] Rundek T, Naini A, Sacco R, et al. Atorvastatin decreases the coenzyme Q10 levels in the blood of patients ar risk for cardiovascular disease and stroke. *Arch Neurol* 2004; 61(6): 889.

[126] Watts GF, Castellucio C, Rice-Evans C et al. Plasma coenzyme Q concentrations in patients treated with simvastatin. *J Clin Pathol* 1993; 46: 1005.

[127] Mortensen SA, Leth A, Agner E et al. Dose related decrease of serum coenzyme Q10 during treatment of HMG-CoA reductase inhibitors. *Mol Aspects Med* 1997; 18 suppl: s137.

[128] Philips PS, Haas RH, Bannykh S et al. Statin-associated myopathy with normal creatine kinase levels. *Ann Intern Med* 2002; 137: 581.

[129] Rosenfeld FL, Pepe S, Ou R et al. Coenzyme Q10 improves the tolerance of the senescent myocardium to aerobic and ischemic stress: studies in rats and in human atrial tissue. *Biofactors* 1999; 9: 291.

[130] Bhuiyan J, Seccombe DW. The effects of HMG-CoA reductase inhibition on tissue levels of carnitine and carnitine acyltransferase activity in the rabbit. *Lipids* 1996; 31: 867.

[131] Gvozdjakova A, Kucharska J, Mizera S et al. Coenzyme Q10 depletion and mitochondrial energy disturbances in rejection development in patients after heart transplantation. *Biofactors* 1999; 9(2-4): 301.

[132] Kucharska J, Gvozdjakova A, Mizera S et al. Participation of coenzyme Q10 in the rejection development of the transplanted heart: a clinical study. *Physiol Res* 1998; 47(6): 399.

[133] Berman M, Erman A, Ben-Gal T et al. Coenzyme Q10 in patients with end stage heart failure awaiting cardiac transplantation: a randomized, placebo-controlled study. *Clin Cardiol* 2004; 27: 295.

[134] Ballantyne CM, Ezetimibe: efficacy and safety in clinical trials. *Eur Heart J Suppl* 2002; 4 suppl J: 9.

[135] Gagne C, Gaudet D, Bruckert E et al. Efficacy and safety of ezetimibe coadministrated with atorvastatin or simvastatin in patients with homozygous familial hypercholesteremia. *Circulation* 2002; 105: 101.

[136] Stein E. Results of phase I/II clinical trials with ezetimibe, a novel selective cholesterol absorbtion inhibitor. *Eur Heart J* Suppl 2001; 3 suppl. E: E11.

[137] Keogh A, Day R, Critchley L et al. The effect of food and cholestyramine on the absorbtion od cyclosporine in cardiac transplant recipients. *Transplant Proc.* 1988; 20: 27.

[138] Jensen RA, Lal SM, Diaz-Arias A et al. Does cholestyramine interfere with cyclosporine absorption? A prospective study in renal transplant patients. *ASAIO J* 1995; 41: 704.

[139] Biossonnat P, Salen P, Guidollet J et al. The long-term effects of the lipid-lowering agent fenofibrate in hyperlipidemic heart transplant recipients. *Transplantation* 1994; 58: 245.

[140] Hidalgo L, Zambrana JL, Blanco-Molina A et al. Lovastatin versus bezafibrate for hyperlipideamia treatment after heart transplantation. *J Heart Lung Transplant* 1995; 14: 461.

[141] Sundararajan V, Cooper DKC, Muchmore J et al. Interaction of cyclosporine and probucol in heart transplant patients. *Transplant Proc* 1991; 23: 2028.

[142] von Schacky C. n-3 fatty acids and the prevention of coronary atherosclerosis. *Am J Clin Nutr* 2000; 71: s224.

[143] Mozzattarian D, Lemaitre RN, Kuller LH et al. Cardiac benefits of fish oil consumption may depend on the type on the type of fish meal consumed. *Circulation* 2003; 107: 1372.

[144] Grimminger F, Grimm H, Fuhrer D et al. Omega-3 lipid infusion in a heart allotransplant model: shift in fatty acid and lipid mediator profiles and prolongation of transplant survival. *Circulation* 1996; 93: 365.

[145] Thiery J, Meiser B, Wenke K et al. Heparin-induced extracorporeal low density lipoprotein plasmapheresis (H.E.L.P) and its use in heart transplant patients with severe hypercholesterolemia. *Transplant Proc* 1995; 27: 1950.

[146] Wenke K, Thiery J, Arndtz N et al. Optimized and safe treatment of hypercholesterolemia after heart transplantation by low dose simvastatin and HELP apheresis. *Thorac Cardiovasc Surg* 1992; 40: 124.

[147] Wenke K, Thiery J, Arndtz N et al. Treatment of hypercholesterolemia and prevention of coronary artery disease after heart transplantation by combination of low dose simvastatin and HELP-LDL-apheresis. *Transplant Proc* 1992; 24: 2674.

[148] Park JW, Vermeltfoort M, Braun P et al. Regression of transplant coronary artery disease during chronic HELP therapy: a case study. *Atherosclerosis* 1995; 115: 1.

[149] Park JW. Regression of transplant coronary artery disease during chronic HELP apheresis: a case report. In: Seidel D, editor. *HELP report* 1994 Germany: MMV Verlag Munchen 1994: 24.

[150] Jaeger BR, Meiser B, Nagel D et al. Aggressive lowering of fibrinogen and cholesterol in the prevention in the prevention of graft vessel disease after heart transplantation. *Circulation* 1997; 96 suppl II: II-154.

[151] Taylor PJ, Kubler PA, Lynch SV et al.Effect of Atorvastatin on cyclosporine pharmacokinetics in liver transplant recipients. *Ann Pharmacother* 2004; 38(2): 205.

In: Cholesterol in Atherosclerosis and Coronary Heart Disease ISBN 1-59454-302-X
Editor: Jean P. Kovala, pp.131-156 

*Chapter VII*

# Postprandial Lipemia and Atherosclerosis: Exercise and Omega 3 Fatty Acids: The Non Pharmaceutical Interventions

***John Q. Zhang****
Department of Health and Kinesiology, University of Texas at San Antonio;
***Bryan K. Smith***
Energy Balance Laboratory & The Center for Physical Activity & Weight Management, University of Kansas
***Tom R. Thomas***
Department of Nutritional Sciences, University of Missouri at Columbia

## Abstract

Prolonged postprandial lipemia (PPL) has been associated with changes in the lipoprotein profile and increased risk for atherosclerosis. Individuals with hypertriglyceridemia tend to have an exaggerated PPL. Evidence suggests that patients with PPL are more susceptible to cardiovascular disease. The syndrome of PPL in the presence of low concentration of high-density lipoprotein cholesterol (HDL-Chol) and high concentration of low-density lipoprotein (LDL)-Chol has been considered as a combined marker of cardiovascular disease. Dietary triglyceride (TG) is carried by chylomicrons and very low density lipoproteins (VLDL) in the blood stream. Lipoprotein lipase (LPL) cleaves the TG to fatty acid from these lipoproteins. There is growing evidence that physical exercise and omega-3 fatty acid (n-3FA) supplementation and are

* Address for correspondence: John Q. Zhang, Ph.D., Department of Health and Kinesiology, University of Texas-San Antonio, 6900 North Loop, 1604 West, San Antonio, TX 78249. Email: jzhang@utsa.edu; Phone: 210 458-7390; Fax: 210 458-5873.

excellent non-pharmaceutical remedies for the treatment of hypertriglyceridemia and PPL. However, the mechanism of how physical activity attenuates PPL still remains unclear. It has been proposed that exercise-induced attenuation of PPL is due to either the elevation of LPL activity or the reduction of VLDL-TG synthesis. The attenuation of PPL by n-3FA supplementation appears to be due to a decrease in chylomicron and VLDL-TG secretion and possibly an increase in fasting LPL activity. This review summarizes the effect of exercise and n-3FA supplementation on plasma lipid metabolism and PPL.

## Introduction

Prolonged or exaggerated postprandial lipemia (PPL) has been associated with changes in the lipoprotein profile and increase risk for atherosclerosis. Exercise has a significant plasma triglyceride (TG) lowering effect, and results in the elevation of high-density lipoprotein (HDL). The mechanism of effects of exercise on PPL still remains elucidated but could relate to the exercise-induced enzymatic changes (Figure 1) such as lipoprotein lipase (LPL), hepatic lipase (HL), lecithin-cholesterol acyltransferase (LCAT), and cholesteryl ester transfer protein (CETP). Supplementation with omega-3 fatty acid (n-3FA), ingested in the form of fish oil, can also independently lower plasma concentrations of chylomicron-TG and very low density (VLDL)-TG. The mechanism for this TG-lowering effect of n-3FA appears to be the inhibition of TG synthesis and/or secretion in the liver but may also due to the increased LPL activity (LPLa) following n-3FA supplementation. The goal of this review is to summarize recent studies that provide evidence in support of the role of exercise and n-3FA on PPL.

## Mechanism of Triglyceride Metabolism

TG is an ester of glycerol with three molecules of fatty acid and also called neutral fat [56]. TG provide more than half the energy requirements of some organs, particularly the liver, heart, and resting skeletal muscles. More than 95% of the TG in plasma is associated with chylomicrons produced in the intestine and VLDL particles secreted by the liver [84]. These particles are buoyant because of the high TG content, which makes up approximately 90% by weight of the chylomicron and 70% by weight of the VLDL [35]. The fatty acid composition of TG in plasma and adipose tissue is determined in large part by the composition of dietary fats. The major fatty acids in plasma are linoleic acid (18:2ω6, 30%), oleic acid (18:1ω9, 20%), palmitic acid (16:0, 20%), and stearic acid (16:0, 7%) [85]. In the digestion system, the dietary fat is first converted from insoluble macroscopic fat particles into finely dispersed microscopic micelles by bile salt. The micelle formation enormously increases the fraction of lipid molecules accessible to the action of water-soluble lipases in the intestine, and the lipases converts TG into monoglycerides, diglycerides, free fatty acids (FFAs) and glycerol [56].

These products of lipase action diffuse into the epithelial cells lining the intestinal surface, where they are reconverted to TG and packaged with dietary cholesterol and incorporate cholesteryl esters, phospholipids, apolipoprotein (apo) A, and apoB48 [14, 35]. ApoC-II and apoE are also incorporated onto the surface of the chylomicron following an interaction with HDL [14, 60]. Chylomicrons move from the intestinal mucosa into the lymphatic system, from which they enter the blood and are carried to muscle and adipose tissue. In the capillaries of these tissues, LPL, the extracellular enzyme, is activated by apo C-II. This enzyme hydrolyzes TG into fatty acids and glycerol which are taken up by cells in the target tissues. In muscle, the fatty acids are oxidized for energy; in adipose tissues, they are reesterified for storage as TG. The remnants of chylomicrons, depleted of most of their TG but still containing cholesterol and apoproteins apo E and apo B-48, travel in the blood to the liver [56].

When the diet contains more fatty acids than are needed immediately for fuel or as precursors, they are converted into TG in the liver, and TG are packaged with specific apolipoproteins into VLDL [56]. Then, the VLDL's are transported out of the liver into the blood stream. As VLDL passes into the peripheral circulation, it comes into contact with LPL, which is located on the surface of capillary endothelial cells [39]. There, TGs are partially removed by lipolysis. After most of the TG has been hydrolyzed, a residual lipoprotein, called a VLDL remnant, is released into the circulation. VLDL remnants can have two fates: they can either be taken up directly by the liver or they can be degraded further to low-density lipoprotein (LDL) [38]. The LDL is the major cholesterol-carrying lipoprotein in plasma. They are rich in cholesterol esters and contain very little TG. They filter readily into the arterial wall and thereby can promote the development of atherosclerosis [39].

## Hypertriglyceridemia and Cardiovascular Disease

Hypertriglyceridemia (HTG, fasting plasma TG > 200 mg/dl) has been proposed as a potential risk factor for CVD [28] because of its effect on lipoprotein metabolism. After dietary intake, the lipids in the diet are absorbed through the digestive system. The function of lipid transport is to facilitate the transfer of exogenous and endogenous TG and cholesterol from their sites of absorption or formation to their sites of storage and utilization. This function is carried out by TG-rich lipoproteins of intestinal and hepatic origin through a series of enzymatic conversion reactions resulting in release of TG fatty acids and generation of cholesterol-rich remnant lipoproteins. Under normal, steady-state conditions, the input and output of TG-rich lipoproteins are balanced with little or no change in their plasma levels. However, an increased influx and /or a decreased efflux of TG-rich lipoproteins from the plasma compartment have been identified as main pathophysiologic mechanism leading to HTG [2, 37].

The catabolism of these TG-rich lipoproteins occurs at the surface of the endothelium by the action of LPL [78]. During the lipolytic process, the TG-rich lipoproteins loose their TG and become remnant particles which are poor in TG and rich in cholesterol. It has been suggested that lipolytic remnants of TG-rich lipoprotein in animals on an atherogenic diet are responsible for the development of atherosclerosis in these animals [4]. Studies on the interaction of VLDL with cultured endothelial cells have indicated that plasma VLDL in certain pathological or physiological states was cytotoxic to the endothelial cells [1] and smooth muscle cells [66]. The hypertriglyceridemic state may influence the metabolism and the composition of intermediate-density lipoprotein (IDL), LDL, and HDL leading to atherosclerosis. Researchers have shown that VLDL in hypertriglyceridemic subjects is modified. Modified VLDL has high affinity for LDL receptors [29]. The apoB contained in VLDL particles may become partially degraded as VLDLs are circulated in plasma, which could enhance their uptake by arterial wall macrophages promoting the development of foam cells [38].

Whether VLDL's are atherogenic may depend in part on their ability to penetrate into the subintimal layers of the arterial wall. Normally, the larger VLDL particles do not pass the endothelial barrier. However, the presence of endothelial injury may facilitate the passage of even the large VLDL species. Furthermore, most of the circulating VLDL's are partially catabolized into VLDL remnants [38]. The VLDL particles present in HTG are probably more atherogenic than normolipemic VLDL, as they have increased affinity to apoB and apoE receptors [10]. The apoB molecules contained in TG rich lipoprotein of certain hypertriglyceridemic subjects may also become partially degraded. This alteration could promote binding to an unregulated macrophage receptor, which is distinct from the B and E receptors [30].

Plasma VLDL is the precursor of plasma LDL [86]. Circumstances associated with the formation of dense LDL, such as over production of VLDL apoB and slow LDL catabolism, may represent the direct atherogenic mechanism. Hypertriglyceridemic LDL has been shown to exhibit lower affinity toward the B, E receptor in cultured human fibroblasts and to be a less efficient regulator of cellular sterol synthesis and receptor activity [74]. LDL cholesteryl ester may also be exchanged for chylomicron and VLDL TG in a reaction mediated by CETP [23]. As a result of this exchange, LDL-TG is hydrolyzed by LPL, resulting in the formation of small, dense LDL particles [23, 74]. These particles appear to be more atherogenic and less likely to bind to LDL receptors than the larger LDL species [28].

Apoproteins characteristics of VLDL and chylomicrons (apoB and apoC) have been identified in lesions of human arteries [49]. Chylomicrons can be taken up by vascular endothelium, followed by degradation of most of their TG [78]. This process appears to take place in most capillary beds and could take place in arterial endothelium or smooth muscle cells if these cells contained LPL. The uptake of chylomicron remnants by the arterial wall also could take place by adsorption of circulating remnants to the arterial surface followed by endocytosis [103]. Arterial smooth muscle cells of the rat take up VLDL remnants rapidly and degrade them relatively poorly [8]. An animal study has shown that the chylomicron remnants are as atherogenic as LDL [73]. Zilversmit [103] suggested that the chylomicron or VLDL remnants could provide the building blocks for arterial lesions due to: 1) Circulating chylomicron or VLDL remnants may bind and penetrate the arterial surface just like plasma LDL's; and 2) chylomicron or VLDL may be adsorbed and then degraded to remnants at the arterial surface. It is possible that the liberation of fatty acid anions during the hydrolysis of chylomicrons on the arterial surface may cause injury.

Studies have shown that lipolytic remnants of TG-rich lipoproteins produced in vitro may induce foam cell formation in macrophages and the cell death in cultured macrophages and endothelial cells. This cell death can be inhibited by HDL. Chung and Segrest [16] reported that *in vitro* the HTG serum lipolyzed by LPL was highly cytotoxic to the cultured macrophages and endothelial cells killing more than 90% of the cells. They also found that the normolipidemic serum, obtained from a fasting subject and lipolyzed under identical conditions as HTG serum, was not cytotoxic to cultured macrophages. However, when this serum was supplemented with preisolated VLDL to a level similar to that of HTG serum, the resultant product was cytotoxic to macrophages. By addition of HDL into the culture dishes the cytotoxicity of the lipolyzed VLDL was inhibited. Based on their findings, the authors hypothesized that: a) lipolytic surface remnants of TG-rich lipoproteins may represent a major class of atherogenic lipoproteins which are exacerbated during postprandial HTG; b) clearance of these surface remnants by HDL *in vivo* may be one important way that HDL prevents atherosclerosis; c) excess surface remnants may be linked to delayed clearance of potentially atherogenic core remnants, directly linked to atherogenicity via surface remnant-mediated cytotoxicity to cells of the artery wall and/or linked to the deposit of unesterified cholesterol-rich vesicles in early atherosclerosis. Gianturco et al. [29] also found that hypertriglyceridemic VLDL was cytotoxic to cultured bovine aortic endothelial cells. Since endothelial cell injury is considered to be an early event in atherosclerosis, the cytotoxic remnants of TG-rich lipoprotein may play an important role in this early process of atherogenesis [90].

## Hypertriglyceridemia and HDL

HDL is synthesized in the liver, the intestine, and also originates from the surface of chylomicrons and VLDL during lipolysis. Nascent HDL particles can take up cholesterol from the peripheral tissues. Once within the HDL particle the cholesterol is esterified into cholesteryl ester by the action of LCAT [35]. The nascent, discoid HDL particles mature into spherical HDL as they add surface components from the TG-rich lipoprotein (chylomicron and VLDL) during the hydrolysis of the latter. The surface components - apolipoproteins, phospholipids, and unesterified cholesterol from the TG-rich lipoproteins - are added to the small $HDL_3$ particles. Generation of cholesteryl esters by LCAT reaction leads to enlargement of the small $HDL_3$ particles, so that they are converted into the larger $HDL_2$ particles (Figure 1) The $HDL_2$ particles are larger in size and contain more lipids than $HDL_3$. Formation of $HDL_2$ increases the cholesterol-carrying capacity of HDL. They can carry about twice as many cholesterol molecules per unit apoprotein compared to $HDL_3$, and are considered as a doubly efficient vehicle for cholesterol transport [68]. This process promotes the so called reverse cholesterol transport in which $HDL_2$ carries cholesterol from peripheral tissue to the liver for excretion [91].

$HDL_2$ is prone to exchange its cholesterol ester for TG with the TG-rich remnants in the condition of sustained HTG [34]. This exchange of insoluble cholesterol ester and TG between HDL and the TG-rich lipoprotein is mediated by the action of CETP [62, 92]. So, $HDL_2$ is converted back into the small $HDL_3$ [69]. When the rate of clearance of TG-enriched remnants is decreased, exchange of cholesterol ester from HDL into the remnants increases. It is well established clinically that patients with permanent or temporary HTG (due to increased levels of VLDL or accumulation of chylomicrons in the course of PPL) tend to have low $HDL_2$-C level. Since the transferred cholesterol esters remain with the TG-rich lipoproteins along their lipolytic cascade and the endocytotic pathways of their remnants (e.g. the LDL-receptor and the scavenger pathways), the heteroexchange may contribute to the atherogenic potential of chylomicron and VLDL [59].

Investigators have shown a strong inverse relationship exists between TG and HDL level [5, 35]. The HDL concentration increases when the concentration of TG decreases due to the uptake of remnant surface particles of chylomicron and VLDL [17]. Overloading chylomicrons and VLDL with TG as a result of HTG may dramatically alter the exchange process between HDL and TG, resulting in TG-rich HDL [88]. TG-rich HDL is converted by HL to smaller, denser HDL, which is more rapidly cleared from the blood stream, resulting in reduced HDL concentration [83]. Researchers have shown that patients with HTG have low concentration of total HDL and $HDL_2$ due to the consequence of exchange of TG for cholesterol esters and reduced concentration of apoA-I and apoA-II [38].

In certain conditions, the cholesteryl ester may be transferred from HDL to LDL, IDL, or VLDL by CETP [35]. In addition, when PPL occurs, or when there is a prolonged elevation of TG-rich lipoprotein, the transfer of TG from TG-rich lipoprotein particles into LDL may also occur in exchange for cholesterol ester. Thus, the metabolic changes associated with HTG may decrease the concentration of HDL and result in small, dense particles of LDL and $HDL_3$, and there will be less $HDL_2$ in the blood stream.

## Postprandial Lipemia

Although fasting HTG condition is associated with the risk of CVD [11], in multivariate analysis adjusted for HDL cholesterol, this association is weakened [13, 100]. The fasting TG level has not yet been defined as an independent factor of CVD. In 1979, Zilversmit [103] postulated a hypothesis that postprandial lipoprotein metabolism might play an essential role in CVD. Humans spend a great deal of time in the postprandial HTG state, and the clearance of these postprandial lipoproteins causes a periodic elevation of lipolytic remnant products, including FFAs in the circulating blood. In people on high-fat, high-cholesterol diets, the arterial wall may be exposed to postprandial lipoproteins for a much longer time than to the postabsorptive lipoprotein pattern [103].

Elevated PPL has been shown to be a characteristic of individuals that have been diagnosed with CVD [54, 67]. Some studies have shown that PPL might be a predictor of future development of CVD [32, 98]. PPL also has been shown to be associated with the intima-media thickness of the carotid artery, an early sign of CVD [9, 18, 53, 75, 82]. The measurement of PPL may have some clinical applications, since it commonly found in CVD patients, it is associated with the progression of CVD, and it might predict future CVD.

In 1992, Patsch et al. [67] compared the PPL response of a group of 61 subjects who had severe CVD and a group of 40 control subjects who were CVD free. Coronary angiography was used to make the diagnosis of CVD. When compared to the control group, the group with severe CVD had significantly higher TG-AUC score (the area under the TG concentration and time curve; high score indicating high TG response) and maximal TG increase. The CVD group also had higher TG values at 6 and 8 h after the meal. Logistic-regression analysis showed that the 6 and 8 h postprandial TG scores were 68% accurate in predicting the presence or absence of CVD. The TG-AUC scores were 75% accurate in predicting the presence or absence of CVD. The addition of HDL-Chol improved the accuracy of the prediction.

Karpe et al. [54] further examined PPL responses in normo- and hypertriglyceridemic post-infarct males to lipid matched healthy males. It was noted that in both groups, the later postprandial plasma TG values (7-9 h) were significantly elevated in the CVD subjects when compared to the controls. Kinetic studies showed that the post-infarct males also had a 27% slower clearance rate than the control subjects.

Both of these reports show that the magnitude of postprandial TG is related to CVD. More importantly, both studies show that the biggest differences in postprandial TG are occurring later during the postprandial period. This would indicate that in individuals that have CVD, the ability to remove the TGs in a timely and efficient manner is altered.

Several groups have reported the relationship between PPL and the intima-media thickness of the carotid artery, a sign of early development of atherosclerosis [18]. Ryu et al. [75] reported that PPL was positively correlated to carotid artery wall thickness in 47 middle aged, moderately hypercholesterolemic individuals. Both the TG-AUC score and the TG peak response were highly correlated to the carotid artery wall thickness. When attempting to predict intima-media thickness with TG peak response and other common risk factors (smoking, age, sex, HDL-Chol, total cholesterol, and waist to hip ratio), the two best predictors were TG peak response followed by smoking.

In 1995, Sharrett et al. [82] compared the PPL response to carotid intima-media thickness in a case-control study. They compared 229 asymptomatic atherosclerosis cases with 373 control subjects who were free of atherosclerosis. Asymptomatic atherosclerosis was defined as having maximum carotid artery thickness greater than 2.5 mm. In this population, the PPL response was associated with case status in white but not black men and women, and only in non-obese individuals (BMI<30 kg/m$^2$). Elevated postprandial TG was associated with the individuals with the greater carotid intima-media thickness. This association was still present even after corrections had been made for coronary risk factors and fasting TGs.

Karpe et al. [53] compared PPL to common carotid artery thickness in 30 healthy normo and hypertriglyceridemic males (fasting TG>265 mg/dl). In the hypertriglyceridemic group the 6 and 7 h postprandial TG values were positively associated with carotid intima-media thickness, even more so than fasting TG values. These correlations were independent of both LDL-Chol and fasting TG concentrations. Only TG-AUC score was positively correlated to carotid intima-media thickness only when the two groups were combined.

Boquist et al. [9] reported that several variables related to PPL were associated with common carotid intima-media thickness in 96 healthy middle-aged men. The plasma TG at 1 to 4 h and TG-AUC values were all significantly related to common carotid intima-media thickness. This is in contrast to Karpe et al. [53] who reported that only TG-AUC score was correlated to intima-media thickness. As with the other studies, these associations were independent of LDL-Chol and the usual CVD risk factors.

The main conclusion of these studies is that PPL is a risk factor for early atherosclerosis, as defined as thickening of the common carotid artery, in addition to being associated with the presence of CVD. These studies also showed that the association of PPL to early atherosclerosis was an independent risk factor, and in some cases, it was a better predictor than some of the common predictors, such as elevated LDL-Chol, fasting TG, obesity, BMI, and smoking.

There also is evidence in the literature that PPL might be associated with a future development of CVD. This has been shown in children of individuals that had been diagnosed with CVD. Some evidence indicates that PPL also may be correlated to the very early stages of CVD.

Uiterwaal et al. in 1994 [98] examined the familial risk of CVD and related it to PPL. They recruited 80 sons of men with severe CVD and compared them to 55 sons of men who were free of CVD. The sons of the men with CVD had prolonged PPL, which was shown by the significantly elevated plasma TG values at 8, 10, and 12 h. The sons of men with CVD also had significantly higher TG-AUC scores.

Ginsberg et al. [32] reported that PPL could be associated with exercise induced myocardial ischemia (EIMI) in individuals without any prior CVD. A total of 50 subjects who had tested positive for EIMI were compared to 95 control subjects. The PPL response for the male case subjects was significantly higher when compared to the control subjects. There was no significant difference in the PPL between the two groups of women subjects. This association between PPL and EIMI was independent of age, race, and smoking status. These results indicate that at least in men, the presence of PPL might be an indicator of the early development of CVD.

There is evidence in the literature that PPL is associated with not only the presence of CVD, but also the progression of CVD, and possibly future development of CVD. In most cases, these relationships are present even when they have been corrected for the major CVD risk factors. Because of this, it has been suggested that PPL is a strong and independent risk factor for CVD.

## Lipoprotein Lipase

LPL is an enzyme responsible for the removal of TG located in chylomicrons and VLDL. LPL is attached to the endothelial layer of the vascular walls of the capillary beds within skeletal muscle and adipose tissue. LPL hydrolyzes the TG contained in chylomicrons and VLDL into FFAs and monoglycerides. These FFAs are then taken up by muscle and adipose tissue [33]. The end result of this process is the reduction of plasma TG concentrations.

The regulation of LPL is complex and can occur at multiple steps in the synthetic pathway. Regardless of where in the synthetic pathway the regulation takes place, the end result will be a change in LPL. To complicate matters, adipose tissue LPL (AT LPL) is regulated differently than skeletal muscle LPL (SM LPL), but in general, they are reciprocally regulated. At this time, the regulation of LPL in adipose tissue is better defined than in skeletal muscle.

Normal eating has been shown to result in a 46% increase in AT LPL and a 32% decrease in SM LPL [57]. It appears that insulin may be responsible for these changes following a meal. Several studies [7, 24, 55, 76, 93] have shown an association between elevated insulin levels and increases in AT LPL. Cell culture studies also have shown that insulin levels were positively correlated to AT LPL [3, 15, 21, 27, 81].

It appears that SM LPL is down regulated by insulin, but the relationship between the two is not as clear as the relationship between AT LPL and insulin. It has been reported that in normal subjects, under euglycemic clamp conditions, increased insulin levels will result in a 14 to 33% decrease in SM LPL [22, 24, 55, 58]. When looking at specific populations, the relationship between insulin and SM LPL is not as clear. Under euglycemic clamp conditions, increased insulin levels resulted in a 41% increase in SM LPL in obese women [22] and a 7% increase insulin resistant subjects [26].

Catecholamines also may be potent regulators of LPL [19, 20, 61, 65, 70]. In rats, perfusions of skeletal muscle with epinephrine will increase SM LPL from 75 to 102%, depending upon the fiber type [61]. Infusion of isoproterenol into rats resulted in a four fold increase in SM LPL and a 50% decrease in AT LPL [19]. The presence of epinephrine in rat adipocytes resulted in 66% decrease of AT LPL [65]. In humans, SM LPL increased 46% following the infusion of isoproterenol [20] and 17% following the infusion of epinephrine [70]. However, the infusion of isoproterenol did not change AT LPL in humans [20]. In humans, catecholamines maybe more important in the regulation of SM LPL than in AT LPL.

A recent article by Greiwe et al. [36] questioned the importance of catecholamines in the expression of SM LPL. Changes in SM LPL protein mass were measured in humans following two bouts of cycling. During one of these cycling bouts, adrenergic receptors were blocked with non-selective adrenergic blockers. This blockade did not prevent the exercise induced increase in SM LPL protein mass. The increase in SM LPL protein mass during the blockade trial was similar to the non-blockade trial. A decrease in SM LPL protein mass would result in a decrease in SM LPL. The authors concluded that the increase in SM LPL protein mass may not be due to increased catecholamines but may be due to alterations in cellular homeostasis that result from the exercise bout. It is speculated that the exercise-induced elevation of LPL might be due to muscle contraction itself rather than EPI stimulation [49]. However, the signaling pathway of muscular contraction induced elevation of LPL remains unknown.

Early studies that compared LPL between trained and untrained subjects showed that both SM LPL and AT LPL were elevated in trained subjects [63, 71, 87]. Nikkila et al. [63] compared SM LPL and AT LPL in sprinters, long distance runners, and sedentary individuals. When compared to the controls, long distance runners exhibited a 2.7 fold increase in SM LPL and a 1.7 fold increase AT LPL. Peltonen et al. [71] compared males that were undergoing a 15 wk training program to sedentary males. After the training program, postheparin LPL was elevated 33% and AT LPL was elevated 56% in the trained subjects. Although postheparin LPL is not a direct measurement of SM LPL, it does contain SM LPL. Postheparin LPL is a measurement of total LPL, which would include AT LPL and SM LPL. In that study, AT LPL accounted for only 2% of the postheparin LPL, therefore, one could conclude that since postheparin LPL increased and AT LPL can only account for 2% of this activity, there must have been an increase in SM LPL. Simsolo et al. [87] reported that following 2 wks of detraining resulted in a 45% decrease in SM LPL. This would indicate that training had significantly elevated SM LPL. In that study, they did report that there was a

90% increase in AT LPL. Thus, it is possible that detraining does not influence AT LPL in the same way that it influences SM LPL.

Recent studies comparing trained and untrained subjects provide conflicting evidence. Thomas et al. [95] have shown that there are no differences in postheparin LPL between trained and untrained subjects when measured 48 h after the last exercise session. Herd et al. [46] reported no differences in postheparin LPL between groups when it was measured 60 h after the last exercise session.

The timing of the last exercise session and the measurement of LPL is a very important point to consider when interpreting the results of these studies. The early studies that compared trained and untrained subjects measured LPL within 24 h of the last exercise session. Based upon the study by Herd et al. [46] it appeared that acute influence of exercise is transient and does not last more than 60 h. The data by Thomas et al. [95] indicated that the acute effect of exercise on LPL may not last more than 48 h.

Based upon the literature, it is difficult to tell what effect training has on SM LPL and AT LPL. Although the early studies clearly show that training increases SM LPL and AT LPL, is the change that was being reported due to the acute effect of the last exercise bout or due to the training? This area of research deserves further investigation. There are numerous unanswered questions about the regulation and expression of LPL and this area of research deserves further investigation. For example, what is the cellular signaling pathway leading to LPL gene expression and what regulates the factors involved in cellular signaling pathway?

## Exercise and PPL

Although PPL is associated with the presence and progression of CVD, it is a condition that can be easily modified. An acute bout of aerobic exercise has been shown to significantly decrease the PPL response [40, 46, 47, 96, 97, 102]. A summary of these studies can be found in Table 1. The magnitude of these reductions appears to be dependent upon the type of exercise, the length of the exercise, the intensity of the exercise, energy expenditure, and the timing of the exercise sessions in relation to a high fat meal (HFM). The association between the exercise and the PPL response may be due to the relationship between exercise and LPL. Exercise has been shown to cause an increase in LPLa [25, 46, 51, 52, 77-80, 101], and it is has been hypothesized that this increase in LPL is primarily responsible for the reductions in PPL when a HFM is preceded by an exercise session. Figure 1 illustrates the adverse effect of PPL and how an acute exercise attenuates this effect.

Kantor et al. [51] has shown that prolonged exercise can increase LPL. They measured LPL in trained men, before and after running a marathon. Following the marathon, LPL was increased 73%. In a later study, Kantor et al. reported that LPL could be modestly increased in both trained and untrained individuals by 10% following a 1-2 h of riding a bicycle ergometer at 80% of maximal heart rate ($HR_{max}$). This increase was just a transient increase. When LPL was determined 48 h after the exercise session it was back to pre-exercise levels. The results of these two studies show that an acute bout of exercise can cause similar increases in both trained and untrained individuals. It also shows that this increase in LPL is only temporary.

**Table 1. Selected Studies on the Effect of Exercise on PPL**

| Authors | Study Design/Purpose | Exercise duration, groups, and time before HFM | Variables Measured | Measurement Time | Changes |
|---|---|---|---|---|---|
| Tsetsonis and Hardman [60] | 6M, 6F. Comparison between different EX intensities, walking at 30 or 60% $VO_{2max}$. | 90 min for both intensities. 1h before HFM | TG-AUC, and max TG increase | Prior to HFM, hourly afterwards for 6h. | 60% trial:TG-AUC ↓, max TG increase, ↓ 30% trial TG-AUC, max TG increase ↔ |
| Tsetsonis and Hardman [61] | 5M, 4F. Comparison between different EX intensities, walking at 30 or 60% $VO_{2max}$. | 30% $VO_{2max}$ trial, 3h. 60% $VO_{2max}$ trial, 1.5h. Similar energy expenditure. 15h before HFM | TG-AUC | Prior to HFM, hourly afterwards for 6h. | 60% trial: TG-AUC ↓. 30% trial: TG-AUC ↓. |
| Herd et al. [27] | 8M. Examine effect of moderate exercise on PPL and LPLa | 90 min cycling. 16h before HFM | TG-AUC, and LPLa | Prior to HFM, 30 min after, then hourly for 6h. | TG-AUC and TG-AUC ↓. LPLa ↔ |
| Zhang et al. [65] | 2M. Examine timing of HFM and EX | 60min running at 60% $VO_{2max}$. 1h post, 1h pre, and 12h pre | TG-AUC, | Prior to HFM, then hourly for 8h, and 24h after. | 1h post: ↔<br>1h pre: ↓<br>12h pre: ↓ |
| Ziogas et al. [66] | 30M, 24F. Examine influence of chronic EX. | No EX. 3 groups: Sedentary, active, and trained | TG-AUC | Prior to HFM then hourly for 8h. | Sedentary: ↔<br>Active: ↓<br>Trained: ↓ |
| Herd et al. [28] | 32M, 20F. Examine influence of chronic EX. | 60min. 3 groups, endurance trained, sprint trained, sedentary. 60h before HFM. | TG-AUC | Prior to HFM, 30 min after, then hourly for 6h. | No difference among groups |
| Herd et al. [26] | 6M, 8F. Examine influence of detraining | 40 min. 2 groups, runners and controls. 15 h, 60 h, and 9 days. | TG-AUC, LPLa | Prior to HFM, hourly afterwards for 6h. | No changes in control group. Runners, 15h ↓, 60h and 9 days ↔. LPLa inversely correlated with PPL |
| Hardman et al. [20] | 9M, 1F. Examine influence of detraining in endurance trained subjects | 30 min. 2 groups, runners and controls. 15 h, 60 h, and 6.5 days. | TG-AUC | Prior to HFM, 30 min after, then hourly for 6h. | 60h and 6.5 days ↑ when compared to 15 h. |

**Note:** ↑ or ↓ = significant increase or decrease, ↔ = no change compared to control. PPL, postprandial lipemia. M, males. F, females. EX, exercise. HFM, high fat meal. TG-AUC, total area under the triglyceride curve. TG-AUC, incremental area under the triglyceride curve. LPLa, lipoprotein lipase.

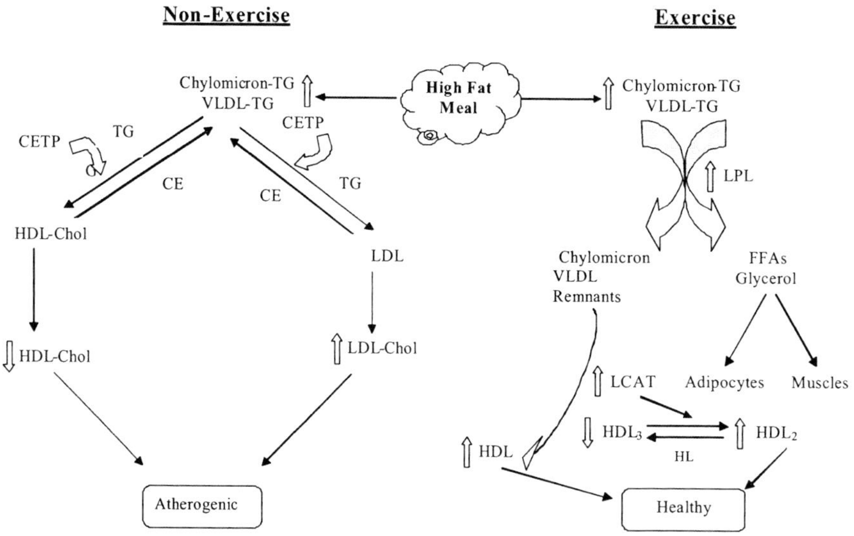


Figure 1. The effect of acute exercise on PHTG response and HDL metabolism.
CE=cholosterylester, CETP=cholesteryl ester transfer protein FFAc=free fatty acids, HDL-Chol=high density lipoprotein cholesterol, HL=hepatic lipase, LCAT=ecithin-cholesterol acyltransferase, LDL-low density lipoprotein, TG=triglyceride, VLDL=very low density lipoprotein.

In 1986, Sady et al. [77] reported that after running a marathon, subjects were able to clear TG at a faster rate when compared to rates obtained before running the marathon. Subjects ingested a 10% solution of soybean oil and the rate of clearance was determined by measuring plasma TG concentrations every 5 min for the 40 min immediately following the meal. This was done 24 h prior to the race and 18 h after the race. The changes in plasma TG concentrations over this time period were used to determine a rate of clearance. Following the marathon, the clearance rate was 76% greater when compared to rates obtained 24 h prior to the race. The increase in clearance rate was associated with a 46% increase in postheparin LPL. These results show that there is an association between TG clearance and LPL.

The PPL response to a bout of running, walking, and cycling has been reported. These studies suggest that the magnitude of the PPL response is dependent upon the intensity and the number of kcal expended during the exercise session.

Tsetsonis and Hardman [96] examined how PPL was influenced by an acute bout of walking at two different exercise intensities. Subjects completed three trials, a control trial (no exercise), and two 90 min bouts of treadmill walking. During these sessions, subjects walked at either 30 or 60% of their VO2max. The PPL response was significantly lower during the 60% exercise session, but was not significantly different from the 30% exercise session. The TG-AUC score and the maximal TG increase during the 30% trial were not significantly different from the control trial. Since the energy expenditure was less during the 30% trial, it was speculated that the differences in energy expenditure during the exercise sessions might explain why there were no differences between the 30% trial and the control trial. The authors concluded that the magnitude of the PPL response might be due to the intensity and/or the energy expenditure due to the acute exercise bout.

In order to determine if the PPL response was more dependent upon the intensity or the energy expenditure of the exercise session, Tsetsonis and Hardman completed a second study, which was similar to the previous study. In this study, the length of time the subjects spent walking was increased so that the energy expenditure was identical between the two exercise sessions [97]. Subjects walked for 3 h during the 30% exercise session and 1.5 h during the 60% exercise session and expended approximately 1000 kcal of energy during both sessions. The TG-AUC score for both exercise sessions was significantly lower than the control trial. There were no significant differences between the two exercise sessions. The authors concluded that during exercise bouts of equal energy expenditure, the exercise intensity does not influence PPL. This would also indicate that energy expenditure might have a significant influence on the PPL response. One could also speculate that these changes in energy expenditure might be associated with change in LPL. These changes in LPL would provide a simple explanation for the differences in PPL that are associated with differences in energy expenditure.

The influence of energy expenditure and LPL was investigated by Ferguson et al. [25]. They measured changes in LPL following exercise bouts that resulted in energy expenditures of 800, 1,100, 1,300, and 1,500 kcal. The exercise sessions were treadmill runs that were completed at 70% of $VO_{2max}$. Subjects were 11 trained males. They reported that LPL was significantly elevated following the 1,100, 1,300, and 1,000 kcal runs. The 1,100 and 1,300 kcal run resulted in a 31% increase in LPL when measured 24 h after the exercise session. At 48 h, LPL was no longer significantly elevated but it had not returned to baseline. LPL was increased 49% following the 1,500 kcal run and it was still increased 47% above baseline when measured 48 h after the exercise session. Although PPL was not determined in this study, one could speculate that there might have been significant differences in PPL between the four trials based upon the results of Tsetsonis and Hardman [96].

Recently Petitt et al. [72] compared the PPL responses following separate bouts of resistance training and aerobic exercise completed 16 h prior to the ingestion of a HFM. Energy expenditure was similar between the two bouts of exercise. The PPL response to the aerobic exercise session was not significantly different from the control trial. The PPL response to the resistance training was significantly lower from both the control trial (14%) and the aerobic exercise trial (18%). The authors concluded that the PPL response to resistance training may not be dependent to the energy expenditure of the exercise session. It was speculated that the higher intensity of the muscular contractions during the resistance training may have stimulated a greater expression of LPL when compared to the lower intensity associated with the aerobic exercise.

Herd et al. [47] examined the effect of an acute bout of exercise on the PPL response in physically active normolipidemic males. An acute exercise bout was completed 15 h prior to the ingestion of a HFM. The exercise bout consisted of a 90 min session of cycling at 62.3% of their $VO_{2max}$. During this exercise session, the subjects expended, on average, 1070 kcal of energy. LPL was determined 16 h after the exercise session. Following the exercise session, the TG-AUC was 28% lower when compared to the PPL response of the control trial (no exercise). There were no significant differences in LPL, but the authors did note that four of the subjects that did have an obvious increase in LPL also had the largest decreases in TG-AUC scores. It was concluded that moderate exercise does reduce PPL and the authors speculated that it might be due to LPL. Although the findings of this study were not significant, it does show that there might be a relationship between increased LPL and reductions in PPL.

The influence of an exercise session on PPL is very dependent upon the length of time between the exercise session and the PPL measurements. This dependence is due to sequence of events that are involved with the production of LPL. The synthesis of LPL is a multiple step process that begins with an increase in LPL gene expression, which increases the amount of LPL mRNA. This is followed by an increase in LPL protein mass. The LPL protein must then undergo post-translational modification before it can be transported to the luminal surface of the vascular endothelium [6]. Due to this multiple step process, there is delay in the increase in post-heparin LPL following an aerobic exercise session.

Evidence for this delay has been reported. LPL mRNA values have been reported to peak 4 h post-exercise, with LPL protein mass peaking 8 h post-exercise [80], and skeletal muscle LPL peaking 14-18 h post-exercise [79]. When these findings are combined with the current data, it can be seen that LPL mRNA, LPL protein mass, skeletal muscle LPL, and post-heparin LPL all have different time courses. Their peaks coincide with their order of appearance in the synthetic pathway of LPL.

Recently Zhang et al. [101] determined the 24 h time course of LPL in humans following an exercise session. Using 12 sedentary male subjects, LPL was determined immediately prior to, and at 4, 8, 12, and 24 h after a 60 min treadmill run at 60% of $VO_{2max}$. They reported significant elevations in LPL only at 24 h following the exercise session. This increase in LPL is in contrast to previous reports. This increase at 24 h was achieved following an exercise session that resulted in an energy expenditure of only 500 kcal. This was less than half of the 1,100 kcal that was required to increase LPL in trained males [25]. This raises the question, is the stimulus for LPL less in sedentary individuals than in trained individuals.

There is a large pool of literature that examines the timing of the last exercise session and the influence that it has on the PPL response. The goals of most of these studies were to show the effects of chronic exercise on PPL, but they also show the importance of the timing of the last exercise session and the PPL response.

Zhang et al. [102] looked at the PPL response to a single 60 min bout of treadmill running at 60% $VO_{2max}$ in recreationally trained males. A HFM was ingested either one hour before, one hour after, or 12 h after the exercise session. Only a non-significant 5% reduction in PPL was seen when the HFM was ingested one hour before the exercise session. A significant 38% reduction in PPL was seen when the HFM was ingested one hour after the exercise session. When the exercise session preceded the HFM by 12 h, the PPL a significant 51% reduction in PPL was reported. There were no significant differences in PPL when the exercise preceded the HFM by one hour or 12 h. In a similar study, Zhang et al. (2004] also found that exercising 12 h prior to a fat-meal significantly reduced PPL response whereas exercising 24 h prior to the meal did not attenuate PPL response in hypertriglyceridemic men. The TG-AUC score in 12 h pre meal exercise trial was 37% than the 24 h pre meal exercise trial and 33% lower than the control trial (meal only). The attenuation of PPL response was accompanied with a significant reduction in insulin response. This phenomenon was also found on normolipemic subjects [31].

These studies show that a greater PPL reduction can be generated when the exercise takes place 12 h before the HFM. Although LPL was not measured in the studies, the increased reduction in PPL which was seen 12 h after the exercise are consistent with the time delay in LPL synthesis [79, 80]. Exercise decreases insulin response and, therefore, removes the insulin inhibition from LPL. On the other hand, the attenuated insulin response may also reduce hepatic secretion of VLDL-TG [50].

The PPL response of three different groups has been reported by Ziogas et al. [104]. Sedentary individuals were compared to recreational exercisers and to endurance trained individuals. Subjects were asked to refrain from vigorous exercise for 36 h prior to the HFM. Compared to the sedentary group, the TG-AUC scores were reduced by 42% and 61% in the recreational trained group and endurance trained group, respectively. There were no significant differences between the two exercising groups. Based upon these results, it was concluded that individuals that participate in regular exercise have a lower PPL response than sedentary individuals. These results should be interpreted with caution. There was only a 36 h time delay between the last exercise and the PPL measurement. It is possible that the last exercise session was still influencing the PPL response.

On the other hand, Herd et al. [48] has reported that there are no differences in PPL between sedentary and trained individuals. PPL responses were determined in trained and untrained individuals 60 h after their last exercise bout. Trained subjects completed a 60 min exercise session 60 h prior to the HFM. There were no significant differences in the TG-AUC score between the trained and sedentary groups. It was concluded that chronic exercise did not have any effect on PPL when it was measured 60 hours after the last exercise bout.

Herd et al. [46] also have examined the effect of detraining on PPL. They took two groups of recreationally trained adults and split them into two groups. One group completed 13 weeks of training and the other group maintained their normal exercise routines. PPL responses were then determined in both groups at the following time points, 15 h, 60 h, and 9 days. The subjects last training session was controlled and consisted of a 40 min treadmill run at a "somewhat hard" to "hard" pace, as determined by ratings of perceived exertion. In the trained group, when compared to 15 h, the PPL response was 37% higher at 60 h and 46% higher at 9 days. The magnitude of the PPL response was correlated with an increase in LPL. The highest values of LPL were seen during the 15 h trial, which also had the largest reduction in PPL. There were no significant differences in the PPL responses or LPL among the control trials and the 60 h and 9 day trials. These trends were the same for both the trained and untrained groups. These data show the importance of regular exercise on PPL and on LPL. It also reveals the relationship between LPL and PPL.

The effect of detraining in endurance trained subjects has been reported by Hardman et al. [40]. They had highly trained endurance athletes complete three PPL trials. The HFM were consumed 15 h, 60 h, and 6.5 days after the last exercise session. The last exercise session was controlled and lasted only 30 min. When compared to the 15 h trial, the PPL response was significantly higher during the 60 h and 6.5 day trials. There were no significant differences between the 60 h and 6.5 day trials. This study showed the importance of regular exercise in even highly trained endurance athletes. It also raises questions in regards to other studies demonstrating that chronic exercise results in lower PPL responses.

It is obvious from the literature that an acute bout of exercise reduces PPL. This is true for running, walking, cycling, and resistance training. The literature also shows that the reduction in PPL is due to an increase in LPL. This increase in LPL is a direct result of the exercise session. Regardless of the mode of exercise, the reduction in PPL is dramatic, but the ability of exercise to cause this reduction is transient. This transient effect of exercise on PPL is present in both trained and untrained individuals and in most cases is gone after 24-36 h. Thus, exercise is very effective in reducing PPL, but the exercise must be done on a regular basis to continually reap the benefits of the exercise.

## Omega-3 Fatty Acid Supplementation and PPL

There is a large pool of literature that shows that omega-3 fatty acids (n-3FA) are effective at lowering fasting and postprandial plasma TG concentrations (Table 2]. The mechanism responsible for the TG lowering influence of n-3FAs is not exactly known. A review of the literature reveals that a decrease in TG synthesis and/or secretion is thought to be the primary mechanism for the reduction in TG following n-3FA supplementation. This decrease in TG synthesis and/or secretion may occur in the gut (chylomicron TG) or in the liver (VLDL-TG).

Although there is abundant evidence pointing to a decrease in chylomicron and VLDL-TG synthesis/secretion, there is also evidence indicating that the increased rates of clearance may contribute to the TG reducing influence of n-3FA supplementation. This increased rate of clearance is most likely due to an increase in LPL. The following section summarizes the literature on the effect of n-3FA supplementation on the reduction of fasting and postprandial plasma TG and the possible mechanisms behind these reductions.

The TG lowering ability of n-3FAs has been known for quite some time. Numerous studies have shown that chronic ingestion of n-3FAs lowers fasting plasma TG concentrations. A comprehensive review of the influence of n-3FAs on fasting TG concentrations can be found in the 1997 review by Harris [41]. Chronic ingestion of n-3FAs also is very effective in lowering the PPL response to a HFM. The reported reductions in the PPL response following n-3FA supplementation are similar in magnitude to the reductions following aerobic exercise.

In 1988, Harris et al. [42] examined how differences in the background diet influenced the PPL response to a HFM. Normolipidemic subjects ingested either a saturated fat, vegetable oil, or n-3FA oil based diet for 4 wk. The n-3FA oil based diet provided approximately 24 g of n-3FA per day. Following these 4 wk, PPL response was then determined following a HFM that contained 50 g of the background diet fat. It was reported that the presence of n-3FA in the background diet reduced the PPL response regardless of the fat composition of the HFM. They also reported that fat absorption was inhibited only when the subjects were on the n-3FA diet. This could have accounted for the reduction in the PPL

**Table 2. Selected Studies on the Effect of Omega-3 fatty Acid Supplementation on PPL**

| Authors | Study Design | n-3FA supplementation, length, source, and dosage | Variables Measured | Measurement Time | Changes (compared to control) |
|---|---|---|---|---|---|
| Harris et al. [22] | 11M, 10F. Compare PPL responses following 3 different background diets. | 24 g n-3FA, salmon oil 4 wk | TG response, LPLa | Prior to HFM then every 2h for next 8h. | n-3FA diet: ↓, other 2 diets. LPLa: ↔ |
| Brown and Roberts [6] | 35M. Examine influence of n-3FA supplementation on PPL | 5 g/day, fish oil, 18% EPA, 12% DHA 6 wk | Plasma TG, TG-AUC, and TG response | Prior to HFM then hourly for 8h. | TG-AUC, and TG response: ↔. Plasma TG: ↓ |
| Harris and Muzio [25] | 8M. Examine influence of n-3FA supplementation on PPL | 5 g/day, fish oil 4 wk | TG-AUC | Prior to HFM, then every 2h for next 14 h and at 24h. | TG-AUC: ↓ |
| Westphal et al. [63] | 12M. Examine influence of n-3FA supplementation on PPL | 3.4g/day, Omacor, 49.1%EPA, 32.2 DHA 6 wk. | TG-AUC | Prior to HFM, then at 4, 6, and 8h. | TG-AUC: ↓ |
| Thomas et al. [58] | 12M. Examine influence of n-3FA supplementation and exercise on PPL | 4g/day, fish oil, 60%EPA 40%DHA 4 wk | TG-AUC, peak TG | Prior to HFM then every 2h for next 8h and 24h | TG-AUC: ↔ peak TG: ↔ |

**Note:** ↑ or ↓ = significant increase or decrease, ↔ = no change. PPL, postprandial lipemia. TG-AUC, total area under the triglyceride curve. TG-AUC incremental area under the triglyceride curve. LPLa, lipoprotein lipase. HLa, hepatic lipase.

response. Increase in LPL could not explain the reduction, because there were no significant changes in LPL following the diets. They concluded that the PPL lowering effect of n-3FA ingestion might be due to decreased TG synthesis or secretion at the level of the gut.

Brown and Roberts [12] investigated the effect of n-3FA supplementation on PPL response following a HFM in two groups of subjects. The control group ingested 5 g of olive oil supplements per day and the other group ingested 5 g of n-3FA per day. Both groups ingested the supplements for 6 weeks. When compared at each time point the chylomicron TG concentrations in the n-3FA supplementation group were always significantly lower than the control group, with the exception of the baseline (0 h) value. The plasma TG concentrations were significantly lower at each time point, including the baseline value. These data suggest that n-3FA supplementation may be altering chylomicron TG metabolism. What is not clear from these results is if the n-3FAs alter chylomicron TG synthesis or clearance.

In 1991, Nozaki et al. [64] provided evidence that n-3FA does not influence the clearance of TG. Changes in plasma TG and LPL were measured in 12 hypertriglyceridemic subjects following the ingestion of 10 g of n-3FA per day for 4 wk. Fasting plasma TG concentrations were reduced 53% following n-3FA supplementation. However, there were no changes in LPL or HL following n-3FA supplementation. These results supported previous results that a decrease in TG synthesis was responsible of the TG lowering effects following n-3FA supplementation.

Harris et al. [43] in a later paper examined how n-3FA supplementation influenced VLDL-TG. Male subjects with a wide range of fasting TG values were selected for this study. VLDL-TG kinetics were measured following 3-5 weeks of ingesting either a n-3FA based diet (10-17 g n-3FA per day) or cocoa butter and peanut oil diet consisting of 20% fat. The VLDL-TG kinetics were determined following the intravenous injection of labeled glycerol. Following the n-3FA diet, plasma TG concentrations fell 66%. This reduction was primarily due to a 78% decrease in VLDL-TG concentrations. The VLDL-TG synthetic rate was reduced 45% when compared to the control diet. The fractional catabolic rate following the n-3FA diet was increased 57%. It was concluded that this decrease in VLDL-TG synthetic rate was the primary reason for the TG lowering effect of n-3FAs. The data also indicated that increased VLDL-TG clearance might also play a small role in the TG lowering effect of n-3FAs. Since LPL (the primary clearing mechanism) was not measured, a definitive conclusion could not be made on the importance of VLDL-TG clearance.

In 1993, Harris and Muzio [45] attempted to determine if an increase in chylomicron clearance was the mechanism responsible for the reduction in PPL following n-3FA supplementation. In a randomized double blind crossover design, eight normolipidemic subjects ingested approximately 5 g per day of either olive oil supplements or n-3FA supplements for 4 wk. Following a washout period the subjects then exchanged their supplements and repeated all experimental trials. Each subject completed an oral fat tolerance test and an intravenous fat tolerance test during each supplementation period. The purpose of the oral fat tolerance test was to compare the changes in TG-AUC, chylomicrons, and VLDL between the two types of supplements. The oral fat tolerance test consisted of four meals over the course of the day and was designed to mimic the eating patterns of a normal adult. The meals contained 43% fat, 44% carbohydrate, and 14% protein. There were significant reductions of 31, 40, and 40% in the TG-AUC, chylomicron, and VLDL, respectively. The purpose of the intravenous fat tolerance test was to examine the lipid removal rates between the two types of supplements. The intravenous fat tolerance test consisted of an injection of a 20% fat Intralipid emulsion (19 ml/m$^2$). The changes in the plasma TG concentration over time were used to calculate the emulsion removal rate. There were no differences in the emulsion removal rates between the two types of supplements. The data indicated that the reduction of chylomicron following n3-FA supplementation is due to the reduced synthesis or secretion rather than the increase in the clearance rate.

Harris et al. [44] attempted to determine if an increased rate of TG clearance was responsible for the reduction in TG following n-3FA supplementation. A randomized double blind cross over design was used to compare endogenous LPL following olive oil or n-3FA supplementation. They also compared a group of healthy subjects to a group of HTG subjects. Healthy subjects ingested 5 g/day of the appropriate supplement for 3 wk. The HTG subjects ingested 5 g/70kg body weight/day for 4 wk. The n-3FA supplementation decreased fasting TG concentrations 18% in the healthy subjects and 35% in the HTG subjects. Endogenous LPL measured in non-heparinized plasma was increased 62% in the healthy subjects and 65% in the HTG subjects. It was concluded that this increase in endogenous LPL could lead to an increased lipolytic rate, which would help explain the TG lowering effects of n-3FA supplementation. The authors noted that the results should be carefully examined, due to the fact that endogenous LPL was measured and not post-heparin LPL. They state that it is unknown if either of these measurements of LPL represent the physiologically active enzyme concentrations. This is one of the few papers that report increases in LPL due to n-3FA supplementation in healthy, normal subjects, but since it is an increase in endogenous LPL the finding should be regarded cautiously.

Westphal et al. [99] further examined changes in plasma TG, chylomicron TG, VLDL-TG, and LPL in HTG subjects. Subjects ingested 3.4 g/day of n-3FA for 6 wk. PPL responses were determined following a HFM prior to and after the n-3FA supplementation period. At the 4, 6, and 8 h time point, plasma TG was reduced 32-39% and VLDL-TG was reduced 36-43%. Chylomicron TG was reduced 49, 58, and 64% at 4, 6, and 8 h, respectively. There were no changes in postheparin plasma LPL following n-3FA supplementation. Despite the fact that there were no changes in LPL, the authors speculated that the reduction in VLDL-TG might be indirectly caused by the increase of the ability of LPL to hydrolyze chylomicron TG. VLDL-TG and chylomicron TG are both substrates for LPL, with chylomicron TG being the preferred substrate. If there were a reduction in VLDL-TG, an increased percentage of LPL would be available to hydrolyze chylomicron TG instead of VLDL-TG. The net result would be an increased rate of removal of chylomicron TG with no apparent increase in LPL. If this were true, it would offer a possible explanation for the results of Westphal et al. [99].

As the literature shows, supplementation with n-3FA is an effective method to reduce PPL. Its effectiveness is equal to the reductions in PPL following a bout of aerobic exercise. There is evidence in the literature that supports an argument for a decrease in chylomicron TG synthesis. There also is evidence that supports the hypothesis that VLDL-TG synthesis is inhibited by the n-3FA supplementation. Together, these two bodies of literature build a strong case for the inhibition of TG production. The literature supporting the claim that n-3FA supplementation increase TG clearance is not as strong. One cannot state confidently that n-3FA increases LPL, but an argument can be made that n-3FA supplementation might increase the efficiency of LPL. The reduction of either VLDL-TG or chylomicron TG decreases the demand placed on LPL following a HFM. Although LPL may not be significantly elevated, the reduction in its primary substrates allows it to remove the TG more efficiently. Together, the decreased TG production and the possible increased efficacy of LPL results in a reduction in PPL following n-3FA supplementation.

## Exercise, n-3FA Supplementation, and PPL

Only two studies have examined the combination of aerobic exercise, n-3FA supplementation, and their combined effects on PPL. Thomas et al. studied this combination in sedentary males [94] and Smith et al. [89] examined this combination in trained males. Since exercise and n-3FA supplementation may work through separate and independent mechanisms, it was hypothesized that when they were combined an additive effect on PPL might be observed. In sedentary males, when exercise and n-3FA supplementation were combined there was no statistically significant difference in PPL between the combined trial and a control trial (no exercise and no n-3FA supplementation [94]. In trained males the reverse was true. The combined treatments reduced PPL to a greater degree than either exercise alone or n-3FA supplementation alone [89].

The contrasting results of these two studies indicate that further research involving the combination of exercise and n-3FA supplementation is warranted. It appears that trained and untrained individuals respond differently to the combined treatments. If interference between these two treatments does occur in sedentary individuals, then there could be important health implications. One question that needs to be answered is how much training does it take to reverse this interference? Since the effect of exercise on PPL is short lived, another question that needs to be answered is how long can one refrain from exercise before they start to behave like an untrained individual.

## References


[1] Abrams A, Speidel MT, Booyse FM, Segrest JP. Cytotoxicity of lipolyzed very low density lipoproteins and inhibition of cytotoxicity by density lipoproteins to endothelial cells *in vitro*. *Fed Proc.* 1988; 5: 4313.

[2] Alaupovic P, Blackenhorn DH, Knight-Gibson C, et al. ApoB-containing lipoprotein particles as risk factors for coronary artery disease. *Adv Exp Med Biol.* 1990; 285: 299-309.

[3] Appel B, Fried SK. Effects of insulin and dexamethasone on lipoprotein lipase in human adipose tissue. *Am J of Physiol.* 1992; 262: E695-699.

[4] Arbogast BW, Lee GM, Raymond TL. *In vitro* injury of porcine aortic endothelial cells by very low density lipoproteins from diabetic rat serum. *Diabetics.* 1982; 31: 593-599.

[5] Austin MA. Plasma triglyceride as a risk factor for coronary heart disease: The epidemiologic evidence and beyond. *Am J Epidemiol.* 1989; 129: 249-259.

[6] Auwerx J, Leroy P, Schoonjans K. Lipoprotein lipase: recent contributions from molecular biology. *Crit Rev Clin Lab Sci.* 1992; 29: 243-268.

[7] Baltzell JK, Wooten JT, and Otto DA. Lipoprotein lipase in rats fed fish oil: apparent relationship to plasma insulin levels. *Lipids.* 1991; 26: 289-294.

[8] Bierman EL, Eisenberg S, Stein D, Stein Y. Very low density lipoprotein "remnant" particles: uptake by aortic smooth muscle cells in culture. *Biochim. Biophys Acta.* 1973; 329: 163-167.

[9] Boquist S, Ruotolo G, Tang R, et al. Alimentary lipemia, postprandial triglyceride-rich lipoproteins, and common carotid intima-media thickness in healthy, middle-aged men. *Circulation.* 1999; 100: 723-728.

[10] Bradley WA, Hwang S, Karlin JB. et al. Low-density lipoprotein receptor binding determining switch from apolipoprtein E to apolipoprotein B during conversion of hypertriglyceridemic very-low density lipoprotein to low-density lipoproteins. *J Biol Chem.* 1984; 259: 14728-14735.

[11] Breier CH, Patsch JR, Munlberger V, Drexel H, Knapp E, Braunsteiner H. Risk factors for coronary artery disease: a study comparing hypercholesterolaemia and hypertriglyceridaemia in angiographically characterized patients. *Eur J Clin Invest.* 1989; 19: 419- 423.

[12] Brown AJ, Roberts DC. Moderate fish oil intake improves lipemic response to a standard fat meal. A study in 25 healthy men. *Arterioscler Thromb.* 1991; 11: 457-466.

[13] Cambien F, Jacqueson A, Richard JL, Warnet JM, Ducimetiere P, Claude JR. Is the level of serum triglyceride a significant predictor of coronary death in "normocholesterolemic" subjects? A Paris prospective study. *Am J Epidemiol.* 1986; 124:624-632.

[14] Castelli WP. The triglyceride issue: a view from Framingham. *Am Heart J.* 1986; 112: 432-437.

[15] Chernick SS, Spooner PM, Garrison MM, Scow RO. Effect of epinephrine and other lipolytic agents on intracellular lipolysis and lipoprotein lipase activity in 3T3-L1 adipocytes. *J Lipid Res.* 1986; 27: 286-294.

[16] Chung BH, Segrest JP. Cytotoxicity of remnants of triglyceride-rich lipoproteins: an atherogenic insult? *Adv Exp Med Biol.* 1990; 285: 341-351.

[17] Chung BH, Segrest JP, Smith K, Griffin FM, Brouliette CG. Lipolytic surface remnants of triglyceride-rich lipoproteins are cytotoxic to macrophages but not in the presence of high density lipoprotein. *J Clin Invest.* 1989; 83: 1363-1374.

[18] Craven TE, Ryu JE, Espeland MA, et al. Evaluation of the associations between carotid artery atherosclerosis and coronary artery stenosis. A case-control study. *Circulation.* 1990; 82: 1230-1242.

[19] Deshaies Y, Geloen A, Paulin A, Marette A, Bukowiecki LJ. Tissue-specific alterations in lipoprotein lipase activity in the rat after chronic infusion of isoproterenol. *Horm Metab Res.* 1993; 25: 13-16.

[20] Eckel RH, Jensen DR, Schlaepfer IR,Yost TJ. Tissue-specific regulation of lipoprotein lipase by isoproterenol in normal-weight humans. *Am J of Physiol.* 1996; 271: R1280-1286.

[21] Eckel RH, Prasad JE, Kern PA, Marshall S. Insulin regulation of lipoprotein lipase in cultured isolated rat adipocytes. *Endocrinology*. 1984; 114: 1665-1671.

[22] Eckel RH, Yost TJ, Jensen DR. Sustained weight reduction in moderately obese women results in decreased activity of skeletal muscle lipoprotein lipase. *Eur J Clin Invest.* 1995; 25: 396-402.

[23] Eisenberg S, Rachmilewitz D. Interaction of rat plasma very low density lipoprotein with lipoprotein lipase-rich (postheparin) plasma. *J Lipid Res*. 1975; 16: 341-344.

[24] Farese RV, Yost TJ, Eckel RH. Tissue-specific regulation of lipoprotein lipase activity by insulin / glucose in normal-weight humans. *Metabolism*. 1991; 40: 214-216.

[25] Ferguson MA, Alderson NL, Trost SG, Essig DA, Burke JR, Durstine JL. Effects of four different single exercise sessions on lipids, lipoproteins, and lipoprotein lipase. *J Appl Physiol.* 1998; 85: 1169-1174.

[26] Ferraro RT, Eckel RH, Larson DE, et al. Relationship between skeletal muscle lipoprotein lipase activity and 24-hour macronutrient oxidation. *J Clin Invest.* 1993; 92: 441-445.

[27] Fried SK, Russell CD, Grauso NL, Brolin RE. Lipoprotein lipase regulation by insulin and glucocorticoid in subcutaneous and omental adipose tissues of obese women and men. *J Clin Invest.* 1993; 92: 2191-2198.

[28] Geurian K, Pinson JB, Weart CW. The triglyceride connection in atherosclerosis. *Ann. Pharmacother.* 1992; 26: 1109-1117.

[29] Gianturco SH, Eskin SG, Navarro LT, Lahart CJ, Smith LC, Gotto AM. Abnormal effects of hypertriglyceridemic very-low-density lipoproteins on 3-hydroxy-3-methylglutaryl CoA reductase activity and viability of cultured bovine aortic endothelial cells. *Biochim Biophys Acta*. 1986; 618: 143-152.

[30] Gianturco SH, Lin A, Hwang S, et al. Distinct murine macrophage receptor pathway for human triglyceride-rich lipoproteins. *J Clin Invest*. 1988; 82: 1633-1634.

[31] Gill JM, Herd SL, Hardman AE. Moderate exercise and post-prandial metabolism: issues of dose-response. *J Sports Sci.* 2002; 20: 961-7.

[32] Ginsberg HN, Jones J, Blaner WS, et al. Association of postprandial triglyceride and retinyl palmitate responses with newly diagnosed exercise-induced myocardial ischemia in middle-aged men and women. *Arterioscler Thromb Vasc Biol.* 1995; 15: 1829-1838.

[33] Goldberg IJ, Merkel M. Lipoprotein lipase: physiology, biochemistry, and molecular biology. *Front Biosci.* 2001; 6: 388-405.

[34] Gotto AM Jr. Hypertriglyceridemia: risks and perspectives. *Am J Cardiol.* 1992; 70: H19-H25.

[35] Gotto AM Jr. Interrelationship of triglycerides with lipoproteins and high-density lipoproteins. *Am J Cardiol.* 1990; 66: 20A-23A.

[36] Greiwe JS, Holloszy JO, Semenkovich CF. Exercise induces lipoprotein lipase and GLUT-4 protein in muscle independent of adrenergic-receptor signaling. *J Appl Physiol.* 2000; 89: 176-181.

[37] Grundy SM. Pathogenesis of hyperlipoproteinemia. *J Lipid Res.* 1984; 25: 1611-1620.

[38] Grundy SM, Vega GL. Hypertriglyceridemia: cause and relation to coronary heart disease. *Seminars in Thrombosis and Hemostasis.* 1988; 14: 149-164.

[39] Grundy SM, Vega GL. Monounsaturated fatty acids, plasma cholesterol, and coronary heart disease. *Am J Clin Nutr.* 1987; 45: 1168-1175.

[40] Hardman AE, Lawrence JEM, Herd SL. Postprandial lipemia in endurance-trained people during a short interruption to training. *J Appl Physiol.* 1998; 84: 1895-1901.

[41] Harris WS. n-3 Fatty Acids and Serum Lipoproteins: Human Studies. *Am J Clin Nutr.* 1997; 65: 1645S-1654S.

[42] Harris WS, Connor WE, Alam N, Illingworth DR. Reduction of postprandial triglyceridemia in humans by dietary n-3 fatty acids. *J Lipid Res.* 1988; 29: 1451-1460.

[43] Harris WS, Connor WE, Illingworth DR, Rothrock DW, Foster DM. Effects of fish oil on VLDL triglyceride kinetics in humans. *J Lipid Res.* 1990; 31: 1549-1558.

[44] Harris WS, Lu G, Rambjor GS, et al. Influence of n-3 fatty acid supplementation on the endogenous activities of plasma lipases. *Am J Clin Nutr.* 1997; 66: 254-260.

[45] Harris WS, Muzio F. Fish oil reduces postprandial triglyceride concentrations without accelerating lipid-emulsion removal rates. *Am J Clin Nutr.* 1993; 58: 68-74.

[46] Herd SL, Hardman AE, Boobis LH, Cairns CJ. The effect of 13 weeks of running training followed by 9 d of detraining on postprandial lipaemia. *Br J Nutr.* 1998; 80: 57-66.

[47] Herd SL, Kiens B, Boobis LH, Hardman AE. Moderate exercise, postprandial lipemia, and skeletal muscle lipoprotein lipase activity. *Metabolism.* 2001; 50: 756-762.

[48] Herd SL, Lawrence JEM, Malkova D, Murphy MH, Mastana S, Hardman AE. Postprandial lipemia in young men and women of contrasting training status. *J Appl Physiol.* 2000; 89: 2049-2056.

[49] Hoff HF, Heideman CL, Jackson RL, Bayardo RJ, Kim H, Gotto AM. Localization patterns of plasma apolipoproteins in human atherosclerotic lesions. *Cir Res.* 1975; 37: 72-75.

[50] Jeppesen J, Hollenbeck CB, Zhou MY, et al. Relation between insulin resistance, hyperinsulinemia, postheparin plasma lipoprotein lipase activity, and postprandial lipemia. *Arterio Thromb Vasc Biol.* 1995; 15. 320-4.

[51] Kantor MA, Cullinance EM, Herbert PN, Thompson PD. Acute increase in lipoprotein lipase following prolonged exercise. *Metabolism.* 1984; 33: 454-457.

[52] Kantor MA, Cullinance EM, Sady SP, Herbert PN, Thompson PD. Exercise acutely increases hight density lipoprotein-cholesterol and lipoprotein lipase activity in trained and untrained men. *Metabolism.* 1987; 36: 188-192.

[53] Karpe F, de Faire U, Mercuri M, Bond MG, Hellenius ML, Hamsten A. Magnitude of alimentary lipemia is related to intima-media thickness of the common carotid artery in middle-aged men. *Atherosclerosis.* 1998; 141: 307-314.

[54] Karpe F, Hellenius ML, Hamsten A. Differences in postprandial concentrations of very-low-density lipoprotein and chylomicron remnants between normotriglyceridemic and hypertriglyceridemic men with and without coronary heart disease. *Metabolism.* 1999; 48: 301-307.

[55] Kiens B, Lithell B, Mikines KJ, Richter EA. Effects of insulin and exercise on muscle lipoprotein lipase activity in man and its relation to insulin action. *J Clin Invest.* 1989; 84: 1124-1129.

[56] Lehninger AL, Nelson DLL, Cox MM. *Principles of Biochemistry*. New York, NY: Worth Publishers; 1993.
[57] Lithell H, Boberg J, Hellsing K, Lundqvist G, Vessby B. Lipoprotein-lipase activity in human skeletal muscle and adipose tissue in the fasting and the fed states. *Atherosclerosis*. 1978; 30: 89-94.
[58] Lithell H, Karlstrom B, Selinus I, Vessby B, Fellstrom B. Is muscle lipoprotein lipase inactivated by ordinary amounts of dietary carbohydrates? *Hum Nutr Clin Nutr*. 1985; 39: 289-295.
[59] Miesenboeck G, Patsch JR. Coronary artery disease: synergy of triglyceride-rich lipoproteins and HDL. *Cardiovasc Risk Factors*. 1991; 1: 293-299.
[60] Miller NF. HDL metabolism and its role in lipid transport. *Eur Heart J*. 1990; 11(supp. H): 1-3.
[61] Miller WC, Gorski J, Oscai LB, Palmer WK. Epinephrine-activation of heparin-nonreleasable lipoprotein lipase in 3 skeletal muscle fiber types of the rat. *Biochem Biophys Res Commun*. 1989; 164: 615-619.
[62] Morton RE, Zilversmit DB. Inter-relationship of lipids transferred by the lipid-transfer protein isolated from human lipoprotein-deficient plasma. *J Biol Chem*. 1983; 258: 11751-11757.
[63] Nikkila EA, Taskinen MR, Rehunen S, Harkonen M. Lipoprotein lipase activity in adipose tissue and skeletal muscle of runners: relation to serum lipoproteins. *Metabolism*. 1978; 27: 1661-1667.
[64] Nozaki S, Garg A, Vega GL, Grundy SM. Postheparin lipolytic activity and plasma lipoprotein response to w-3 polyunsaturated fatty acids in patients with primary hypertriglyceridemia. *Am J Clin Nutr*. 1991; 53: 638-642.
[65] Ong JM, Saffari B, Simsolo RB, Kern PA. Epinephrine inhibits lipoprotein lipase gene expression in rat adipocytes through multiple steps in posttranscriptional processing. *Mol Endocrinol*. 1992; 6: 61-69.
[66] Parks J, Speidel MT, Segrest JP. The effect of lipolyzed hypertriglyceridemic lumen serum and lipolyzed very low density lipoprotein on smooth muscle cells *in vitro*. *Fed Proc*. 1988; 4: 4114 (abstr.).
[67] Patsch JR, Miesenbock G, Hopferwieser T, et al. Relation of triglyceride metabolism and coronary artery disease. studies in the postprandial state. *Arterioscler Thromb*. 1992; 12: 1336-1345.
[68] Patsch JR, Patsch W. Exercise, high density lipoproteins, and fat tolerance. *Comp. Ther*. 1984; 10: 29-37.
[69] Patsch JR, Prasad S, Gotto AM Jr., Patsch W. High density lipoprotein$_2$: Relationship of the plasma levels of this lipoprotein species to its composition, to the magnitude of postprandial lipemia, and to the activities of lipoprotein lipase and hepatic lipase. *J Clin Invest*. 1987; 80:341-347.
[70] Pedersen SB, Bak JF, Holck P, Schmitz O, Richelsen B. Epinephrine stimulates human muscle lipoprotein lipase activity in vivo. *Metabolism*. 1999; 48: 461-464.
[71] Peltonen P, Marniemi J, Hietanen E, Vuori I, Ehnholm C. Changes in serum lipids, lipoproteins, and heparin releasable lipolytic enzymes during moderate physical training in man: a longitudinal study. *Metabolism*. 1981; 30: 518-526.

[72] Petitt DS, Arngrimsson SA, Cureton KJ. Effect of resistance exercise on postprandial lipemia. *J Appl Physiol.* 2003; 94: 694-700.

[73] Ross AC, Minick CR, Zilversmit DB. Equal atherosclerosis in rabbits fed cholesterol-free, low-fat diet or cholesterol-supplemented diet. *Atherosclerosis.* 1978; 29: 310-304.

[74] Ross R, Glomset JA. The pathogenesis of atherosclerosis. *N Engl J Med.* 1976; 295: 369-372.

[75] Ryu JE, Howard G, Craven TE, Bond MG, Hagaman AP, Crouse JR, 3rd. Postprandial triglyceridemia and carotid atherosclerosis in middle-aged subjects. *Stroke.* 1992; 23: 823-828.

[76] Sadur CN, Eckel RH. Insulin stimulation of adipose tissue lipoprotein lipase. Use of the euglycemic clamp technique. *J Clin Invest.* 1982; 69: 1119-1125.

[77] Sady SP, Thompson PD, Cullinane EM, Kantor MA, Domagala E, Herbert PN. Prolonged exercise augments plasma triglyceride clearance. *JAMA.* 1986; 256: 2552-2555.

[78] Scow PO, Brachet-Machie EJ, Smith LC. Role of capillary endothelium in the clearance of chylomicrons: a model for lipid transport from blood by lateral diffusion in cell membranes. *Circ Res.* 1976; 39: 149-162.

[79] Seip RL, Angelopoulos TJ, Semenkovich CF. Exercise induces human lipoprotein lipase gene expression in skeletal muscle but not adipose tissue. *Am J Physiol.* 1995; 268: E229-E236.

[80] Seip RL, Mair K, Cole TG, Semenkovich CF. Induction of human skeletal muscle lipoprotein lipase gene expression by short-term exercise is transient. *Am J Physiol.* 1997; 272: E255-261.

[81] Semenkovich CF, Wims M, Noe L, Etienne J, Chan L. Insulin regulation of lipoprotein lipase activity in 3T3-L1 adipocytes is mediated at posttranscriptional and posttranslational levels. *J Biol Chem.* 1989; 264: 9030-9038.

[82] Sharrett AR, Chambless LE, Heiss G, Paton CC, Patsch W. Association of postprandial triglyceride and retinyl palmitate responses with asymptomatic carotid artery atherosclerosis in middle-aged men and women. The Atherosclerosis Risk in Communities (ARIC) Study. *Arterioscler Thromb Vasc Biol.* 1995; 15: 2122-2129.

[83] Shepherd J, Krauss RM. Pathophysiology of triglyceride-rich particles. *Am J Cardiol.* 1991; 68: 5A-7A.

[84] Shepherd J, Packard CJ. Metabolic consequences of hypertriglyceridemia. In: *Atherosclerosis Review*, A. M. Gotto and R. Paoletti (Eds.). New York, NY: Raven Press; 1991.

[85] Siguel EN, Chee KM, Gong J, Schaefer EJ. Criteria for plasma essential fatty acid deficiency as assessed by capillary column gas liquid chromatography. *Clin Chem.* 1987; 33: 1869-1873.

[86] Sigurdsson G, Nicoll A, Lewis B. Conversion of very low density lipoprotein to low density lipoprotein. A metabolic study of apolipoprotein B kinetics in human subjects. *J Clin Invest.* 1975; 65: 1481-1485.

[87] Simsolo RB, Ong JM, Kern PA. The regulation of adipose tissue and muscle lipoprotein lipase in runners by detraining. *J Clin Invest.* 1993; 92: 2124-2130.

[88] Sirtori CR, Mancini M, Paoletti R. Consensus: hypertriglyceridemia as a risk factor. *Eur Heart J.* 1990; 11(suppl H): 44-48.

[89] Smith BK, Sun GY, Donahue OM, Thomas TR. Exercise plus n-3 fatty acids: Additive effect on postprandial lipemia. *Metabolism.* 2004; In Press.

[90] Speidel MT, Booyse FM, Abram A, Moore MA, Chung BH. Lipolyzed hyertriglyceridemic serum and triglyceride-rich lipoprotein cause lipid accumulation in and are cytotoxic to cultured human endothelial cells. High density lipoproteins inhibit this cytotoxicity. *Thromb Res.* 1990; 58: 251-264.

[91] Stein Y, Glangeaud MC, Fainaru M, Stein O. The removal of cholesterol from aortic smooth muscle cells in culture and Landschutz ascites cells by fraction human high-density apolipoproteins. *Biochim Biophys Acta.* 1975; 380: 106-118.

[92] Tall AR. Plasma lipid transfer proteins. *J Lipid Res.* 1986; 27: 361-367.

[93] Taskinen MR, Nikkila EA. Effect of acute vigorous exercise on lipoprotein lipase activity of adipose tissue and skeletal muscle in physically active men. *Artery.* 1980; 6: 471-483.

[94] Thomas TR, Fischer BA, Kist WB, Horner KE, Cox RH. Effects of exercise and n-3 fatty acids on postprandial lipemia. *J Appl Physiol.* 2000; 88: 2199-2204.

[95] Thomas TR, Horner KE, Langdon MM, et al. Effect of exercise and medium-chain fatty acids on postprandial lipemia. *J Appl Physiol.* 2001; 90: 1239-1246.

[96] Tsetsonis NV, Hardman AE. Effect of low and moderate intensity treadmill walking on postprandial lipaemia in healthy young adults. *Eur J Appl Physiol.* 1996; 73: 419-426.

[97] Tsetsonis NV, Hardman AE. Reduction in postprandial lipemia after walking: influence of exercise intensity. *Med Sci Sports Exerc.* 1996; 28: 1235-1242.

[98] Uiterwaal CS, Grobbee DE, Witteman JC, et al. Postprandial triglyceride response in young adult men and familial risk for coronary atherosclerosis. *Ann Intern Med.* 1994; 121: 576-583.

[99] Westphal S, Orth M, Ambrosch A, Osmundsen K, Luley C. Postprandial chylomicrons and VLDLs in severe hypertriacylglycerolemia are lowered more effectively than are chylomicron remnants after treatment with n-3 fatty acids. *Am J Clin Nutr.* 2000; 71: 914-920.

[100] Wilhelmsen L, Wedel H, Tibblin G. Multivariate analysis of risk factor for coronary heart disease. *Circulation.* 1973; 48:950-958.

[101] Zhang JQ, Smith B, Langdon MM, et al. Changes in LPLa and reverse cholesterol transport variables during 24-h postexercise period. *Am J Physiol Endocrinol Metab.* 2002; 283: E267-274.

[102] Zhang JQ, Thomas TR, Ball SD. Effect of exercise timing on postprandial lipemia and HDL cholesterol subfractions. *J Appl Physiol.* 1998; 85: 1516-1522.

[103] Zilversmit DB. Atherogenesis: a postprandial phenomenon. *Circulation.* 1979; 60: 473-485.

[104] Ziogas GG, Thomas TR, Harris WS. Exercise training, postprandial hypertriglyceridemia, and LDL subfraction distribution. *Med Sci Sports Exerc.* 1997; 29: 986-991.

In: Cholesterol in Atherosclerosis and Coronary Heart Disease ISBN 1-59454-302-X
Editor: Jean P. Kovala, pp.157-185 

*Chapter VIII*

# Lipid-lowering Drugs: Pharmacoepidemiological Studies of Prescription Patterns in General Practice

***John Larsen****

University of Southern Denmark, Odense, Denmark

## Abstract

The present study has shown that LLD use was low in the beginning of the nineties in the general population but has increased substantially over the period 1993 1998. The use of statins has increased nearly exponentially and now makes up more than 90% of the lipid-lowering drugs used. After publication of especially the 4S study in 1994, utilisation has at least quantitatively approached a level corresponding to the number of people in the general population, who need treatment according to current recommendations. The majority of patients treated with LLDs had drug indicators of cardiovascular risk factors. General practitioners issued 73% of the total number of LLD prescriptions. The present study has shown good compliance with statin treatment in a Danish population measured by persistence as well as by continuity. However, a high percentage of the youngest group of patients without drug indicators of cardiac disease or diabetes discontinued treatment before obtaining the full benefit in terms of decreased risk of coronary heart morbidity and mortality. Contrary to Denmark, LLD use in Italy was characterised by high consumption, prevalence and incidence but low persistence in the period 1994 to 1996. Among patients with a history of myocardial infarction who met the criteria for LLD reimbursement, far too few were actually treated. Therefore, more attention is needed to initiate treatment in these patients.

* Address of correspondence: General Practitioner, Assistant Professor, PhD, Research Unit of General Practice & Clinical Pharmacology, University of Southern Denmark, Winsloewparken 19, DK-5000 Odense, Denmark. E-mail: jlarsen@health.sdu.dk; Phone: +45 2166 1795

# Introduction

In 1948, blood cholesterol levels were not believed to be causally related to coronary artery disease. Peters and VanSlyke's *Quantitative Clinical Chemistry*, one of the most respected clinical biochemistry textbooks of its era, stated that "[t]here is no satisfactory evidence that the incidence of atherosclerosis bears any relation to the concentration of cholesterol in the blood" [1]. As late as in 1989 T.J. Moore stated that "there is no evidence at all that lowering your cholesterol level will lengthen your life" [2]. However, during the last decade the role of elevated serum cholesterol as a risk factor for coronary heart disease (CHD) has become well established [3-6], although still controversial in the elderly [7-10]. Approximately 15% of adults in the US and Europe have hypercholesterolaemia and are therefore at increased risk of cardiovascular mortality and morbidity [11]. Also, the effect of lipid-lowering drugs (LLDs) on coronary heart disease is now well documented through several large clinical trials [12-22]. The goal of lipid-lowering therapy in patients with hypercholesterolaemia is to reduce the risk of CHD (primary prevention) or, in those with existing CHD, reduce the likelihood of a recurrent vascular event (secondary prevention). However, several studies have demonstrated that although overall use of LLD may be high, only a small fraction of people eligible for LLD treatment are actually treated [23-25]. In Denmark, as opposed to most other western countries, the use of these drugs has been shown to be low [26]. This information was based on aggregated sales data from the pharmacies [27], not on detailed knowledge of the utilisation in terms of consumption and compliance on an individual level. Also, referring to current guidelines, it has been claimed that too few patients with risk factors for CHD are treated with LLDs [28]. We do not know, however, whether this holds true or if it is true for certain parts of the population. Several studies that have addressed the extent of non-compliance with LLD treatment [29-34] have found a considerable problem. These studies have, however, been based on rather crude measures of compliance. The measurement of serum cholesterols is now regarded a useful tool in the decision of whether the patient should be treated with LLDs, and is, therefore, widely used in the guidelines for prevention of CHD. As with LLD treatment, the meaningfulness of measuring serum cholesterol in older people, even those with established coronary heart disease, is controversial [10;35;36]. A recent study demonstrated that even in patients prescribed LLDs, recommended serum lipid target levels were only achieved in 38% of cases [37]. Whether this is due to lack of effect or lack of compliance remains unknown.

In order to take the full advantage of these drugs it is important to identify population groups and factors associated with potential underuse and poor compliance.

The results presented in this chapter are based on a PhD study [38] (five papers published 2000-2003 in clinical pharmacological and cardiovascular journals [39-43]) and supplementary comments.

# Background

## Lipid-lowering Drugs and their Role in Reducing Cardiovascular Risk

### *Evidence for Effect of Lipid-Lowering Drugs*

Over the past decades, a considerable number of large scale clinical trials have provided clear evidence that cholesterol-lowering is an important risk-reduction strategy for secondary and primary prevention of CHD. Unlike the older studies with fibrates, the most recent trials of cholesterol-lowering therapies with 3-hydroxy-3-methylglutaryl coenzyme A (HMG-CoA) inhibitors (statins) have clearly shown that their use can reduce the risk of CHD and total mortality, as well as the need for expensive hospitalisation and revascularisation procedures. Studies such as the Scandinavian Simvastatin Survival Study (4S) [12], the West of Scotland Coronary Prevention Study (WOSCOPS) [13], the Cholesterol and Recurrent Events (CARE) trial [16], the Long-Term Intervention with Pravastatin in Ischaemic disease (LIPID) [17], the Air Force/Texas Coronary Atherosclerosis Prevention Study (AFCAPS/TEXCAPS) [18], as well as numerous other investigations have established the role of these drugs in reducing cholesterol levels, resulting in a reduction in CHD morbidity and mortality in primary as well as secondary prevention. The relative risk reduction in cardiovascular outcomes for many of these studies was similar. However, the number of persons needed to treat (NNT) for one year to prevent one person from experiencing an event varied from 63 in 4S to 256 in AFCAPS/TexCAPS and was intermediate in WOSCOPS (217) and CARE (167) [44].

### *Guidelines for Treatment with Lipid-lowering Drugs*

According to guidelines agreed upon by a number of medical societies, including the European Societies on Coronary Prevention, individuals with a high risk of cardiovascular heart disease (CHD) should be identified and targeted for lifestyle intervention and, when appropriate, LLD therapy [12;16;45;46]. Recommendations for the use of lipid-lowering drugs derive mainly from the results of large clinical trials and are often presented for the clinician as a set of guidelines meant to be a practical help in the daily work. These guidelines are frequently changed reflecting new knowledge in the field. Years ago, patients were not considered "hypercholesterolemic" unless their levels exceeded 7.76 mmol/L (300 mg/dl) [1]. Current Danish recommendations as of March 2002 [47] target at a total cholesterol of 4.5 mmol/L in patients with established ischemic heart disease.

As illustrated in Figure 1, patients' as well as doctors' attitude towards drug treatment are, among other things, determined by a combination of guidelines and reimbursement rules for the drugs in question [48]. For society and for the individual patient to benefit from these rather expensive drugs, it is, however, of utmost importance that patients who may benefit from the treatment actually receive treatment, e.g. patients with pre-existing coronary heart disease and elevated serum cholesterol according to current recommendations [45].

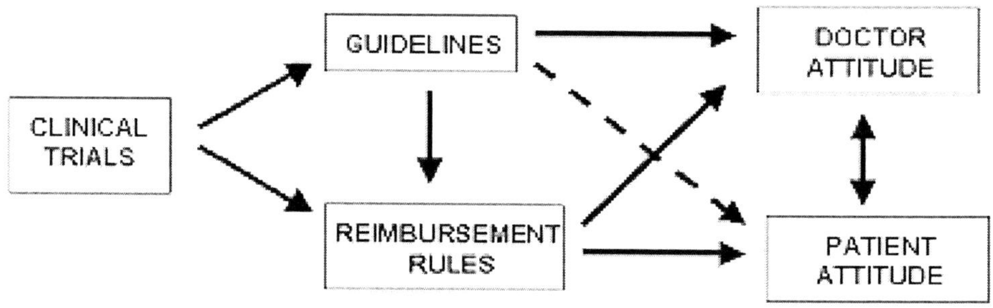


Figure 1. Factors affecting adherence to guidelines.

### *Reimbursement of Lipid-lowering Drugs*

The results of clinical trials widely constitute the basis for the development of guidelines and reimbursement rules (Figure 1). However, political interests weigh heavily in the decision whether a drug should be reimbursed or not. The rising costs for pharmaceuticals are of great concern to most payers (patients, governments, insurance companies), and different attempts have been introduced to combat this development. With a limited health budget, priority decisions have to be made by the politicians. The aim of health care professionals is to make sure that the resources provided are used in the most effective way. However, a study to assess the impact of reference pricing in New Zealand [49] showed that switching from one lipid-lowering drug to another (cheaper) resulted in lipid elevations due to both lesser potency and underdosing. It was concluded that the responsibility to the taxpayer should be weighed carefully against the ethical responsibility to the individual patient and the potential to do harm. In Denmark, it was feared that unrestricted reimbursement of the use of lipid-lowering drugs would lead to an overuse [27].

From 1993 until December 1998, reimbursement rules as to LLD treatment in Denmark remained unchanged from 1993 in the sense that these drugs were reimbursed to the extent of 75% of the cost only after individual application from the patient's physician to the Danish National Board of Health under certain conditions, which until January 1998 were: 1) known ischemic heart disease, e.g. former myocardial infarction, angina pectoris and serum cholesterol above 5.4 mmol/l despite diet, 2) inherited hyperlipidemia, 3) high serum cholesterol and concurrent important risk factor for developing ischemic heart disease (family disposition or diabetes mellitus). No reimbursement was given for the cause of primary prevention. Furthermore, following the publication of the 4S study the Danish National Board of Health issued a letter to all physicians in January 1995 stressing that reimbursement could not be obtained for the purpose of primary prevention. As from January 1998, a set of new directions was issued [50], according to which reimbursement could be obtained for secondary prevention in case of total cholesterol above the level of 4.5 mmol/l. This also counts for patients with diabetes and triglyceride (TG) >2.5 mmol/l. Further, reimbursement could now be obtained for primary prevention upon application, if the person had a total cholesterol above 6.5 mmol/l, LDL-cholesterol above 4.5 mmol/l, and one cardiovascular risk factor, or total cholesterol above 7-8 mmol/l and LDL-cholesterol above 5 mmol/l and one risk factor, or HDL-cholesterol <1mmol/l in combination with TG >5 mmol/l and at least one risk factor. Risk factors for cardiovascular disease were defined as: male sex, familial disposition for ischemic heart disease, hypertension, smoking, peripheral arterial insufficiency and cerebrovascular disease. Two differentiated serum cholesterol measurements after two months of diet were now required. As of December 1998, the mandatory individual applications for secondary prevention were abandoned.

# Lipid-lowering Drug Utilization

## Patterns of Lipid-lowering Drug Consumption

Before 1994, wholesale figures showed that LLD use in Denmark was below 2 Defined Daily Doses per 1,000 inhabitants per day (DDD/TID) [27]. In most other countries, however, use of LLDs was higher, albeit with a considerable variation in the development of consumption in various countries [26]. In their comparative study of Australia, Finland, Italy, Norway and Sweden, Magrini et al found that Australia had the highest therapeutic intensity: 11.9 DDD/TID in 1994 (increased from 5.3 DDD/TID in 1992), whereas the utilisation in Nordic countries ranged from 4.0 (Finland) to 5.6 DDD/TID (Sweden) in 1994 [26]. In 1993, LLD use in Germany was as high as 14.7 DDD/TID [51]. In Spain, the overall consumption of LLDs multiplied by 7.8 from 1986 to 1998 reaching nearly 15 DDD/TID [52].

### *Compliance as Detected in Claims Databases*

Here, *compliance* shall be used as the overall term covering the doctor's adherence to guidelines and the patient's persistence and continuity with the prescribed treatment (see below for definitions).

The actual treatment of a patient relies on the doctor's capability and willingness to follow current guidelines in the field, as well as the patient's capability and willingness to follow the treatment suggested by the doctor. The cooperation between doctor and patient is essential for obtaining overall compliance (*Figure 1*). The doctor may have several reasons not to treat according to guidelines: he may not be familiar with the guidelines, he may not believe in them, or considerations towards the individual patient may force him not to do so. On the other hand, the patient may – perhaps with a good reason - not want to be treated at all or with the dose recommended, or for the course of time required to obtain the real benefit from the treatment. A combination of the doctor's and the patient's arguments may also lead to non-adherence to guidelines, leading to detection of non-compliance in database studies.

The term *compliance* in a drug utilisation context usually means "the willingness of the patient to take a drug as prescribed" [53]. This, however, is also a very wide definition as the term includes aspects as different as: the patient filling the prescription at the pharmacy (primary compliance), taking the drug as prescribed (secondary compliance), and the patient with a chronic disease getting a new package of the drug either by refilling the prescription at the pharmacy or by seeing the doctor for a refill prescription (refill compliance). By using data solely from prescription databases, it is only possible to investigate the prescriptions the patients actually did fill, but not the number of tablets the patients really ingested. Also, it is not possible to detect the drugs the doctors prescribed but were not redeemed by the patients.

Thus, although the term *compliance* was used differently in this chapter, one must be aware that it is actually only possible to describe what may be termed *apparent compliance.*

As hyperlipidemia is considered a condition needing lifelong treatment [54], compliance was in this study overall defined as the detection in prescription databases of the patients' actual filling of a set of prescriptions reasonably considered (under specified assumptions) to cover a continuous treatment. The 4S study [12] showed that a biochemical effect of simvastatin may already be observed after a few weeks, but the effect on ischemic heart disease (IHD) related morbidity and mortality was observed after approximately two years at the earliest. Data from the WOSCOPS study [13] showed that mortality risk from coronary heart disease was significantly influenced by the degree of compliance. Several studies that have addressed the extent of non-compliance with LLD treatment [29-34] have found a considerable problem but these studies have been based on rather crude measures of compliance.

### Setting

A very short summary of the setting therefore is:

- Cholesterol lowering is an important risk-reduction strategy for secondary and primary prevention of CHD. Statins can reduce the risk of CHD morbidity and mortality as well as the need for hospitalisation and revascularisation procedures.
- According to international guidelines, individuals with high risk of CHD should be identified and targeted for lifestyle intervention and, when appropriate, cholesterol lowering therapy.
- Based on the results of the 4S study, an effect on cardiovascular morbidity and mortality may not be expected before at least 1½ to 2 years of treatment.
- Compliance with lipid-lowering drug treatment has been shown to be low in selected populations. Our knowledge about use and compliance with guidelines is, however, inadequate.
- The use of lipid-lowering drugs in Denmark appears to be low compared with most other countries.

## Aims

The objective of the study was:

- to analyse the development in LLD utilisation (prevalence, incidence and compliance) over a six year period on an individual level in the general population, with special emphasis on prescribing in general practice
- to compare LLD utilisation in two different health care systems (Denmark and Italy)

- to investigate measurements of serum cholesterol among people with a history of MI and to analyse the utilisation of LLDs for secondary prevention in individual patients.

# Own Studies

## Material and Methods

### *Databases and Study Population*

The *Odense University Pharmacoepidemiologic Database (OPED)* (Denmark), established 1990 and providing complete coverage of the region since 1993 [55], covers all individuals living in Funen County (approximately 470,000 inhabitants). The population of the county is considered representative of the total Danish population for a number of important factors including drug consumption [55]. The database contains information about filled prescriptions for reimbursed drugs and provides the following information for each prescription: identification of the dispensed product according to the ATC-classification [56], number of packages and number of Defined Daily Doses (DDD) dispensed, code of the prescriber, anonymous code of the patient, date of prescription. The prescribed daily dose and the indication for prescription are not relevant to the processing of refunds and are, therefore, not recorded. Likewise, the database does not contain data on drugs sold over the counter (OTC). For patients receiving at least one prescription for an LLD in the period 1993 to 1998 in Funen County, Denmark, data were retrieved on all filled prescriptions (n = 286,707) for LLDs (ATC code C10, formerly B04), cardiovascular (ATC codes B01 and C01 to C09) and anti-diabetic medication (ATC code A10). The total Danish study population comprised approximately 470.000 inhabitants (465,239-471,873 inhabitants 1993-1998).

For the Danish-Italian comparative part of the study (1994-1996), data were also retrieved from the *Emilia Romagna Health Care Database* [57,58], covering approximately 4 million inhabitants and providing the same information as OPED. For this part, the study cohort comprised 420,731 persons in Funen and 334,935 persons in Bologna at the beginning of the study period (1994).

For the study of patients with a history of myocardial infarction, the study population comprised all people (213,868 inhabitants by January 1996) resident in the municipality of Odense and four surrounding municipalities (Munkebo, Otterup, Tommerup and Vissenbjerg) (demographic information from OPED). The *Patient Registry of Funen County* contains information on all contacts to hospitals, in- and outpatient- as well as emergency ward contacts. Patients are registered individually by way of their CPR (central person registration) number. The registry was established 1973 and has had complete coverage of Funen County since 1985 (personal communication with Poul Lund Poulsen, Department of Computer Technology, *Sygehus Fyn*, June 2001). Information about patients hospitalised due to acute MI (codes I21.0-I21.9 according to the ICD-10 coding system) in the period 1994 to 1997 was retrieved from this registry. For these patients, information on hospital, period of hospitalisation, diagnosis, residency and, where applicable, patients' date of death was obtained. A database containing serum cholesterols measured within the study period existed at the Department of Clinical Chemistry at Odense University Hospital, which analyses samples from the involved municipalities. Together with one other department in the county, this department keeps data on serum cholesterol values for all patients in the county.

### *Analysis of Lipid-lowering Drug Use*

The extent of LLD use (ATC code C10, formerly B04) was analysed as the therapeutic intensity (number of Defined Daily Doses per 1,000 inhabitants per day (DDD/TID)) according to the ATC/DDD methodology [56], and as the annual prevalence of use (number of individuals receiving at least one prescription in one calendar year per 1,000 inhabitants). An incident LLD user was defined as a user who had not purchased any LLD 12 months prior to the first prescription captured within the study period. Incidence was calculated as the number of new users per 1,000 inhabitants per year. Data from Bologna July 1995 concerning new users were missing. Therefore, the sex- and age specific incidence was for this month estimated as the average incidence for the rest of 1995. The waiting time distribution, as described by Hallas et al [59], recording the first occurrence of an LLD prescription for a given patient after 1 January 1993, was used to visualize the change in incidence over time. Data were broken down by sex and age classes in ways that ensured comparability with similar previous studies.

To estimate the amount of LLDs purchased without reimbursement, information on wholesale data on statin use 1994-1998 in Funen County was provided by the Statistical Department of the Danish Medicines Agency.

### *Analysis of Cardiovascular Risk Factors*

Cardiovascular disease or risk factors were identified for incident users of LLD if in the preceding year they received at least one prescription for one or more drugs belonging to the following ATC groups: A10 (insulins and oral anti-diabetics) as a marker for diabetes and B01 (anti-thrombotics), C01 (cardiac glycosides, anti-arrhythmics, nitrates), C02 (anti-hypertensives), C03 (diuretics), C07 (beta-blockers), C08 (calcium antagonists) and C09 (ACE inhibitors and angiotensin II antagonists) as markers for cardiovascular disease.

### *Compliance*

For the Danish Compliance Study [42], analyses were restricted to cover only statins. The intention was to describe two aspects of compliance by investigating persistence (treatment period as defined below) and continuity (compliance within the treatment period). Compliance was calculated for incident statin users only. An incident user was defined as a patient who filled his first statin prescription after a one-year run-in period from 1 January 1993. Compliance was calculated for a patient's first period of treatment only. A treatment period was considered discontinued, if the interval between two prescriptions exceeded a period covered by the number of tablets prescribed (one tablet per day) plus 30 days. Patients were allowed to save tablets for later use, whereas an excess of tablets received later in the period could not be included backwards.

*Persistence* of statin use was measured as the period from the date of the first prescription to the date of discontinuation. Observations were censored if they exceeded the end of the study period or at the time the patient died or moved out of the county, whichever event came first.

*Continuity* was measured as the number of days with treatment (= number of tablets) divided by the total number of days in the period of persistence. A limit between good and poor compliance in relation to continuity was set at 80% [29].

In the Danish-Italian Comparative Study [40], analyses of compliance were undertaken by way of simpler methods, the terms persistence and continuity being defined slightly differently. Identifying all individuals treated in 1994 who were still on a lipid-lowering drug in 1995 and in 1996 assessed persistence of LLD use during 1994-1996. In a more detailed analysis, the total number of DDDs received by each individual in one year was evaluated. This number reflects both persistence of treatment and within-treatment adherence to the recommended regimen (continuity). Continuity was further investigated under the assumption that 1 DDD represents an average day of treatment. A fully compliant long-term user should grossly receive 365 DDDs in one year. For practical purposes, the limit was put at 300 DDD/year (i.e. 82%). This analysis was performed in the subgroups of individuals who received one or more prescriptions for LLDs in the first month (January) of each year. This was done in order to capture prevalent users in three complete one-year periods.

### *Database Linkage*

For the IHD-study [43], information from the regional patients' registry, the OPED, and Department of Clinical Chemistry were linked by means of the unique Danish personal identification number system.

Patients hospitalised at Odense University Hospital and still alive at their discharge from hospital were registered by the date of discharge and followed until the end of the study period. Only patients for whom MI was the main diagnosis were included in the study as were only patients who were not treated with LLDs in the year prior to the hospitalisation. One year of non-use was considered an adequate period to ensure the capture of incident LLD use in OPED. For survival time estimates, observations were censored if they exceeded the study period, at the date of death or if the patient moved out of the defined study area, whichever event came first. The total observation period was 1993-1998.

1,296 people out of the total population of 213,868 in the municipality of Odense and four surrounding municipalities were hospitalised at Odense University Hospital because of an MI in the period 1994 to 1997, the average annual incidence being 1.5 MIs per 1,000 inhabitants. 20% died during hospitalisation.

Observed was the number of patients starting LLD treatment in relation to their first and second consecutive serum cholesterol value above 5.4 mmol/L and the course of time to initiation of LLD treatment after discharge after their first MI registered.

### *Ethics*

The Danish Data Protection Agency has approved the use of Odense University Pharmacoepidemiologic Database. For the present study, the Agency also approved the use of information from the regional patients' registry in the County of Funen and from the Department of Clinical Chemistry at Odense University Hospital. In all analyses, arbitrary consecutive numbers substituted the personal identifier and no patients were contacted. Therefore, according to law the project needed no approval from the regional scientific ethical committee. The committee was, however, notified.

## Results

### *Use of Lipid-lowering Drugs in the General Population*

Of the total population of 470,000, 5,600 objects received one or more prescriptions for LLDs in the period from 1993 to 1998. A total of 82,738 prescriptions were analysed and a nearly exponential increase in the consumption of LLDs was observed with statins making up the vast majority (*Figure 2*). *Figure 3* shows the development in age-specific 1-year prevalence. *Figure 4* demonstrates by way of the waiting time distribution [59] the monthly number of new users over the study period and Table 1 shows the incidence of LLD use for 1994 and 1998 stratified according to gender and age. Utilisation of statins registered in OPED compared with wholesale data from Funen County and the whole of Denmark can be seen in Table 2. The difference between wholesale data and OPED data showed that an average of 3% of statins used during the period 1994-1998 was purchased without reimbursement. In the year prior to their first LLD prescription, 77% of the 4,387 incident LLD users had a prescription indicating the presence of manifest cardiovascular disease or diabetes. General practitioners wrote 73% of the LLD prescriptions, and 55% of the LLD treatments were initiated in general practice.

**Table 1. Stratified incidence of lipid-lowering drug users 1994 and 1998 in Funen County, Denmark (Number of New Users per 1,000 Inhabitants per Year)**

| | 1994 | | | 1998 | | |
|---|---|---|---|---|---|---|
| | N | Background population | Incidence | n | Background population | Incidence |
| Females | 120 | 236177 | 0.51 | 561 | 238814 | 2.35 |
| Males | 218 | 230390 | 0.95 | 717 | 233059 | 3.08 |
| Age <65 | 245 | 390780 | 0.63 | 816 | 396978 | 2.06 |
| Age >=65 | 93 | 75787 | 1.23 | 462 | 74895 | 6.17 |
| Females <65 | 81 | 192116 | 0.42 | 338 | 195175 | 1.73 |
| Females >=65 | 39 | 44061 | 0.89 | 223 | 43639 | 5.11 |
| Males <65 | 164 | 198664 | 0.83 | 478 | 201803 | 2.37 |
| Males >=65 | 54 | 31726 | 1.70 | 239 | 31256 | 7.65 |
| Total | 338 | 466567 | 0.72 | 1278 | 471873 | 2.71 |

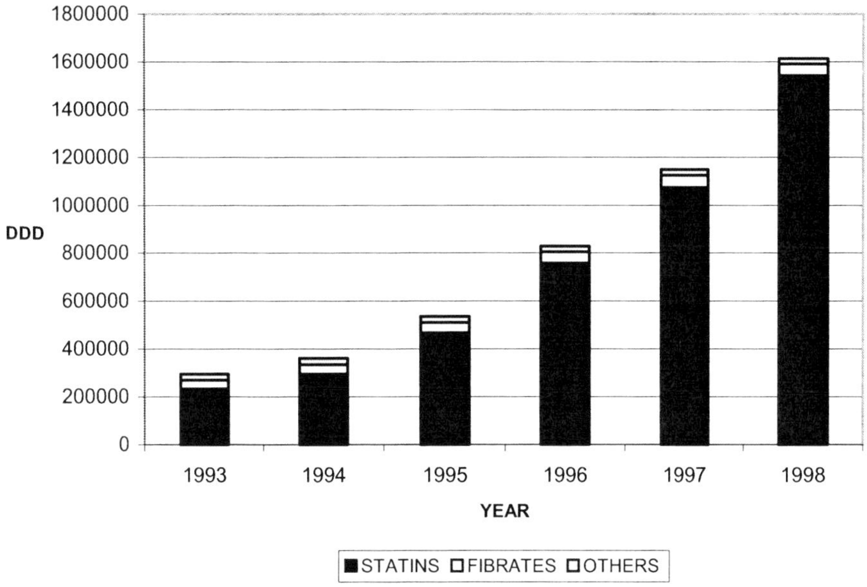


Figure 2. Development in consumption (DDD) of lipid-lowering drugs 1993-1998 in Funen County, Denmark.

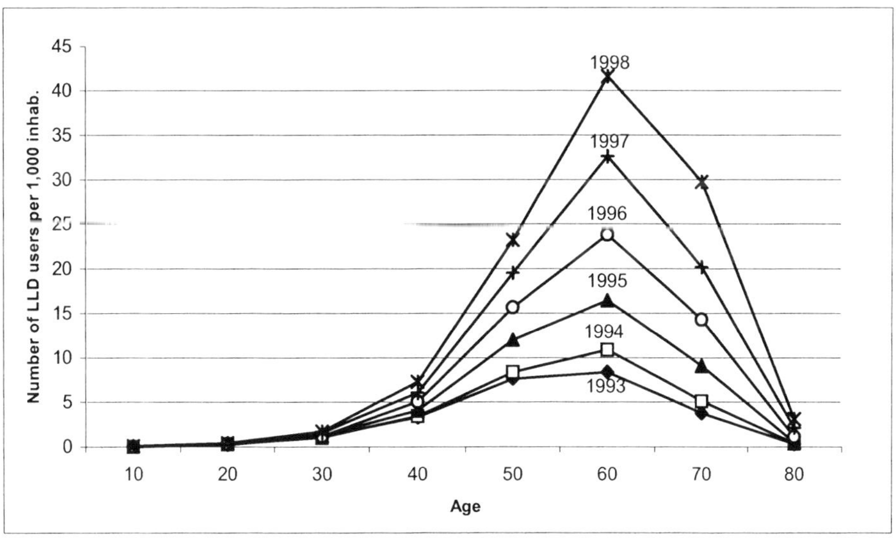


Figure 3. Age specific one-year prevalence of lipid-lowering drug use 1993-1998 in Funen County, Denmark

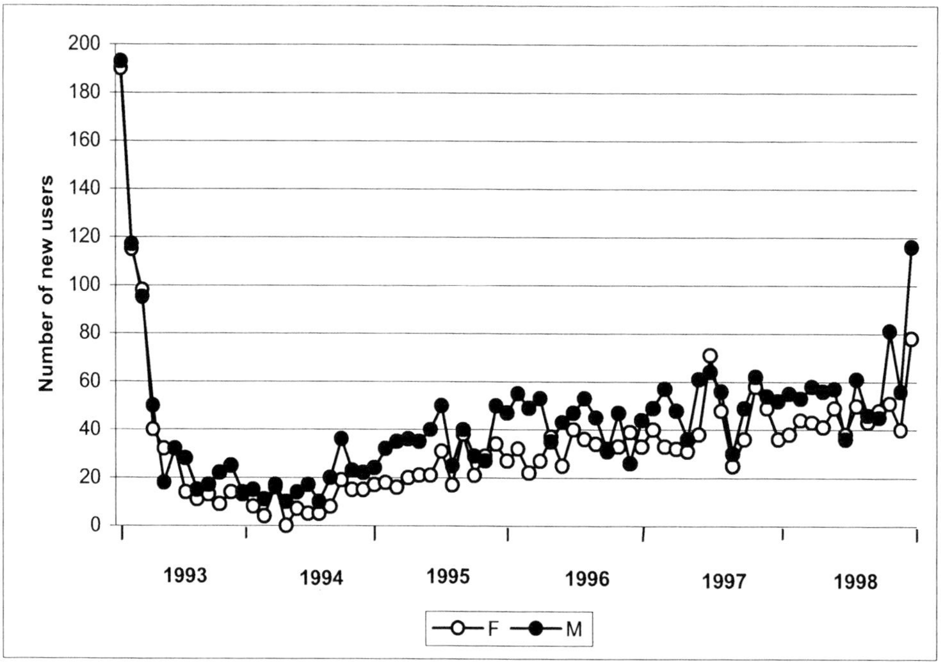


Figure 4. Number of lipid-lowering drug users (females and males) registered when they purchased the drugs for the first time in the period 1993-1998 in Funen County, Denmark. The columns represent prevalent as well as incident users. As a plateau is reached, they represent true incident users. This presentation justifies the use of a 12-month run-in period before a steady level of new users per month is reached.

**Table 2. Utilization of Statins in DDD per 1,000 Inhabitants per Day (DDD/TID) 1994-1998**

| | 1994 | 1995 | 1996 | 1997 | 1998 |
|---|---|---|---|---|---|
| Funen (reimbursed) | 1.7 | 2.7 | 4.4 | 6.2 | 9.0 |
| Funen (wholesale) | 1.7 | 2.9 | 4.5 | 6.5 | 9.2 |
| Denmark (wholesale) | 2.2 | 3.1 | 4.4 | 6.0 | 8.4 |

Data from Funen (reimbursed) compared to wholesale data from Funen and total Denmark

Among 3,623 incident statin users, 406 (11.2%) filled only one prescription in the study period. *Figure 5* shows the overall survival curve for statin treatment (persistence) for patients filling more than one prescription in their first period of treatment. Median persistence was 41 months. Table 3 shows the effect of six independent variables on persistence. The middle age group was used as reference. When adjusted for the other variables, there was no significant difference between males and females nor between the age group above 75 years and the reference group, whereas age <45 years predicted low persistence. *Figure 6* demonstrates the survival curves for persistence of statin treatment for patients stratified according to age and risk factor co-medication. Patients starting statin treatment in 1994 showed significantly lower persistence than patients starting in any of the following years. 95.1% of the incident statin users were 80% or more continuant within their first treatment period. When adjusted for the other variables, young age (<45 years) predicted a significantly lower continuity than the reference group (Table 3).

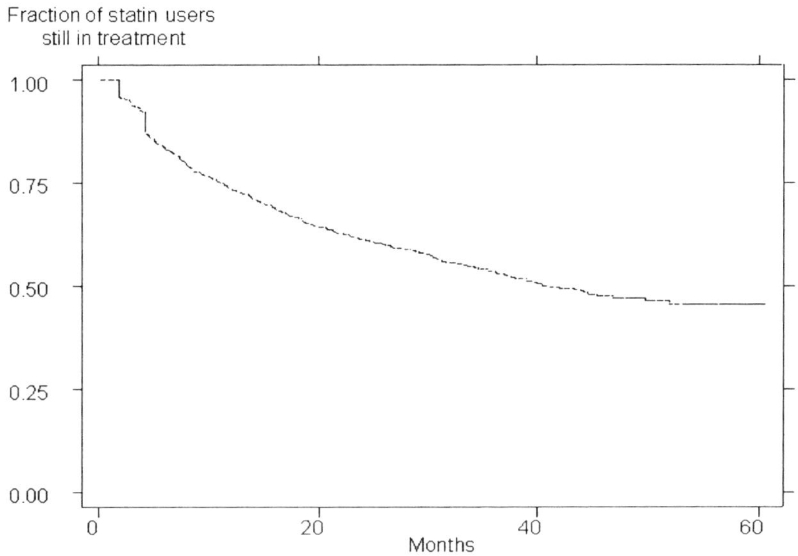


Figure 5. Overall persistence of statin treatment 1994-1998 in Funen County, Denmark (Kaplan-Meier survival estimate).

**Table 3. Persistence and continuity of statin treatment analysed by Cox's proportional hazards model and a logistic regression model. Relative risk of discontinuation and odds ratio of continuity <80% by sex, age <45 years, age 75+ years and risk factor co-medication**

| Variable | N | Persistence: Relative Risk of discontinuation | | P | Continuity: OR for low continuity (<80%) | | P |
|---|---|---|---|---|---|---|---|
| Sex | 3623 | 1.00 | (0.89 - 1.13) | 0.98 | 1.10 | (0.79 - 1.53) | 0.57 |
| Age 0-44 | 247 | 2.24 | (1.86 - 2.71) | <0.001 | 0.46 | (0.27 - 0.78) | <0.01 |
| Age 75+ | 168 | 1.15 | (0.87 - 1.53) | 0.323 | 1.17 | (0.47 - 2.92) | 0.74 |
| Cardiovascular co-med. | 2823 | 0.88 | (0.77 - 1.01) | 0.07 | 1.33 | (0.91 -1.95) | 0.14 |
| Insulin | 98 | 1.43 | (1.03 - 1.98) | 0.032 | 0.62 | (0.26 - 1.45) | 0.27 |
| Oral antidiabetics | 193 | 1.05 | (0.80 - 1.38) | 0.732 | 0.67 | (0.35 -1.27) | 0.22 |

The middle age group (i.e. 45-74 years) served as reference. (95% confidence intervals shown in brackets)

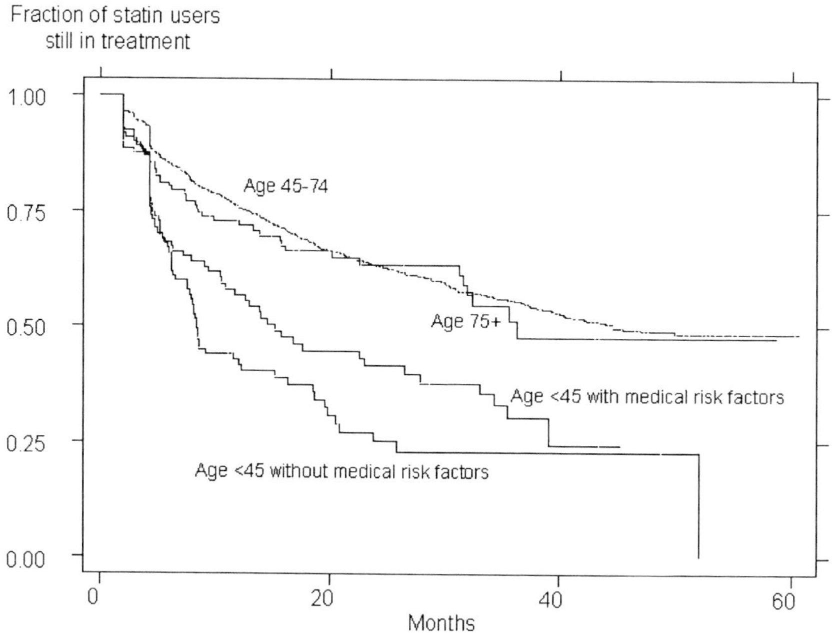


Figure 6. Persistence of statin treatment grouped by age >45 years without risk factor co-medication, age >44 years with risk factor co-medication and age 75+ years with and without risk factor co-medication compared with age group 45-74 years (Kaplan-Meier survival estimate).

Table 4 shows the average number and percentage of users over the years 1994-1996 specified by LLD group in Bologna, Italy and Funen, Denmark as average of the 3 years and the dose officially recommended in Denmark [60]. *Figure 7* shows the development in age-specific 1-year- prevalence for the two regions. Trends were similar for females and males in both regions. The waiting time distribution, showing similar patterns for the gender and age groups described, demonstrates a higher incidence in Bologna than in Funen (*Figure 8*), whereas the incidence in Funen increased, the incidence in Bologna showed a slightly decreasing trend. In Bologna, the number of patients who were co-treated with drugs indicating cardiovascular or diabetic co-morbidity was 62.2% in 1996. Table 5 shows persistence with LLDs in 1994-1996 in Funen and Bologna. The average number of DDD used per patient per year was closer to the expected 365 DDD/year for 100% continuity in Funen than in Bologna (*Figure 8*).

**Table 4. Average Number and Percentage of Users over the Years 1994-1996 Specified by LLD Group in Bologna, Italy and Funen, Denmark**

| | | Bologna | | Funen | | Recommended Dose | |
|---|---|---|---|---|---|---|---|
| | | N | % | N | % | mg | DDD |
| C10AA01 | Simvastatin | 6721 | 43.4 | 915 | 42.8 | 10 | 0.67 |
| | | | | | | 10-40* | 0.67-2.67* |
| C10AA02 | Lovastatin | | | 517 | 24.2 | 30 | 1.00 |
| C10AA03 | Pravastatin | 2383 | 15.4 | 314 | 14.7 | 15-20 | 0.75-1.00 |
| C10AA04 | Fluvastatin | 593 | 3.7 | 57 | 2.7 | 40 | 1.00 |
| *C10AA* | *Statins* | *9696* | *62.5* | *1803* | *84.4* | | |
| C10AB01 | Clofibrat | | | 7 | 0.3 | 2000 | 1.00 |
| C10AB02 | Bezafibrat | 1696 | 10.9 | 95 | 4.4 | 600 | 1.00 |
| C10AB04 | Gemfibrozil | 3022 | 19.6 | 96 | 4.5 | 1200 | 1.00 |
| C10AB05 | Fenofibrate | 388 | 2.5 | | | 300* | 1.00† |
| C10AB06 | Simfibrate | 1 | 0,0 | | | 750-1500* | 0.75-1.50† |
| *C10AB* | *Fibrates* | *5107* | *33.0* | *198* | *9.3* | | |
| C10AC01 | Colestyramin | 488 | 3.2 | 99 | 4.6 | 16000 | 1.14 |
| C10AC02 | Colestipol | | | 22 | 1.0 | 20000 | 1.00 |
| C10AC03 | Detaxtran | 181 | 1.2 | | | 2000-3000* | 0.80-1.20† |
| *C10AC* | *Resins* | *669* | *4.4* | *121* | *5.6* | | |
| C10AD05 | Nicotinyl alcohol | | | 4 | 0.2 | 900 | 0.96 |
| C10AD06 | Acipimox | | | 10 | 0.5 | 500 | 1.00 |
| *C10AD* | *Others* | | | *14* | *0.7* | | |
| *C10* | | *15473* | *100.0* | *2136* | *100.0* | | |

*Italian recommendations.

†DDD created by DURG-Italia, as no information was available from the WHO.

Doses recommended in official drug catalogues and corresponding number of DDD as of 1998 in Denmark

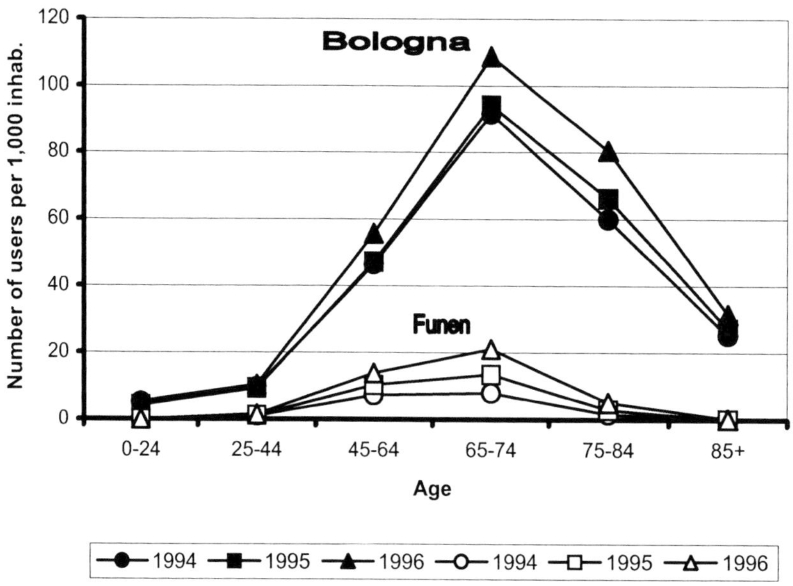


Figure 7. Age specific 1 year prevalence of LLD use in Bologna (closed symbols) and Funen (open symbols 1994-1996.

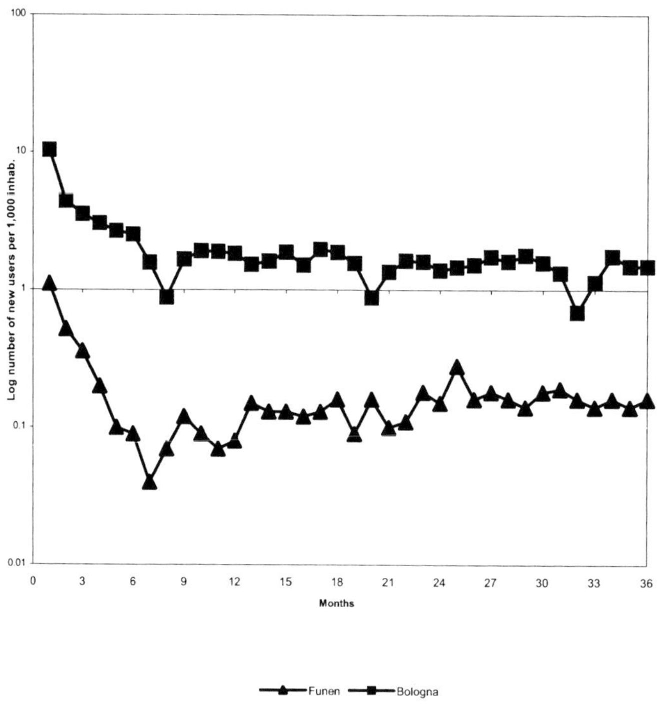


Figure 8. Waiting time distribution for LLD users, Funen and Bologna 1994-1996. Users were counted the first time they appeared in the time window. In the first 6 months, the curve represents prevalent users, and after 12 months, it represents incident users. Note that the scale for Funen figures is lower than that for Bologna figures by a factor of 10.

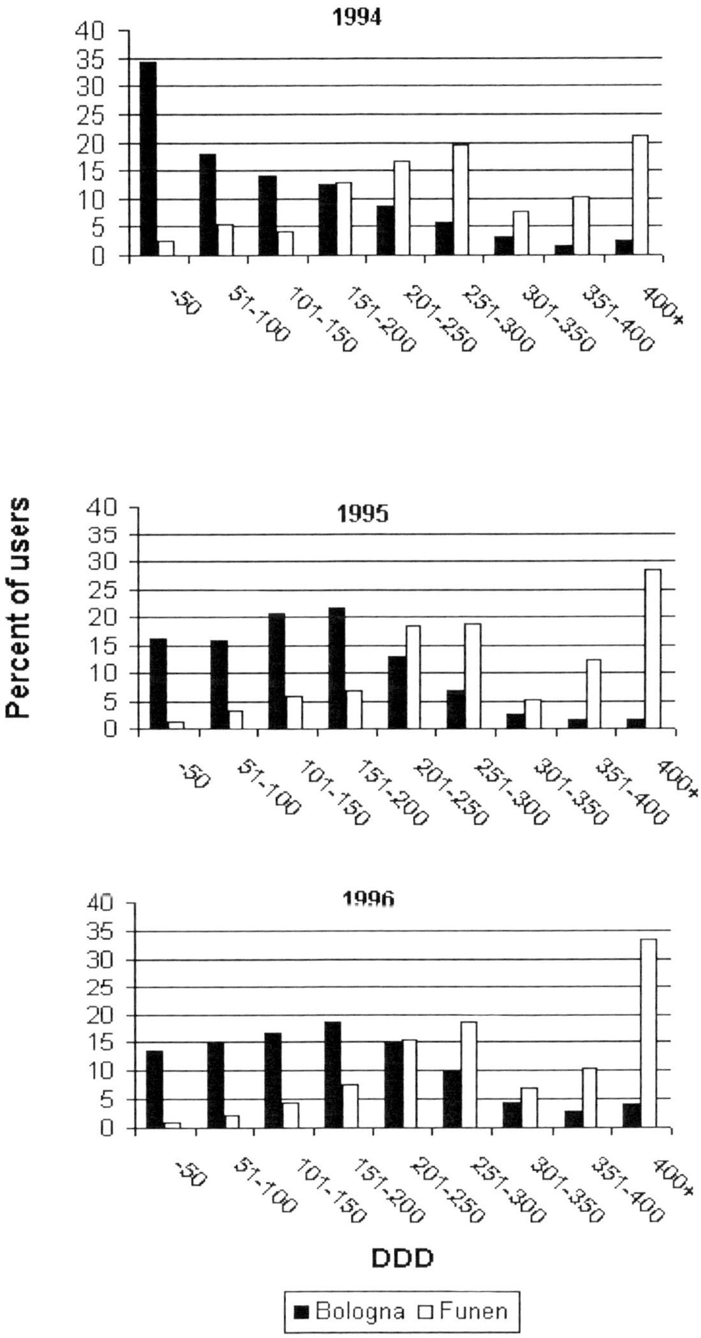
1994
1995
1996
Percent of users
0
5
10
15
20
25
30
35
40
-50
51-100
101-150
151-200
201-250
251-300
301-350
351-400
400+
DDD
Bologna
Funen

Figure 9. Distribution of annual LLD use (DDD/user/year) for selected populations prescribed a LLD in January for each of the years 1994-95-1996 in Bologne (n=3550-3434-4280) and Funen (n=517-635-1024).

**Table 5. Persistence with Lipid Lowering Drugs 1994-1996 in Funen and Bologna in Total and in Selected Strata**

| Variable | Funen | | | Bologna | | |
|---|---|---|---|---|---|---|
| | Persistent n | Total N | % Persistent (CI95%) | Persistent n | Total N | % Persistent (CI95%) |
| Total | 1204 | 1326 | 90,8 (89,1 - 92,3) | 5870 | 12360 | 47,5 (46,6 - 48,4) |
| Females | 552 | 604 | 91,4 (88,9 - 93,5) | 3861 | 7844 | 49,2 (48,1 - 50,3) |
| Males | 652 | 722 | 90,3 (87,9 - 92,4) | 2009 | 4616 | 43,5 (42,1 - 45,0) |
| 0-44 | 122 | 151 | 80,8 (73,6 - 86,7) | 200 | 1162 | 17,2 (15,1 - 19,5) |
| 45-64 | 750 | 809 | 92,7 (90,7 - 94,4) | 2356 | 4848 | 48,6 (47,2 - 50,0) |
| 65-74 | 298 | 324 | 92,0 (88,5 - 94,7) | 2618 | 4680 | 55,9 (54,5 - 57,4) |
| 75+ | 34 | 42 | 81,0 (65,9 - 91,4) | 696 | 1670 | 41,7 (39,3 - 44,1) |
| - Co-prescription | 462 | 524 | 88,2 (85,1 - 90,8) | 2200 | 5259 | 41,8 (40,5 - 43,2) |
| + Co-prescription | 742 | 802 | 92,5 (90,5 - 94,2) | 3670 | 7101 | 51,7 (50,5 - 52,9) |

Co-prescription with anti-diabetic or cardiovascular drugs.

## *Use of Lipid-lowering Drugs among Patients with Myocardial Infarction*

Among 1,296 patients who were hospitalised with an MI, 1,041 survived and were discharged (*Figure 10*). Twenty-three of these patients received LLDs before admission. A total of 265 (26%) of the remaining 1,018 started LLD treatment after their MI. *Figure 11* demonstrates time till initiation of LLD treatment as "Kaplan Meier survival plots", stratified according to age over and under 70. There was no difference between females and males in the time till initiation of LLD treatment.

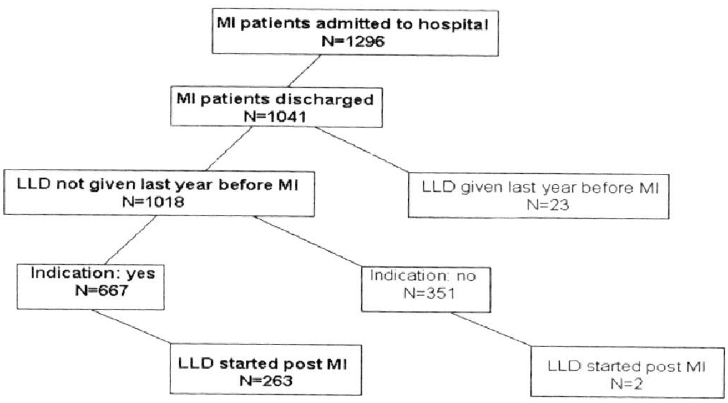


Figure 10. Number of patients admitted to and discharged from Odense University Hospital following myocardial infarction 1994-1997. Lipid-lowering drug treatment was considered to be indicated according to current reimbursement rules if the patient had at least one serum cholesterol value above 5.4 mmol/L from three months prior to MI and throughout the study period.

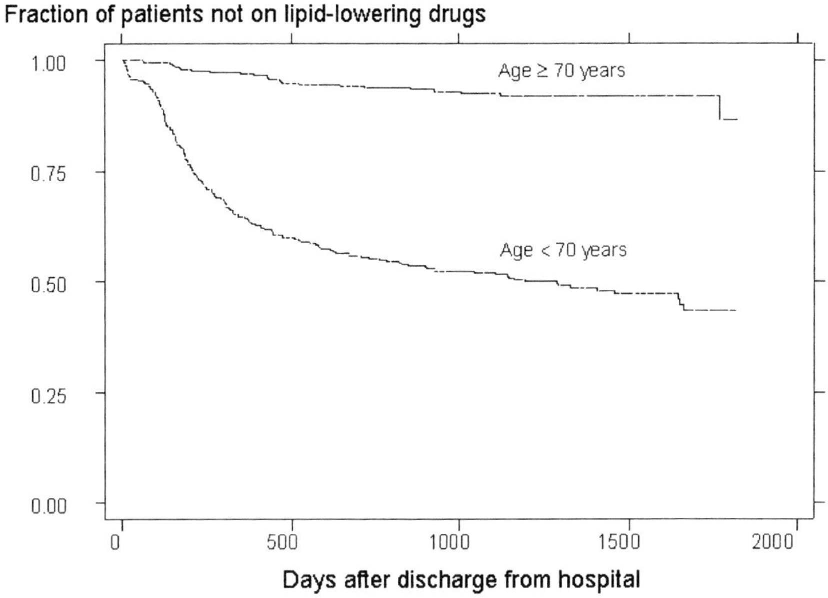


Figure 11. Time till initiation of lipid-lowering drug treatment among 1,018 patients discharged from hospital after myocardial infarction (Kaplan-Meier plot). Data were stratified by age under and over 70 years.

# General Discussion

The present study describes on an individual level and by means of population-based register data the long-term development of LLD utilisation in large populations covering the use and compliance of these drugs in specified subgroups of the populations studied.

## Principal Findings

The use of LLDs increased rapidly during the period 1993-1998, and statins accounted for more than 90% of the total LLD consumption. General practitioners prescribed the majority of LLDs. Compliance with statin use was high. 50% of the incident users stayed on the drugs continuously for more than three years. Younger patients without drug indicators of cardiovascular disease or diabetes presented the lowest compliance, their median persistence being less than one year. Among people with MI, total use of LLDs was low. The majority of the patients had their serum cholesterol measured, but only 39% of those having serum cholesterol above 5.4 mmol/L (lower limit for reimbursement) started treatment. In Bologna, LLD use was considerably higher than in Funen, and compliance substantially lower, indicating a higher degree of sporadic use in Italy.

## Strengths and Weaknesses of the Study

Drug utilisation studies provide a reasonably accurate view of usage patterns in everyday practice, which may differ from official recommendations [61]. Information on drug utilisation can be extracted from various sources: patients, pharmacy wholesale data, and individualised prescription databases. Allowing easy access to unbiased and detailed data, individualised prescription databases provide useful knowledge of drug utilisation. However, using this information, one must be aware of the strengths and weaknesses of the databases. This section addresses the advantages and disadvantages of the use of register data in the description of drug utilisation in general and the problems found in this study specifically: the advantages of using the Danish CPR register, the quality of the prescription data and other register data used in the study, and methodological problems concerning for example the definition of compliance and the measurement of duration of treatment.

### *Quality of Data*

From birth every Danish citizen is provided with a unique personal identification code, the CPR (Central Personal Registration) number, which is used to identify the individual for all kinds of public administrative purposes. Also, upon application, certain research registries are allowed to include people's CPR number. For instance, this is the case for regional prescription registries, and enables the study of prescription data over time on an individual level, which compared with studies based on aggregated data yields the option of describing drug utilisation more detailed. Furthermore, the CPR number makes it possible to link various registries of relevance to the study of drug utilisation, e.g. data on diagnoses on patients discharged from hospital, results of blood sample values, and data on prescriptions filled by individuals. Prescription databases usually cover large populations, enabling the research of even more rarely used drugs. Data are not subject to recall or interviewer bias; it allows the study of large and representative populations; the study can cover a relatively long observation time without high costs. The prescribing practice, holding a provider identification number, can be determined as well as the specialty of that provider.

A limitation of claims data with respect to characterising drug exposure is lack of information on indications for prescribing and prescribed daily doses. Other weaknesses include the fact that access to primary medical records is missing. A major point is the completeness of these databases. Completeness of drug data varies: for some databases, data are delivered by different health maintenance organisations (HMOs) covering various patient groups. In some databases, only reimbursed drugs are included, i.e. the possibility of studying various kinds of drugs varies with the specific reimbursement rules of the area/country studied. A drug that can be purchased OTC in Italy may qualify for reimbursement in Denmark. A drug may be reimbursed for the use on one indication and not on another. Individual subsidies for certain population groups not specified in the database can be difficult to handle. The individual physician within a certain practice cannot be identified as more physicians may share one provider number. The use of individualised prescription databases as opposed to wholesale statistics has made it possible to describe LLD utilisation in large populations in a natural setting. It was possible to describe duration of treatments as well as the amount of the drug collected by each individual.

All results in this study are based on register data. The validity of a register study highly depends on the completeness of data. Information on all LLD prescriptions filled in the study period in the whole of the Funen County could be retrieved. Data were delivered directly from all pharmacies in the county, and less than 1% of the study population filled LLD prescriptions outside the county [41]. The high validity of the OPED prescription database has previously been described in detail by Gaist et al. [55]. However, the use of LLDs may have been underestimated, since only reimbursed prescriptions are detected in the OPED database. The difference between wholesale data and OPED data showed that an average of 3% of statins used in the period 1994-1998 was purchased without reimbursement, and the problem is therefore negligible. The use of anti-diabetic drugs and cardiovascular co-medication as indicators of diabetes and cardiovascular diasease revealed some limitations. Using only anti-diabetic drugs leads to an underestimation of the LLDs used for secondary prevention, as no estimate of the number of diabetics that were dietarily controlled was available. On the other hand, the use of some of the co-medication as being used for cardiovascular purposes may have been overestimated. For instance, diuretics may have been intended for leg oedema of non-cardiac origin. Unfortunately, it was not possible to determine the specific use of the drugs, as information on indications was not available, nor did any of the two prescription databases used in this study hold information on prescribed daily dose (PDD), which information together with a count of the number of doses ingested by patients within a particular time-frame would be the ideal for compliance studies. As no such data were available, results had to rely on approximations. Further, using DDD as a measure in the compliance calculations in the Funen-Bologna comparison presents a weakness, as DDD may poorly reflect an actual daily use of a certain drug. This method clearly underestimated LLD compliance in both regions. The variations of DDD for the various drugs cannot, however, possibly account for the entire six-fold higher compliance calculated in Funen. If serum cholesterols were generally lower in Bologna this would probably lead to more prescribing of smaller than recommended doses. However, as the mortality rate from cardiovascular diseases is even slightly higher in Bologna than in Funen (5.51 versus 4.82/ 1,000 inhabitants/year) there is no reason to believe that this should be so. As the compliance results based on the DDD methodology may be regarded somewhat artificial, and as tablets come in all clinically relevant strengths, it seemed unlikely that a patient took for instance half a tablet or two tablets a day and compliance with statin use was therefore calculated under the assumption of the use of one tablet a day as the basic unit, whatever strength.

Information about hospitalisation due to acute MI (codes I21.0-I21.9 according to the ICD-10 coding system) 1994 to 1997 was retrieved from the regional patients' registry. The validity of these data depends on the correct coding by hospital personnel. Since 1977 data from this register have been included in The Danish National Hospital Register [54], and are, hence, subject to the quality demands in force for this register. A validation study showed that 75-90% of the diagnoses registered were correct [55]. In the present study, the assumption was that misclassification would tend to leave out real MIs rather than to include other diseases as MIs. As only those, but all of them, coded as MIs were included in the calculations, a misclassification was not assumed to present a problem for the results.

Valid data on serum cholesterols were available only from one of the two departments of clinical chemistry analysing serum cholesterols in Funen County, i.e. the department at Odense University Hospital. Within the uptake area of the hospital, completeness is nearly 100%, also covering serum samples sent in by the general practitioners of the area (personal communication with head of the department Palle Wang, March 2000). However, follow-up may be missing and the total number of serum cholesterol measurements may thus have been underestimated, as patients could have moved from their original municipality to one, where doctors had serum cholesterols analysed at the laboratory not included in this study.

### *Definitions of Compliance*

A serious problem concerns the definition of compliance, especially when it comes to comparing results from one study with another, as definitions vary substantially between studies. In this study, definitions were chosen that were 1) "handy" to work with according to the options of the databases used, 2) at most comparable with recent major studies of compliance, and 3) as close to a natural setting as possible.

In order to obtain a realistic setting, it seemed reasonable to define *discontinuation* of a treatment period from a clinical point of view. The effect of simvastatin on serum cholesterol has been reported to return to pre-treatment level 5 weeks after withdrawal [64]. Thus, a 30-day period without statin supply was chosen to define discontinuation of treatment. This, naturally, underestimates persistence compared with a method using a longer period without supply.

For practical reasons, more crude measures of persistence and continuity were used in the Funen-Bologna comparative study: identifying all individuals treated in 1994 who were still on a lipid-lowering drug in 1995 and 1996 assessed persistence of LLD use during 1994-1996.

## Results Compared with Other Studies

Despite the marked increase in prevalence during the study period reaching about 1% of the total population, this constitutes only two thirds of the level expected by the expert group in 1997 (secondary prevention only) [28]. This expert estimate, based on the assumption that 250,000 Danish persons out of the total population of approximately 5 million were suffering from ischaemic heart disease in 1994, was subject to considerable uncertainty and may have been overestimated in order to create a 'worst case scenario' for the decision about general reimbursement of LLDs in Denmark. In this study, a relatively higher number of younger than elderly persons and more males than females started LLD treatment. Few old patients received lipid-lowering drugs. This contrasts the data from Italy [40] and Germany [51], where more people above the age of 80 were treated. Lipid-lowering treatment in the elderly is still controversial [65], although the elderly have been shown to benefit from cholesterol lowering in both 4S and WOSCOPS [12;13]. The findings regarding sex differences are consistent with results reported from the US [66], Ireland [67] and Finland [68], but contradictory to results from South Africa [69]. In the past, the difference in coronary risk between the sexes has meant that treatment of women has often been withheld, but there is no reason why the effect of lowering serum lipids should be different in women and men [9]. In contrast to the present study, Juul et al found in 1995 that 15% of all LLDs were purchased without reimbursement [27], but they did not take into account the number of prescriptions reimbursed retroactively. The fraction of LLD prescriptions issued by general practitioners was 20% lower than that estimated from total drug prescribing (number of prescriptions and DDD) in general practice [55;70], probably as a consequence of the treatments being started during hospitalisation. It is noteworthy that general practitioners initiated relatively more LLD treatments in females and in elderly patients than hospital doctors did. The difference observed may be due to a high female to male and elderly to younger persons contact ratio in general practice [63], so that the finding may not express a real difference in the attitude towards starting LLD treatment in females and the elderly.

According to the definition of the study cohort in the Funen-Bologna study, only persons staying alive during the whole study period were included. This selection may have biased the results leading to overestimation of compliance and underestimation of prevalence as persons treated with LLDs are supposed to live longer. Considering this fact, Italian results may differ even more from the North American results.

Of all lipid-lowering drugs, Avorn et al found the highest one-year continuation rate for statins (64% days covered) [29]. In Australia, Simons et al found a 60% discontinuation after 12 months [31], contrasting the discontinuation rate of 30% after 6 to 7 months recently found by the same main author [34]. In a controlled trial, Eriksson et al [33] found nearly 90% continuation of pravastatin treatment in a two-year closely followed-up study in Sweden. The study cohort was highly selected, and furthermore, it is well-known that patients participating in controlled trials comply better with medication compared with patients observed in a natural setting.

Although the incidence of ischaemic heart disease has declined over the past 20 years [72], this study still shows an average incidence of MI of 1.5 per 1.000 inhabitants per year. In countries with higher use of lipid-lowering drugs than in Denmark, it has previously been shown that use in patients with ischaemic heart disease was low [23-25;73-75], indicating that LLD use in those countries is not targeted at high risk patients. This study showed that a very low fraction of elderly patients started treatment, which may reflect the current controversy of monitoring serum cholesterol and treating this part of the population [7-10;35;36].

Not surprisingly, the status of reimbursement regimens tends to influence consumption of LLDs to a considerable extent. In Italy after changing full reimbursement up till 1993 to co-payment for prescriptions exceeding a number of 16 per year, consumption decreased from 11.5 to 10.4 DDD/1,000 inhabitants/day [26]. Again, after restricting the fully reimbursed part of LLDs to the indication of familial hyperlipidemia with high levels of cholesterol or triglycerides and full patient's payment for other indications, consumption further decreased to 6.7 DDD/1,000 inhabitants/day. The influence of the restrictions was, however, rather transient, as consumption increased again to reach 9.2 (12.5 in Bologna) DDD/1,000 inhabitants/day in 1996 without any change of the reimbursement rules. In Denmark, consumption has been low compared to other countries. Reimbursement (75%) – remaining unchanged until December 1998 – has been restricted to secondary prevention of ischaemic heart disease, failing effect of dietary intervention and only after individual application from the patient's physician. In Italy, restrictions with reimbursement rules showed only temporary impact on consumption, a pattern also seen in other countries [68]. It is not certain that one could assume the same reaction to change of reimbursement rules in Danish patients (and doctors) as in Italian. It is possible that the low Danish consumption is due to the rather restrictive reimbursement rules, and also that consumption may increase if restrictions were eased. As of mid December 1998 reimbursement rules have been eased in Denmark, so that no individual application is needed for the use of LLDs for secondary prevention, although still needed for primary prevention.

Usually, it is estimated that general practitioners issue 90% of all prescriptions (all drugs). In the present study general practitioners prescribed approximately only 70% of the LLDs. This may be explained by the fact that treatment with these drugs is relatively often initiated during hospitalisation.

## Conclusion

The present study has shown:

- that LLD use was low in the beginning of the nineties in the general population but has increased substantially over the period 1993-1998. The use of statins has increased nearly exponentially and now makes up more than 90% of the lipid-lowering drugs used. After publication of especially the 4S study in 1994, utilisation has at least quantitatively approached a level corresponding to the number of people in the general population, who need treatment according to current recommendations. The majority of patients treated with LLDs had drug indicators of cardiovascular risk factors. General practitioners issued 73% of the total number of LLD prescriptions. The present study has shown good compliance with statin treatment in a Danish population measured by persistence as well as by continuity. However, a high percentage of the youngest group of patients without drug indicators of cardiac disease or diabetes discontinued treatment before obtaining the full benefit in terms of decreased risk of coronary heart morbidity and mortality;
- that contrary to Denmark, LLD use in Italy was characterised by high consumption, prevalence and incidence but low persistence in the period 1994 to 1996;
- that among patients with a history of myocardial infarction who met the criteria for LLD reimbursement, far too few were actually treated. Therefore, more attention is needed to initiate treatment in these patients.

## Unanswered Questions and Future Research

We need to examine to what extent non-compliance influences morbidity and mortality of CHD and to assess expenses for society. We need further clinical investigations to uncover the degree to which the apparent compliance problems are due to doctors' non-compliance with guidelines or due to patients' non-compliance with the prescribed medicine. We need studies concentrating on compliance with LLDs under other compliance definitions in natural settings (primary non-compliance by comparing doctors' prescriptions with patients' fillings from prescription registries, and secondary non-compliance, e.g. from patient interviews etc.). We further need to analyse LLD consumption and compliance following the changes in reimbursement rules, especially concerning LLD treatment for secondary prevention, and to investigate diverging compliance in different health care systems.

# References


[1] Steinberg D, Gotto AM, Jr. Preventing coronary artery disease by lowering cholesterol levels: fifty years from bench to bedside. *JAMA* 1999;282:2043-2050.

[2] Moore TJ. The Cholesterol Myth. *The Atlantic Monthly* 1989;264:37-66.

[3] Rose G, Shipley M. Plasma cholesterol concentration and death from coronary heart disease: 10 year results of the Whitehall study. *Br Med J Clin Res Ed.* 1986;293:306-307.

[4] Martin MJ, Browner WS, Hulley SB, Kuller SH, Wentworth W. Serum cholesterol, blood pressure, and mortality. *Lancet* 1986;ii:933-936.

[5] Anderson KM, Castelli WP, Levy D. Cholesterol and mortality. 30 years of follow-up from the Framingham study. *JAMA* 1987;257:2176-2180.

[6] Kromhout D, Bosschieter EB, Drijver M, de-Lezenne CC. Serum cholesterol and 25-year incidence of and mortality from myocardial infarction and cancer. The Zutphen Study. *Arch Intern Med* 1988;148:1051-1055.

[7] Forrester JS, Shah PK. Using serum cholesterol as a screening test for preventing coronary heart disease: the five fundamental flaws of the American College of Physicians Guidelines. *Am J Cardiol* 1997;79:790-792.

[8] Krumholz HM, Seeman TE, Merrill SS, Mendes-de LC, Vaccarino V, Silverman DI *et al.* Lack of association between cholesterol and coronary heart disease mortality and morbidity and all-cause mortality in persons older than 70 years. *JAMA* 1994;272:1335-1340.

[9] Bhatnagar D. Lipid-lowering drugs in the management of hyperlipidaemia. *Pharmacol.Ther.* 1998;79:205-230.

[10] Haycox A, Barton S, Walley T. Cost effectiveness of lowering cholesterol. Study did not take account of confounders. *BMJ* 1996;313:1142-1143.

[11] Plosker GL, Wagstaff AJ. Fluvastatin: a review of its pharmacology and use in the management of hypercholesterolaemia. *Drugs* 1996;51:433-459.

[12] The Scandinavian Simvastatin Survival Study Group. Randomised trial of cholesterol lowering in 4444 patients with coronary heart disease: the Scandinavian Simvastatin Survival Study (4S). *Lancet* 1994;344:1383-1389.

[13] Shepherd J, Cobbe SM, Ford I, Isles CG, Lorimer AR, MacFarlane PW *et al.* Prevention of coronary heart disease with pravastatin in men with hypercholesterolemia. West of Scotland Coronary Prevention Study Group. *N.Engl J Med* 1995;333:1301-1307.

[14] Davis BR, Cutler JA, Gordon DJ, Furberg CD, Wright JT, Cushman WC, et al. Rationale and Design for the Antihypertensive and Lipid Lowering Treatment to Prevent Heart Attack Trial (ALLHAT). *AJH* 1996;9:342-60.

[15] Lindholm LH, Ekbom T, Dash C, Isacsson Å, Scherstén B. Changes in cardiovascular risk factors by combined pharmacological and nonpharmacological strategies: the main results of the CELL Study. *J Int Med* 1996;240:13-22.

[16] Sacks FM, Pfeffer MA, Moye LA, Rouleau JL, Rutherford JD, Cole TG *et al.* The effect of pravastatin on coronary events after myocardial infarction in patients with average cholesterol levels. Cholesterol and Recurrent Events Trial investigators. *N Engl J Med* 1996;335:1001-1009.

[17] The Long-Term Intervention with Pravastatin in Ischaemic Disease (LIPID) Study Group. Prevention of cardiovascular events and death with pravastatin in patients with coronary heart disease and a broad range of initial cholesterol levels. *N Engl J Med* 1998;339:1349-1357.

[18] Downs JR, Clearfield M, Weis S, Whitney E, Shapiro DR, Beere PA *et al.* Primary prevention of acute coronary events with lovastatin in men and women with average cholesterol levels: results of AFCAPS/TexCAPS. Air Force/Texas Coronary Atherosclerosis Prevention Study. *JAMA* 1998;279:1615-1622.

[19] Sever PS, Dahlöf B, Poulter NR, Wedel H, Beevers G, Caulfield M, et al. Prevention of coronary and stroke events with atorvastatin in hypertensive patients who have average or lower-than-average cholesterol concentrations, in the Anglo-Scandinavian Cardiac Outcomes trial – Lipid Lowering Arm (ASCOTT-LLA): a multicentre randomised controlled trial. *Lancet* 2003;361:1149-58.

[20] Kristianson K, Fyhrquist F, Devereux RB, Kjeldsen SE, Lindholm LH, Lyle PA, et al. An Analysis of Cholesterol Control and Statin Use in the Losartan Intervention for Endpoint Reduction in Hypertension Study. *Clin Ther* 2003;(?):1186-99.

[21] Heart Protection Study Collaboratory Group. MRC/BHF Heart Protection Study of cholesterol lowering with simvastatin in 20536 high-risk individuals: a randomised placebocontrolled trial. *Lancet* 2002;360:7-22.

[22] Shepherd J, Blauw GJ, Murphy MB, Bollen ELEM, Buckley BM, Cobbe SM, et al. Pravastatin in elderly individuals at risk of vascular disease (PROSPER): a randomised controlled trial. *Lancet* 2002;360:1623-30.

[23] Majumdar SR, Gurwitz JH, Soumerai SB. Undertreatment of hyperlipidemia in the secondary prevention of coronary artery disease. *J Gen Intern Med* 1999;14:711-717.

[24] Primatesta P, Poulter NR. Lipid concentrations and the use of lipid lowering drugs: evidence from a national cross sectional survey. *BMJ* 2000;321:1322-1325.

[25] Khan M, Mukkamala A, Taylor DK, Espinosa A, Duff J. Use of lipid lowering drugs with acute myocardial infarction patients: An examination of physician prescribing behaviors. *J Cardiovasc Pharmacol Ther* 1998;3:217-222.

[26] Magrini N, Einarson T, Vaccheri A, McManus P, Montanaro N, Bergman U. Use of lipid-lowering drugs from 1990 to 1994: an international comparison among Australia, Finland, Italy (Emilia Romagna Region), Norway and Sweden. *Eur J Clin Pharmacol* 1997;53:185-189.

[27] Aarup A-L, Juul KV. Consumption of cholesterol-lowering drugs. The Danish Medicines' Agency's drug data November 1995. *Copenhagen: Danish Medicines' Agency*, 1995.

[28] Hvidberg E, Haghfelt T, Husted SE, Jensen G, Nielsen I. [Report on cholesterol lowering drugs in relation to national insurance reimbursement.]. 2nd edition, *Copenhagen: Danish Medicines' Agency*, 1997.

[29] Avorn J, Monette J, Lacour A, Bohn RL, Monane M, Mogun H *et al*. Persistence of use of lipid-lowering medications: a cross-national study. *JAMA* 1998;279:1458-1462.

[30] Andrade SE, Walker AM, Gottlieb LK, Hollenberg NK, Testa MA, Saperia GM *et al*. Discontinuation of antihyperlipidemic drugs--do rates reported in clinical trials reflect rates in primary care settings? *N Engl J Med* 1995;332:1125-1131.

[31] Simons LA, Levis G, Simons J. Apparent discontinuation rates in patients prescribed lipid-lowering drugs. *Med J Aust* 1996;164:208-211.

[32] Beck P, Downey W, Butler-Jones D, Lueck L. Pharmaceutical costs of patient non-adherence to lipid-lowering drug therapy. Presented at the *Third Annual International Meeting of the International Society for Pharmacoeconomics and Outcomes Research (ISPOR)* May 27-30, 1998.

[33] Eriksson M, Hadell K, Holme I, Walldius G, Kjellstrom T. Compliance with and efficacy of treatment with pravastatin and cholestyramine: a randomized study on lipid-lowering in primary care. *J Intern Med* 1998;243:373-380.

[34] Simons LA, Simons J McManus P Dudley J. Discontinuation rates are high. *BMJ* 2000; 321:1084.

[35] Mendelson G, Aronow WS. Underutilization of measurement of serum low-density lipoprotein cholesterol levels and of lipid-lowering therapy in older patients with manifest atherosclerotic disease. *J Am Geriatr Soc* 1998;46:1128-1131.

[36] Garber AM. Cholesterol screening should be targeted. *Am J Med* 1997;102:26-30.

[37] Pearson TA, Laurora I, Chu H, Kafonek S. The lipid treatment assessment project (L-TAP): a multicenter survey to evaluate the percentages of dyslipidemic patients receiving lipid- lowering therapy and achieving low-density lipoprotein cholesterol goals. *Arch Intern Med* 2000;160:459-467.

[38] Larsen J. Lipid-lowering drugs. Pharmacoepidemiological studies on prescription patterns in general practice. (PhD-dissertation) Copenhagen 2002.

[39] Bergman U, Andersen M, Vaccheri A, Larsen J, Montanaro N. Marked differences in lipid-lowering drug use in Bologna, Italy and Funen Denmark. *Eur Heart J* 1999;20: 1135.

[40] Larsen J, Vaccheri A, Andersen M, Montanaro N, Bergman U. Lack of adherence to lipid-lowering drug treatment. A comparison of utilisation patterns in defined populations i Funen, Denmark and Bologna, Italy. *Br J Clin Pharmacol* 2000;49:463-471.

[41] Larsen J, Andersen M, Gram L, Kragstrup J. Changes in the utilization of lipid-lowering drugs over a six-year period (1993-1998) in a Danish population. *Eur J Clin Pharm* 2001;57:343-348.

[42] Larsen J, Andersen M, Kragstrup J, Gram LF. High persistence of statin use in a Danish population: Compliance study 1993-1998. *Br J Clin Pharmacol* 2002;53(4): 375-378.

[43] Larsen J, Andersen M, Bjerrum L, Kragstrup J, Gram LF. Insufficient use of lipid lowering drugs correlated to serum cholesterol values among people with myocardial infarction 1994-1997 in a Danish population. *J Cardiovasc Risk* 2003;10(1):61-4.

[44] *www.uptodate.com*. Last updated April 21 2001, Ed: Rosenson, RS, Northwestern University School. 2001.

[45] Wood D, Backer Guy de, Faergeman O, Graham I, Mancia G, Pyörälä K et al. Prevention of coronary heart disease in clinical practice. Recommendations of the Second Joint Task Force of European and other Societies on Coronary Prevention. *Eur.Heart J.* 1998;19:1434-1503.

[46] Rosser WW, Palmer WH. Dissemination of guidelines on cholesterol. Effect on patterns of practice of general practitioners and family physicians in Ontario. Ontario Task Force on the Use and Provision of Medical Services. *Can Fam Physician* 1993;39:280.

[47] Hansen HS, Haghfelt T. [Drug treatment of dyslipidaemia] Medikamentel behandling af dyslipidæmi. Lægemiddelhåndbogen, Odense University Press. *Odense* 2002.

[48] Bjerrum L, Larsen J, Kragstrup J. Guidelines accompanied by changes of reimbursement rules. Effects on lipid-lowering drug prescribing. *Scand J Prim Health Care* 2001;19:158-162.

[49] Oliver MF. Statins prevent coronary heart disease. *Lancet* 1995;346:1378-1379.

[50] Nielsen PE, McNair A, Rasmussen S, Pedersen FH. [The Medical Products Agency's new guidelines on complements to medical treatment of hypercholesterolemia] Laegemiddelstyrelsens nye retningslinjer for tilskud til medikamental behandling af hyperkolesterolaemi. *Ugeskr Laeger* 1998;160:4665-4667.

[51] Krappweis J, Aumann D, Rentsch A, Kirch W. The Prescribing of lipid lowering drugs during a 1-year period: Analysis of 7490 health insurance files. *Pharmacoepidemiology and Drug Safety* 2000;9(2):119-125.

[52] Carvajal A, del Pozo JG, Rodriguez MB, Arias LHM, de Castro AMR. Utilisation of lipid-lowering drugs in Spain between 1986 and 1998. *Clinical Drug Investigation* 2000;20:197-201.

[53] Holm-Nielsen N. ed. [*Clinical dictionary*] Klinisk Ordbog. 15th edition, Copenhagen: Munksgaard, 1999.

[54] Zwisler JE, Larsen J, Kragstrup J, Gram LF. Discontinuation of drug therapy started in general practice – Recommendations and evidence. *Odense*, 2004 (Manuscript).

[55] Gaist D, Sorensen HT, Hallas J. The Danish prescription registries. *Dan Med Bull* 1997;44:445-448.

[56] WHO Collaborating Centre for Drug Statistics Methodology, Oslo Norway. *ATC index with DDDs*, 1998.

[57] Montanaro N, Vaccheri A, Magrini N, Battilana M. FARMAGUIDA: a databank for the analysis of the Italian drug market and drug utilization in general practice. *Eur J Clin Pharmacol* 1992;42:395-399.

[58] Web site of the Regional Government of Emilia Romagna by February 1999: *www.regione.emilia-romagna.it/sas/statistica/*. 1999.

[59] Hallas J, Gaist D, Bjerrum, L. The waiting time distribution as a graphical approach to epidemiologic measures of drug utilization. *Epidemiology* 1997;8:666-670.

[60] Aldershvile J, Hansen MS, Kampmann JP, Vej-Hansen B. Lægeforeningens Medicinfortegnelse 1998. *Copenhagen: Lægeforeningen*, 1998:213.

[61] Leufkens HG, Urquhart J. Variability in patterns of drug usage. *J Pharm Pharmacol* 1994;46 Suppl 1:433-437.

[62] Andersen TF, Madsen M, Jørgensen J, Mellemkjær L, Olsen JH. The Danish National Hospital Register. A valuable source of data for modern health sciences. *DMB* 1999;46:263-272.

[63] Mosbech J, Jørgensen J, Madsen M, Rostgaard K, Thornberg K, Poulsen TD. The national patient registry. Evaluation of data quality. [Landspatientregisteret. Evaluering af datakvaliteten]. *Ugeskr.Laeger* 1995;157(26):3741-3745.

[64] Sampietro T, Galetta F, and Bionda A. Behavior of Lp(a) and apoproteins (A1, B, C2, C3, E) during and after therapy with simvastatin. *Cardiovasc Drugs Ther.* 1995;9:785-789.

[65] Corti MC, Guralnik JM, Salive ME, Harris T, Ferrucci L, Glynn RJ, Havlik RJ. Clarifying the direct relation between total cholesterol levels and death from coronary heart disease in older persons. *Ann Intern Med* 1997;126:753-760.

[66] Lemaitre RN, Furberg CD, Newman AB, Hulley SB, Gordon DJ, Gottdiener JS *et al.* Time trends in the use of cholesterol-lowering agents in older adults: the Cardiovascular Health Study. *Arch Intern Med* 1998;158:1761-1768.

[67] Feely J, McGettigan P, Kelly A. Growth in use of statins after trials is not targeted to most appropriate patients. *Clin Pharmacol Ther* 2000;67:438-441.

[68] Martikainen J, Klaukka T, Reunanen A, Peura S, Wahlroos H. Recent trends in the consumption of lipid-lowering drugs in Finland. *J Clin Epidemiol* 1996;49:1453-1457.

[69] Truter I,.Kotze TJ. A drug utilisation study investigating prescribed daily doses of hypolipidaemic agents. *S Afr Med J* 1996;86:1397-1401.

[70] Website of the Danish Medicines Agency June 2000*: www.medicinpriser.dk/docushare/dscgi/ds.py/View /Collection-154*. 2000.

[71] Hollnagel, H., Nørrelund, N., and Schroll, H. eds. [General health problems. A textbook in family medicine.]. *Copenhagen-Aarhus-Odense FADL*: 1987.

[72] Osler M, Sorensen TI, Sorensen S, Rostgaard K, Jensen G, Iversen L *et al.* Trends in mortality, incidence and case fatality of ischaemic heart disease in Denmark, 1982-1992. *Int J Epidemiol* 1996;25:1154-1161.

[73] Abookire, SA, Karson, AS, Fiskio, J, and Bates, DW. Use and monitoring of "statin" lipid-lowering drugs compared with guidelines. *Arch Intern Med* 2001;161(1):53-58.

[74] Silber S, Krischke I, and Prohaska M. Undertreatment in secondary prevention of patients with coronary heart disease after revascularization. *Herz* 2000;25(6):623-626.

[75] Ergin A, Abaci A, Sakalli A, Eryol NK, Oguzhan A, Unal S, Cetin S. Pharmacological profile of survivors of acute myocardial infarction at Turkish academic hospitals. *Int J Cardiol.* 1999;68(3):309-316.

In: Cholesterol in Atherosclerosis and Coronary Heart Disease ISBN 1-59454-302-X
Editor: Jean P. Kovala, pp.187-213 

*Chapter IX*

# The Cholesterol Lowering Effect of Plant Sterols

***Elizabeth J. Brink and Henk F.J. Hendriks****

TNO Nutrition and Food Research, Physiological Sciences Department, the Netherlands

## Abstract

Products enriched with plant sterols and plant stanols either in its esterified or unesterified form have demonstrated to be effective in cholesterol lowering. This paper presents a review of literature on cholesterol lowering effects of plant sterols and plant stanols. Dosages of 1.5-2.5 per day reduce total cholesterol up to 10% and LDL cholesterol up to 16%. The mean reduction in LDL cholesterol is about 10% which on a population basis may result in a 20% risk reduction for coronary heart disease. Sterols and stanols seem to be equally effective. Factors possibly influencing the magnitude of the cholesterol lowering effect being esterification, food matrix, composition of the background diet, moment of consumption and blood cholesterol concentration are addressed. Plant sterols and stanols are not only effective in normo- and mildly hypercholesterolaemic subjects, but also in hypercholesterolaemic subjects receiving cholesterol lowering therapies. No effects are observed on HDL cholesterol and triacylglycerol level. Plant sterols and stanols are poorly absorbed and plasma concentrations are low, except in subjects with a rare inherited disorder phytosterolaemia. Safety of plant sterols and stanols has been extensively tested and no adverse effects seem to be present, although there is a lack of chronic exposure data. Consumption of plant sterols and stanols results in a substantial reduction of carotenoid levels. The implication of this reduction for human health on the long term is not clear. With the growing number of enriched products entering the market the consumption of plant sterols and stanols should be monitored. An intake not exceeding 1-3 g per day is

---

* TNO Nutrition and Food Research, Physiological Sciences Department, P.O. Box 360, 3700 AJ Zeist, The Netherlands. Tel.: +31 69 44 144; fax: +31 69 44 928; e-mail: L.Brink@voeding.tno.nl

adviced. A follow-up of samples from the general population eating plant sterol and stanol enriched foods by post marketing surveillance techniques is important to evaluate both the beneficial as well as the adverse effects on the very long term.

# Introduction

One of the major modifiable risk factors for coronary heart disease mortality is blood cholesterol concentration [Stamler et al., 2000]. Several large scale intervention trials have shown that cholesterol lowering drug therapy in hypercholesterolaemic patients beneficially affects coronary heart disease mortality risk [Gould et al., 1998]. Blood cholesterol concentrations also may be modulated by changes in the intake of dietary fat and cholesterol [Tang et al., 1998]. Mildly hypercholesterolaemic subjects usually have dietary guidelines prescribed as a first treatment to lower their blood cholesterol. The National Cholesterol Education Program diet used in the US typically lowers LDL-concentrations by 3-10% [taken from Maki et al., 2001]. Also normocholesterolaemic subjects may apply such diets as a part of a healthy life-style. However, the percentage reduction in blood cholesterol attributable to dietary advice is modestly effective in free-living subjects and may be not a sufficient reduction for persons with mild-to-moderate hypercholesterolaemia to reach their LDL cholesterol goal. A well established dietary factor that lowers blood cholesterol concentrations is linoleic acid when compared with other more saturated types of fatty acids or carbohydrates [Keys et al., 1965; Mensink & Katan, 1992; Katan et al., 1994]. Since the 1950s the cholesterol lowering properties of plant sterols have been known [Pollak, 1953; Farquhar et al., 1956].

Plant sterols are naturally occurring plant compounds that are not synthesized by the human body. Plant sterols and stanols are structurally related to cholesterol, but contain an extra methyl or ethyl group on the cholesterol side chain. The major plant sterols found in nature are β-sitosterol, campesterol and stigmasterol, from which β-sitosterol is the most abundant one (comprising 90% of the total). The hydrogenation of unsaturated bounds in plant sterols results in plant stanols. Plant sterols and stanols occur naturally in food as free alcohol, esterified with long chain fatty acids (25-80% of total plant sterols) or conjugated as glycosides (usually in small amounts).

The main sources of plant sterols in the basic diet are cooking oils and margarine. Bread and cereals can also contribute significantly to total plant sterol intake [Morton et al., 1995]. Plant sterols are present in Western diets in amounts similar to those for dietary cholesterol. For the United States, average daily intakes of plant sterols are reported between ca. 180-250 mg [Connor, 1968]. In the Netherlands an average daily intake of plant sterols of 263 (women) to 307 mg (men) has been estimated [Normén et al., 2001]. For the United Kingdom, this intake is estimated to vary between on average 150-200 mg [Morton et al., 1995] and for Japan about 400 mg [Hirai et al., 1986]. The Tarahumara Indians of Mexico, who consume a diet containing unusually high amounts of beans and corn, ingest over 400 mg of phytosterols per day [Cerqueira et al., 1979]. In general the intake of adult vegetarians and their children is higher (up to 40%) than the average for the population as a whole [Nair et al., 1984; Miettinen et al., 1990; Ling and Jones, 1995].

The practical use of plant sterols as cholesterol lowering agents was limited for many years due to the poor solubility in fat and high amounts (10 to 20 g per day) that were needed to obtain substantial reductions in serum cholesterol levels. Esterification of plant sterols and stanols with fatty acids increases this solubility in fat. Additionally, newly developed technologies improve solubility of unesterified plant sterols and stanols. These processes allow lower concentrations to be incorporated in foods and increasing the cholesterol reducing effect at lower dietary intakes. This renewed the interest in plant sterols and stanols as blood cholesterol lowering agents. Plant sterol mixtures from various sources have been isolated and modified, i.e. hydrogenated and or esterified, for application as a functional food ingredient. At present many plant sterol and plant stanol enriched food products are on the market and claim cholesterol lowering activity.

# Metabolism of Plant Sterols and Mechanism of Cholesterol Lowering

## Plant Sterols Metabolism

Intestinal absorption of plant sterols is low compared to absorption of cholesterol. Heinemann et al. [1993] reported in a study with human volunteers percentages absorption for campestanol, campesterol, stigmasterol, and sitosterol which were, respectively 12.5%, 9.6%, 4.8%, and 4.2%. Sitostanol absorption was negligible whereas cholesterol absorption in the same study was 31%. Ostlund et al. [2002] reported absorption of plant sterols varying from 0.4-3.5% whereas intestinal absorption of plant stanols varied from 0.02%-0.3%. Sitosterol absorption in patients suffering homozygous phytosterolaemia is typically 15% to 25% [taken from Katan et al., 2003].

Plant sterols and stanols are cleared from the plasma and preferentially taken up by the liver and to a lesser extent distributed to other tissues. Results from rat studies indicate that of the other tissues, the adrenals showed the highest levels on the basis of tissue weight followed by the testes [Subbiah and Kuksis, 1973]. No accumulation of plant sterols has been observed in dogs and rats [Shipley et al., 1958]. For humans, only little information is available regarding the distribution of plant sterols in various tissues of the body. Only trace amounts of plant sterols have been determined in the liver and liver microsomes of healthy subjects [Ling and Jones, 1995]. High levels of plant sterols in liver microsomes have been found in subjects suffering from sitosterolemia.

Consumption of plant sterols and stanols has shown to increase plasma levels in healthy subjects. Weststrate and Meijer [1998] demonstrated that plant sterol esters from soy, which have a high content of both sitosterol and campesterol, raised the concentration of both plant sterols in the plasma. Hendriks et al. [2003] showed that after consumption of plant sterol esters-enriched spread during one year the concentrations of campesterol and β-sitosterol in red blood cells were increased as compared to control. The relative increase in red blood cells was similar to the increase in serum suggesting that plant sterols did not accumulate in cell membranes. Hallikainen et al. [2000] compared the effect of margarines enriched with plant sterol esters and plant stanol esters. Both plant sterol and plant stanol concentrations in plasma increased. Consumption of plant stanols reduced plasma sterol concentrations [Hallikainen et al., 2000]. Concentrations of plant sterols in plasma in subjects consuming sterol esters-enriched margarines are within the range of 11-30 umol/L which is about 20-100 times lower than patients with phytosterolaemia. Whether such an increase in plasma plant sterol concentrations might be a risk factor for coronary heart disease is not known.

### Mechanism of Cholesterol Lowering

The main mechanism of the cholesterol lowering action of plant sterols and plant stanols is by inhibiting dietary cholesterol absorption as well as biliary cholesterol absorption [Grundy and Mok, 1976; Heinemann et al., 1991; Gylling et al., 1997]. The postulated mechanism is that plant sterols and stanols are able to displace cholesterol in bile acid micelles due to competition for micellar solubilization [Grundy and Mok, 1976; Ikeda et al., 1989]. As plant sterols and stanols are more hydrophobic than cholesterol, they have a higher affinity for micelles. As a consequence the micellar cholesterol concentration will be reduced thus resulting in a decrease of cholesterol absorption.

In addition some other mechanisms for the cholesterol lowering effect have been proposed. It has been suggested that plant sterols and stanols influence the cholesterol metabolism in the enterocyte, resulting in an increased excretion of cholesterol by the enterocyte back into the intestinal lumen [Plat and Mensink, 2002]. At present, scarce evidence for this effect is available. Also effects of plant sterols and stanols on cholesterol excretion via the enterohepatic cycle have been suggested. However, no consistent evidence is available. Bile salt excretion was reduced in transgenic mice after consumption of plant stanols [Volger et al., 2001] but remained unchanged after consumption of plant stanols by colectomized patients [Miettinen et al., 2000] or plant sterols in ileostomy patients [Normen et al., 2000].

## Cholesterol Lowering Action of Plant Sterols

### Studies in Healthy Volunteers

There is abundant evidence that plant sterols and plant stanols lower blood total and LDL cholesterol under a wide range of different study conditions. This review will focus on studies published from mid 1990s until end 2003. Table 1 presents an overview of 44 clinical trials investigating the effects of plant sterols and plant stanols, either as esters or in free form, on blood cholesterol concentrations. Of these, 30 studies were with plant sterols and 14 studies were with plant stanols. In 13 of the 44 reviewed studies plant sterols or stanols were in the unesterified form. The dosages of plant sterols and plant stanols given in the studies ranged from 0.7 to 3.4 g per day. From Table 1 it can be concluded that plant sterols and plant stanols consistently lower total cholesterol concentrations up to 13% and LDL cholesterol concentrations up to 16.0 %. In two out of the 44 reviewed studies the cholesterol lowering effect of either unesterified plant stanols [Denke, 1995] or unesterified plant sterols

[Jones et al., 2003] could not be demonstrated. In all studies levels of serum HDL cholesterol and triacylglycerols remained more or less unchanged.

Studies presented in Table 1 indicate that in most cases daily consumption of plant sterols and plant stanols in doses of 0.8-1 g results in LDL cholesterol reductions of 5% or more compared to a control treatment [Pelletier et al., 1995; Hendriks et al., 1999; Sierksma et al., 1999; Meguro et al., 2001; Volpe et al., 2001]. In one case only a slight reduction in LDL cholesterol (1.7%) was observed after treatment with 0.8 g/day plant stanols [Hallikainen et al., 2000]. Increasing dosages to 1.5-2.5 g per day substantially increases the cholesterol lowering effect of plant sterols and plant stanols. The mean reduction in LDL cholesterol compared to control treatment at these intakes was about 9.3% (c.f. Table 1; 39 treatment periods). Daily consumption of plant sterols and plant stanols of dosages >2.5 g slightly further increased this LDL cholesterol lowering effect to about 10.9% (c.f. Table 1; 21 treatment periods).

Plant sterols and plant stanols are effective in lowering plasma lipoproteins within a few weeks, the effect remaining stable in studies during 1 year. Hendriks et al. [2003] showed a sustained cholesterol lowering effect of daily consumption of 20 g spread enriched with 1.6 g plant sterol esters during one year in Dutch normocholesterolaemic and mildly hypercholesterolaemic men and women. This cholesterol lowering effect was consistent throughout the study, namely cholesterol was reduced on average by about 4% and LDL cholesterol on average by about 6%. Another long-term study conducted by Miettinen et al. [1995] reported a reduction 8.5 % of LDL cholesterol in a hypercholesterolaemic Finnish population after consumption of 1.8 g/day plant stanol esters during one year. The differences in response between both studies are most likely not caused by differences in efficacy between sterols and stanols but by differences in for example blood cholesterol levels between study populations.

As illustrated in Table 1, there is a wide range in efficacies over the various studies either testing sterols or stanols. Since β-sitostanol has shown to be more effective than β-sitosterol in the inhibition of cholesterol absorption [Heineman et al., 1988; Ntanios & Jones, 1998; Heinemann et al., 1991], it has been suggested that plant stanols are more effective in cholesterol lowering than plant sterols. Also Katan et al. [2003] suggested a higher efficiency of plant stanols. They performed a meta analysis and demonstrated that mean reduction in LDL cholesterol level was 10.1% (95% confidence interval 8.9%-11.3%) in 27 trails testing stanols (mean dosage 2.5 g/day) and 9.7% (95% confidence interval 8.5%-10.8%) in 21 trials testing sterols (mean dosage 2.3 g/day). They indicated that although this difference in LDL lowering capacity between plant stanols and sterols was not statistically significant 'the comparison lacked the statistical power to detect a moderate difference'. However, straightforward conclusions on the cholesterol lowering effect of plant sterols and plant stanols can only be drawn from a direct comparison in the same study. Several studies have been performed so far [Weststrate and Meijer, 1998; Hallikainen et al., 2000; Jones et al., 2000; Normén et al., 2000]. These short-term human trials, either dietary controlled or in free living conditions, showed a similar [Weststrate and Meijer, 1998; Hallikainen et al., 2000; Normén et al., 2000] or better [Jones et al., 2000] efficacy in cholesterol lowering for plant

**Table 1. Effects of Esterified and Unesterified Plant Sterols and Plant Stanols on Total and LDL Cholesterol in Different Populations**

| Reference | Design | Duration | Subjects & age | Sterol, stanol esterification | Matrix | Dose g/day | Serum cholesterol % change vs control Total | LDL |
|---|---|---|---|---|---|---|---|---|
| *Cleghorn et al., 2003* | Randomised, double-blind, placebo-controlled, cross-over | 4 weeks | 50 normo- and mildly hypercholesterolaemic adults (47 y) | Sterol esters | Spread 64% fat | 2 | -4.5% | -7.2% |
| *Hendriks et al., 2003* | Randomised, double-blind, placebo-controlled, parallel | 1 year | 89 normo- and mildly hypercholesterolaemic adults (48 y) | Sterol esters | Spread 35% fat | 1.6 | -4% | -6% |
| *Jones et al., 2003* | Randomised, double-blind, placebo-controlled, cross-over | 21 days | 15 moderately hyperholesterolaemic adults (22-68 y) | Unesterified sterols | Beverage, no-fat, low-fat 1% | 1.8 | -3.1, no – 1.6, low | -5.4, no – 3.5, low |
| *Maki et al., 2003* | Randomised, double-blind, placebo controlled, parallel | 6 weeks | 57 hypercholesterolaemic adults (59 y) | Unesterified sterols | Beverage no-fat | 1.8 g | - 2.1% | -3.7% |
| *Naumann et al., 2003* | Randomised, double-blind, placebo-controlled, cross-over | 3 weeks | 44 normocholesterolaemic adults (32/37 y) | Sterol and stanol esters | Spread 47% fat or 62% fat | 1 sterol 1 stanol 1.5 ster 0.5 stan | -3.4% - 2.7% | -6.0% - 6.7% |
| *Admundsen et al.*, 2002 | Randomised, double-blind, placebo-controlled, cross-over | 8 weeks | 38 hypercholesterolaemic patients (11y) | Sterol esters | Spread 35% fat | 1.6 | -7.4% | -10.2% |
| *De Graaf et al., 2002* | Randomised, double-blind, placebo-controlled, parallel | 4 weeks | 31 patients with primary hypercholesterolaemia (56 y) | Unesterified sterol/stanol mixture | Chocolate 48% fat | 1.8 | - 6.4% | -10.3% |
| Judd et al., 2002 | Randomised, double-blind, placebo-controlled, cross-over | 3 weeks | 53 normo- and mildly hypercholesterolaemic adults (47 y) | Sterol esters | Dressing 27% fat | 2.2 | -6.8% | -9.7% |

**Table 1. Effects of Esterified and Unesterified Plant Sterols and Plant Stanols on Total and LDL Cholesterol in Different Populations (Continued)**

| Reference | Design | Duration | Subjects & age | Sterol, stanol esterification | Matrix | Dose g/day | Serum cholesterol % change vs control Total | LDL |
|---|---|---|---|---|---|---|---|---|
| *Matvienko et al., 2002* | Randomised, triple-blind, placebo controlled, parallel | 4 weeks | 17 normo- and mildly hypercholesterolaemic adults (24 y) | Sterol mixture 67% esters, 33% unesterified | Ground beef 10-15% fat | 2.7 | -9.3% | -14.6% |
| *Mussner et al., 2002* | Randomised, double-blind, placebo-controlled, cross-over | 3 weeks | 63 normo- and mildly hypercholesterolaemic adults (42 y) | Sterol esters | Margarine 60% fat | 1.82 | -3.4% | -5.4% |
| *Noakes et al., 2002* | Randomised, double-blind, placebo-controlled, cross-over | 3 weeks | 46 mildly hypercholesterolaemic adults (56-58 y) | Sterol esters or stanol esters | Spread 34% fat or 31% fat | 2.3 ster 2.5 stan | -6.1% - 7.3% | -7.7% - 9.5% |
| *Noakes et al., 2002* | Randomised, double-blind, placebo-controlled, cross-over | 3 weeks | 35 mildly hypercholesterolaemic adults (56-58 y) | Sterol esters | Spread 64% fat | 2 | -6.4% | -9.6% |
| *Ntanios et al., 2002* | Randomised, double-blind, placebo-controlled, cross-over | 3 weeks | 53 normo- and mildly hypercholesterolaemic adults (45 y) | Sterol esters | Spread 70% fat | 1.8 | -5.8% | -9.1% |
| *Temme et al.*, 2002 | Randomised, double-blind, placebo-controlled, cross-over | 4 weeks | 42 normo- and mildly hypercholesterolaemic adults (55 y) | Sterol esters | Spread 35% fat | 2 | -7% | -10% |
| *Vanstone et al., 2002* | Randomised, double-blind, placebo-controlled, cross-over | 3 weeks | 15 hypercholesterolaemic patients (48 y) | Unesterified sterols & stanols | Butter | 1.8 ster 1.8 stan 1.8 mix | -7.8% - 11.9% - 13.1% | -11.3% - 13.4% - 16.0% |
| *Christiansen et al., 2001* | Randomised, double-blind placebo controlled, parallel | 6 months | 89 hypercholesterolaemic adults (51 y) | Unesterified sterols | Spread 64% fat | 1.5 3 | -8.9% - 8.3% | -11.3% - 10.6% |

**Table 1. Effects of Esterified and Unesterified Plant Sterols and Plant Stanols on Total and LDL Cholesterol in Different Populations (Continued)**

| Reference | Design | Duration | Subjects & age | Sterol, stanol esterification | Matrix | Dose g/day | Serum cholesterol % change vs control Total | LDL |
|---|---|---|---|---|---|---|---|---|
| *Davidson et al., 2001* | Randomised, double blind, placebo controlled, parallel | 8 weeks | 21 normo- and mildly hypercholesterolaemic adults (44 y) | Sterol esters | Spread 48% fat Dressing 28% fat | 3 | -5% | -5% |
| *Maki et al., 2001* | Randomised, double-blind placebo controlled, parallel | 5 weeks | 132 mild to moderately hypercholes-terolaemic adults (59/60 y) | Sterol esters | Spread 40% fat | 1.1 (n=92) 2.2 (n=40) | -5.2% - 6.6% | -7.6% - 8.1% |
| *Meguro et al.*, 2001 | Randomised, double-blind, placebo-controlled, cross-over | 2 weeks | 12 normo- and moderate hypercholesterolaemic adults (36 y) | Unesterified sterols in TAG or DAG | Mayonaise | 0.5 TAG 0.5 DAG | -- -4.7% | - 3.6 % ns - 7.6% |
| Neil et al., 2001 | Randomised, double-blind, placebo-controlled, cross-over | 8 weeks | 29 familiar hypercholesterolaemic adults (53 y) | Sterol esters | Spread 70% fat | 2.5 | -7.8% | -10% |
| *Nestel et al., 2001* | Randomised, single-blind, placebo-controlled, cross-over | 4 weeks | 22 hypercholesterolaemic adults (60 y) | Sterol esters & unesterified stanols | Cereal Bread Spread 70% fat | 2.4 sterol 2.4 stanol | -8.5% - 3.6% | -13.6% - 8.3% |
| *Nestel et al., 2001* | Randomised, single-blind, placebo-controlled, cross-over | 4 weeks | 15 hypercholesterolaemic adults (60 y) | Sterol esters | Spread 80% fat | 2.4 | -8.5% | - 12.2% |
| Nigon et al., 2001 | Randomised, double-blind, placebo-controlled, cross-over | 8 weeks | 53 hypercholesterolaemic patients (58 y) | Sterol esters | Spread | 1.6 | - 6.4% | -8.8% |
| *Tikkanen et al., 2001* | Randomised, double-blind, placebo-controlled, parallel | 15 weeks | 36 hypercholesterolemic adults (56 y) | Unesterified sterols | Bread, meat, jam yoghurt All low fat | 0.91, 5 wk 1.86, 5 wk 4.17, 5 wk | -5% (15 wk) | -8% (15 wk) |

**Table 1. Effects of Esterified and Unesterified Plant Sterols and Plant Stanols on Total and LDL Cholesterol in Different Populations (Continued)**

| Reference | Design | Duration | Subjects & age | Sterol, stanol esterification | Matrix | Dose g/day | Serum cholesterol % change vs control Total | LDL |
|---|---|---|---|---|---|---|---|---|
| *Volpe et al., 2001* | Randomised, double-blind, placebo-controlled, cross-over | 4 weeks | 30 moderate hypercholesterolaemic adults (51 y) | Sterol esters | Yoghurt 1% fat | 1 (n=30) | -4.4% | -6.2% |
| *Hallikainen et al. 2000* | Randomised, double-blind, placebo-controlled, cross-over | 4 weeks | 34 hypercholesterolaemic adults (49 y) | Sterol esters & stanol esters | Margarine 70% fat | 2 sterol 2 stanol | -7.3% - 9.2% | -10.4% - 12.7% |
| Jones et al., 2000 | Randomised, double-blind, placebo-controlled, cross-over | 3 weeks | 15 hypercholesterolaemic adults (52 y), | Sterol esters & stanol esters | Margarine | 1.84 sterol 1.84 stan | -13.4% - 10.2% | -12.9% - 7.9% |
| *Vissers et al.*, 2000 | Randomised, double-blind, placebo-controlled, cross-over | 3 weeks | 60 normocholesterolaemic adults (23 y) | Sterol esters | Spread 82% fat | 2.1 | -4.5% | -8.5% |
| Hendriks et al., 1999 | Randomised, double-blind, placebo-controlled, cross-over | 3.5 weeks | 80 normo- and mildly hypercholesterolaemic adults (37 y) | Sterol esters | Spread 70% fat | 0.83 1.61 3.24 | -4.9% - 5.9% - 6.8% | -6.7% - 8.5% - 9.9% |
| *Jones et al., 1999* | Randomised, double-blind, placebo-controlled, parallel | 30 days | 16 hypercholesterolaemic adults (50 y) | Unesterified sterol-stanol mixture | Spread | 1.7 | - 9.1% | - 15.5% |
| Sierksma et al., 1999 | Randomised, double-blind, placebo-controlled, cross-over | 3 weeks | 76 normocholesterolaemic adults (44 y) | Unesterified sterols | Spread 71% fat | 0.8 | -3.8% | -6% |
| Westrate and Meijer, 1998 | Randomised, double-blind, placebo-controlled, cross-over | 3.5 weeks | 80 normo- and mildly hypercholesterolaemic adults (45 y) | Sterol esters or stanol esters | Spread 71-73% fat | 3.2 sterol 1.7 sterol 3.0 sterol 2.7 stanol | -8.3% - 1.1% - 0.7% - 7.3% | -13% - 1.5% - 0.9% - 13% |

**Table 1. Effects of Esterified and Unesterified Plant Sterols and Plant Stanols on Total and LDL Cholesterol in Different Populations (Continued)**

| Reference | Design | Duration | Subjects & age | Sterol, stanol esterification | Matrix | Dose g/day | Serum cholesterol % change vs control Total | LDL |
|---|---|---|---|---|---|---|---|---|
| *Pelletier et al., 1995* | Randomised, double-blind, placebo-controlled, cross-over | 4 weeks | 12 normocholesterolaemic adults (23 y), | Sterol esters | Butter | 0.740 | -10% | -15% |
| *Spilburg et al., 2003* | Randomised, double-blind, placebo-controlled, parallel | 4 weeks | 24 mildly hypercholesterolaemic adults (51 y) | Unesterified stanols | Beverage Non fat | 1.9 | -10.1% | -14.3% |
| *Mensink et al., 2002* | Randomised, double-blind, placebo-controlled, cross-over | 4 weeks | 20 normocholesterolaemic adults (36 y) | Stanol esters | Yoghurt, low-fat | 3 | -8.7% | -13.7% |
| *Hallikainen et al., 2000* | Randomised, double-blind, placebo-controlled, cross-over | 4 weeks | 22 hypercholesterolaemic adults (51 y) | Stanol esters | Spread 68-70% fat | 0.8 1.6 2.4 3.2 | -2.8% - 6.8% - 10.3% - 11.3% | -1.7% - 5.6% - 9.7% - 10.4% |
| *Plat and Mensink, 2000* | Randomised, double-blind, placebo-controlled, parallel | 8 weeks | 70), normocholesterolaemic adults (33 y | Stanol esters | Spread 74% fat Shortening 82% fat | 4.0 3.8 | -7.6% - 7.8% | -12.8% - 14.6% |
| *Plat et al., 2000* | Randomised, double-blind, placebo-controlled, cross-over | 4 weeks | 39 normocholesterolaemic adults (31 y) | Stanol esters | Spread 68% fat | 2.5 | -6.6% | -10.4% |
| *Gylling and Miettinen, 1999* | Randomised, double-blind, placebo-controlled, cross-over | 6 weeks | 23 moderately hypercholesterolaemic women (53 y) | Stanol esters | Margarine | 3.2 (tall) 3.2 (veg) | -4% -6% | -8% -10% |
| *Gylling and Miettinen, 1999* | Randomised, double-blind, placebo-controlled, cross-over | 5 weeks | 21 moderately hypercholesterolaemic women (53 y) | Stanol esters | Butter | 2.4 | -8% | -12% |

**Table 1. Effects of Esterified and Unesterified Plant Sterols and Plant Stanols on Total and LDL Cholesterol in Different Populations (Continued)**

| Reference | Design | Duration | Subjects & age | Sterol, stanol esterification | Matrix | Dose g/day | Serum cholesterol % change vs control Total | LDL |
|---|---|---|---|---|---|---|---|---|
| *Nguyen et al., 1999* | Randomised, double-blind, placebo-controlled, parallel | 8 weeks | 238 mildly hypercholesterolaemic adults (36-46 y) | Stanol esters | Spread 66-72% fat | 2 (n=82) 3 (n=77) 3 (n=79) | -4.9% - 6.9% - 5.2% | -4.2% - 10.2% - 5.3% |
| *Hallikainen and Uusitupa, 1999* | Randomised, double-blind, placebo-controlled, parallel | 8 weeks | 38 hypercholesterolaemic adults (41/43 y) | Stanol esters | Spread 40% fat | 2.3 (wood) 2.2 (veg) | -10.6% - 8.1% | -13.7% - 8.6% |
| *Gylling & Miettinen, 1996* | Randomised, double-blind, placebo-controlled, cross-over | 7 weeks | 8 hypercholesterolaemic adults with NIDDM (60 y) | Stanol esters | Margarine | 3 | -11% | -14% |
| *Denke, 1995* | Not blinded or controlled | 3 months | 33 moderate hypercholesterolaemic adults | Unesterified sitostanol | Capsule | 3 | No change | No change |
| *Miettinen et al., 1995* | Randomised, double-blind, placebo-controlled, parallel | 1 year | 51 mildly hypercholesterolaemic adults (56 y) | Stanol esters | Margarine | 2.6 | -10.2% | -14.1% |
| *Gylling and Miettinen, 1994* | Randomised, double-blind, placebo-controlled, cross-over | 6 weeks | 11 hypercholesterolaemic adults with NIDDM (58 y) | Stanol esters | Margarine | 3 | -5.8% | -9.3% |
| *Vanhanen et al.*, 1993 | Randomised, double-blind, placebo-controlled, parallel | 6 weeks | 34 hypercholesterolaemic adults (48 y) | Stanol esters | Mayonaise | 3.4 | -7.5% | -10% |

Figures represent characteristics of subjects receiving the plant sterol treatment sterol esters-enriched spread as compared to plant stanol esters-enriched spread. Although it is difficult to draw firm conclusions from these results most probably there is no difference in cholesterol lowering effect of plant sterols compared to plant stanols.

Thus, depending on the dosage, reductions in total and LDL cholesterol varying from 0.3% to 16 % can be obtained by consumption of plant sterols or plant stanols. Most common dosage given in different trials is about 1.5-2.5 g/day resulting in a mean decrease of LDL cholesterol of about 10%. Such a decrease may, on a population basis, substantially contribute to the prevention of coronary heart disease [Law et al., 1994]. Analysis of cohort studies by Law et al. [1994] indicated that the longer term risk reduction would be about 20%.

## Factors Possibly Interfering with Cholesterol Lowering

Besides above described factors dosage and hydrogenation (sterols versus stanols) also other factors have been suggested to influence the efficacy of plant sterols and stanols. Below the possible influence of esterification, food matrix, background diet, moment of consumption and baseline cholesterol concentration are discussed.

### *Esterification*

Most commonly plant sterols and plant stanols are applied in spreads in esterified form. Esterification of plant sterols and stanols increases solubility thus providing a technically feasible way of introducing plant sterols into edible fats and oils [Wester, 2000]. It has been suggested that the physical state (esterified versus unesterified) of plant sterols and plant stanols influences their cholesterol reducing capacity. From a review by Jones and Raeini-Sarjaz [2001] it was concluded that unesterified sterol and stanols can have the same effect on plasma cholesterol as sterol and stanol esters. The trials presented in Table 1 show a great cholesterol lowering potential of unesterified sterols and stanols when incorporated in high fat products. In hypercholesterolaemic subjects a decrease in total cholesterol concentrations up to 13.1% and LDL cholesterol concentrations up to 16% was observed after consumption of unesterified plant sterols and stanols [Christiansen et al., 2001; De Graaf et al., 2002; Vanstone et al., 2002]. The mean reduction in LDL cholesterol after consumption of plant sterol and stanol esters calculated from data presented in Table 1 is about 9% (26 treatment periods). Although these reductions seem to be somewhat lower than after consumption of unesterified plant sterols no hard conclusion can be drawn on differences in efficacy between the esterified and unesterified plant sterols. For instance baseline blood cholesterol concentrations were about 10% higher in subjects participating in trials with the unesterified plant sterols. In a recent study by Richelle et al. [2004] in normocholesterolaemic subjects, milk enriched with plant sterol esters induced a similar decrease in cholesterol absorption as milk enriched with free plant sterols. Whether or not there are in differences in blood cholesterol lowering action of esterified and unesterified plant sterols should be confirmed by a direct comparison within the same study.

### Food Matrix

Since the supposed mechanism for cholesterol lowering is inhibition of cholesterol absorption from the intestine plant sterols and plant stanols should be consumed in a matrix or with a meal stimulating biliary flow to exert their efficacy. The influence of fat content of the spread on the magnitude of cholesterol reduction was evaluated by splitting-up the spreads used in the trials presented in Table 1 into three fat levels: 30-50%, 50-70% and ≥ 70% (as far as data were given in the papers). The mean reductions in total cholesterol and LDL cholesterol calculated from these studies were respectively 6.7% and 8.6% at a fat level of 30-50% (10 treatment periods), 6.6% and 8.3% at a fat level of 50-70% (13 treatment periods) and 7.4% and 10.8% at fat levels ≥ 70% (20 treatment periods). This suggests that plant sterols and stanols are more effective in cholesterol reduction when incorporated in spreads containing high fat levels. It should be noted that these calculated means were not balanced for other factors possibly influencing the efficacy of plant sterols and plant stanols like dosage and blood cholesterol concentration.

Especially for unesterified sterols and stanols the matrix seems to be important. As indicated above (3.2.1), unesterified sterols are very effective in cholesterol lowering when incorporated in a high fat matrix. When incorporated in a non-fat or low fat beverage, consumption of unesterified plant sterols did not exert a greater hypocholesterolaemic effect than consumption of a non fat placebo beverage [Jones et al., 2003]. On the other hand, plant sterol and plant stanol esters have shown to be effective in cholesterol lowering when incorporated into low fat products such as bread and cereals or low fat yogurt [Nestel et al., 2001; Mensink et al., 2002; Clifton et al., 2004], although a matrix effect was demonstrated. Clifton et al. [2004] compared the relative effects of each of four plant sterol esters-enriched low fat foods. They showed that for all foods there was a significant reduction in total cholesterol and LDL cholesterol. However, plant sterols in low fat milk appeared to be almost three times more effective (LDL reduction 15.9%) than in bread (LDL reduction 6.5%) and cereals (LDL reduction 5.4%). Most probably solubility or dispergation of plant sterols and plant stanols in a low fat matrix determines their effectiveness.

### Background Diet

It has been suggested that composition of the diet might influence the cholesterol lowering capacity of plant sterols and plant stanols. Mussner et al. [2002] demonstrated that the LDL cholesterol lowering capacity of plant sterol esters enriched margarine was more pronounced at higher cholesterol and fat intake. Furthermore, Denke [1995] could not demonstrate a cholesterol lowering effect of 3 g/d sitostanol in hypercholesterolaemic subjects when supplemented to a diet low in cholesterol. However, many evidence became available the recent years that plant sterols and plant stanols are effective in cholesterol lowering in hypercholesterolaemic subjects consuming low cholesterol or low fat diets [Hallikainen et al., 2000; Maki et al., 2001; Cleghorn et al., 2003; Shin et al., 2003].

### Moment of Consumption; Number of Servings

Since the supposed mechanism for cholesterol lowering is inhibition of cholesterol absorption from the intestine it may be expected that a constant presence of plant sterols in the intestine may be needed for an optimal effect. It can therefore be hypothesized that for the best effect, plant sterols should be ingested simultaneously with meals containing cholesterol in order to block the absorption of exogenous cholesterol from the intestinal lumen [Pollak and Kritchevsky, 1981]. In most trials the total daily intake of plant sterols and stanols is divided over 2 or 3 portions per day. In our study [Hendriks et al., 2003] it appeared that after 13 weeks the majority of the volunteers consumed all spread with breakfast. Since we considered the consumption of the plant sterol esters-enriched spread with at least two meals per day relevant, a request was issued half-way the study, to eat 10 g of spread with both breakfast and lunch. The request resulted in a clear increase in the proportion of volunteers consuming spread with two meals (from about 40% to about 70%), but the cholesterol lowering efficacy did not dramatically change. This is in accordance with the results of Plat et al. [2000]. They showed that 2.5 g plant stanols taken at lunch produced the same LDL lowering effect as 2.5 g of plant stanols divided over the three meals. Although both results suggest that eating moment is not essential in the cholesterol lowering effect of plant sterols and plant stanols more research is required to draw firm conclusions with respect to this topic.

### *Blood Cholesterol Concentration of the Population under Study*

Efficacy of plant sterols and plant stanols may be higher at high blood cholesterol concentrations. Mussner et al. [2002] investigated the cholesterol lowering effects of three week consumption of plant sterol esters-enriched margarine. They demonstrated that the efficacy was more pronounced at higher basal cholesterol absorption. The correlation between initial cholesterol concentration and the degree of cholesterol reduction was demonstrated by our own results [Hendriks et al., 2003]. For both, total cholesterol and LDL cholesterol, the cholesterol lowering after consumption of plant sterol esters-enriched spread tended to be higher when baseline cholesterol concentration was higher. Dividing the study population into quartiles based on baseline cholesterol concentration mean total cholesterol lowering during the study was 0.2% for the lowest quartile and 5.1% for the highest quartile. Percentage reduction of LDL cholesterol was 1.5% for the lowest quartile and 7.2% for the highest quartile.

## Cholesterol Lowering in Patients and Role of Genotype

Plant sterols and stanols are not only effective in normo- and mildly hypercholesterolaemic subjects, but are also in hypercholesterolaemic subjects, subjects with familial hypercholesterolaemia receiving cholesterol lowering therapies, and in type II diabetic hypercholesterolaemic patients. Maki et al. [2001] studied the effect of daily consumption of low fat spreads (40%) enriched with 1.1 or 2.2 g plant sterol esters in low to mildly hypercholesterolaemic subjects on a cholesterol reducing diet. After two weeks LDL cholesterol was reduced with respectively 7.6 % and 8.1 % compared with control treatment. Also Hallikainen et al. [2000] studied the cholesterol lowering capacity of margarines enriched with plant sterols and plant stanols in hypercholesterolaemic subjects. Thirty-four patients consumed during 4 weeks a control spread, a spread enriched with plant sterols and a spread enriched with plant stanols. Sterols lowered LDL cholesterol with 10.4% and stanols

with 12.7% compared with the control product. Comparable cholesterol lowering effects were found by Blair et al. [2000] and Vuori et al. [2000]. Both groups demonstrated that consumption of plant stanol esters in hypercholesterolaemic patients receiving statin therapy lowered LDL cholesterol levels by 10% or more compared to consumption of placebo. Neil et al. [2001] investigated the cholesterol lowering effect of daily consumption of margarine enriched with 2.5 g plant sterols in hypercholesterolaemic patients with heterozygous familial hypercholesterolaemia receiving either statin therapy or no therapy. In both groups LDL cholesterol concentrations decreased with 10-15%. There was no difference in response between hypercholesterolaemic patients prescribed statins and those not taking lipid lowering drug.

Also in diabetic patients plants stanols have shown to be effective in reducing LDL. Gylling and Miettinen [1994] showed a reduction in LDL cholesterol of 9% in diabetic patients after consumption of plant stanols, which was comparable with the observed effect in non diabetic subjects. In patients with diabetes type 2 receiving a statin therapy LDL cholesterol was lowered by an additional 14% after consumption of stanol esters [Gylling and Miettinen, 1996].

The apolipoprotein E polymorphism may influence the absorption of cholesterol from the intestine and thus the response of serum cholesterol to diet. Some studies [Miettinen & Vanhanen, 1994; Vanhanen et al., 1993] indicated that subjects with apoE4 genotype responded to sitostanol consumption with a greater reduction in total cholesterol and LDL-cholesterol than individuals with the apoE3 genotype. Others concluded that the serum cholesterol response to plant sterols is not affected by the apolipoprotein E polymorphism in healthy subjects who consume a low-cholesterol diet [Geelen et al. 2002, Ishiwata et al., 2002].

## Additional Physiological Effects of Plant Sterols

Besides the cholesterol lowering potential, animal studies have shown that plant sterols and plant stanols may reduce development of atherosclerotic lesions [de Jong et al., 2003]. The potency of reduction of development and progression of atherosclerotic lesions ideally should be confirmed in very large intervention trials. Smaller and shorter-term trials with surrogate end points like flow mediated dilatation, pulse wave velocity or intima media thickness might help in proving the efficacy of plant sterols and stanols in reducing cardiovascular disease.

In addition to the effects on CHD risk, effects of plant sterols and plant stanols on risk on colon cancer and prostate cancer are suggested.

Compared with the general population, Seventh-day Adventists have lower rates of cancer at many sites, including colorectal cancer, and higher dietary intakes of plant sterols [Nair et al., 1984]. Since bile acids are reported to be tumor promoters in colon cancer [Cohen and Raicht, 1981] a proposed mechanism is that plant sterol consumption reduce bile acid excretion and thus the risk on colon cancer. On the other hand, increased consumption of plant sterols and plant stanols results in increased presence of cholesterol in the large intestine, which in turn can be converted into mutagenic metabolites (4-cholesten-3-one).

Wolfreys and Hepburn [2002] investigated the mutagenic potential of plants sterols and plant sterol esters as well as 4-cholesten-3-one in a bacterial mutation assay and an in vitro chromosome aberration assay. None of the components did show any evidence of mutagenic activity in any of these assays. Moreover, studies with mice and rats showed a decreased mucosal cell proliferation after consumption of different dosages of β-sitosterol [Janezic and Rao, 1992; Awad et al., 1997]. However, results of a prospective cohort study by Normen et al. [2001] indicated that high dietary intake of plant sterols was not associated with a lower risk of colon and rectal cancers in the Netherlands Cohort Study on Diet and Cancer.

It has also been suggested that plant sterols may beneficially affect prostate cancer. Dietary supplementation of sitosterol has been shown to improve the clinical symptoms of prostatic hyperplasia in humans [Berges et al., 1995]. Awad et al. [1998] showed that among other things plant sterol feeding in rats reduced serum testosterone concentrations. They concluded that dietary plant sterols may reduce risk of prostate cancer by stimulating the activities of the enzymes of testosterone metabolism. However, Hendriks et al. [2003] could not demonstrate an effect of one year consumption of plant sterol esters-enriched spread on serum testosterone concentrations in healthy men.

# Safety of Plant Sterols

## Plant Sterols and Sitosterolaemia

Subjects suffering from the rare inherited metabolic disease phytosterolaemia (sitosterolaemia) have serum plant sterol concentrations approximately 20-100 times higher than healthy subjects [Bhattacharyya and Connor, 1974; Salen et al, 1985; Ling and Jones, 1995]. These elevated concentrations of plant sterols have been implicated as a risk factor for premature atherosclerosis and coronary heart disease. The estimated frequency in the population of the homozygous state is in the order of one in 5 to 10 million. Increased dietary sitosterol absorption and decreased excretion are believed to be responsible for the accumulation of sitosterol in plasma and tissues. Since cholesterol absorption in phytosterolaemic subjects seems to be normal, there may be an intestinal defect to discriminate between cholesterol and plant sterols, resulting in excessive plant sterol absorption. Recent literature suggests that intestinal ABCG5 and ABCG8 transporters are involved in absorption of plant sterols but not cholesterol [Sehayek 2003]. Mutations in these genes are suggested to be responsible for at least some forms of phystosterolemia [Sehayek 2003].

Whether increased plasma concentrations of plant sterols or plant stanols might be a risk factor for coronary heart disease (CHD) in non phytosterolaemic subjects has not been established.

## Endpoints of in Vitro and Animal Experiments

Numerous studies on toxicity of plant sterols and plant stanols have been performed. The acute toxicity of plant sterols and plant stanols is low [Robinson et al., 1998]. There are no reports in literature of allergic reactions associated with plant sterols and plant stanols. For sub-acute and semichronic toxicity of various plant sterols or plant stanols holds that in general, the test substances did not reveal any adverse toxicological effects. No observed adverse effect levels (NOAEL) for plant sterols and plant stanols were established by Turnbull et al. [1999a] and Hepburn et al. [1999]. Plant sterols and stanols are not genotoxic [Turnbull et al., 1999b] or teratogenic [Slesinski et al., 1999]. It has been suggested that plant sterols or stanols have estrogenic activity. However, in vitro and in vivo assays did not reveal any estrogenic or uterotrophic activity of either stanol esters, free stanol fatty acids [Turnbull et al., 1999c] or plant sterols sourced from a variety of edible vegetable oil distillates [Baker et al., 1999].

## Human Studies

### *Clinical safety*

As described in this chapter many clinical studies with plant sterols and stanols, with both sexes, in both children and adults, with both healthy volunteers and hypercholesterolaemic patients have been performed. The aim of most of these studies was mainly to demonstrate the reduction of serum cholesterol levels by the addition of plant sterols in the diet. In general, the occurrence of adverse events associated with the use of plant sterols and plant stanols is rare and the adverse events reported are mild and not considered to be treatment related. Studies investigating effects of plant sterols or plant stanols on blood chemistry and haematology parameters did not show adverse effects in these parameters after short term consumption [Weststrate & Meijer, 1998; Plat & Mensink, 1998; Plat et al., 1999]. Two studies were conducted to evaluate long term effects of consumption of plant stanol esters and plant sterol esters. Miettinen et al. [1995] studied in a randomized double-blind placebo-controlled parallel trial the effects of daily consumption of a sitostanol enriched margarine (1.8 g sitostanol/day) in mildly hypercholesterolaemic subjects during one year. No adverse effects on body weight were observed and no adverse clinical signs were reported. Hendriks et al. [2003] evaluated the clinical and safety parameters after daily consumption of plant sterol esters-enriched spread (1.6 g/d) during one year in a randomized double blind parallel placebo controlled study in healthy volunteers. No adverse side effects, defined as reported adverse events or undesirable changes in clinical chemical parameters, haematological parameters and urinalysis, were observed. In addition, hormone levels in males and females were unaffected.

### *Nutritional Safety*

Since plant sterols and plant stanols decrease the absorption of cholesterol, they may also interfere with the absorption of fat-soluble components. Studies investigating the effect of plant sterols and plant stanols on carotenoids and fat-soluble vitamins are presented in Table 2. A substantial decrease in carotenoids was observed in most studies. After adjustment for the decrease in cholesterol still in many studies plant sterol and plant stanol consumption resulted in a significant decrease in lipid adjusted alpha- and beta-carotene up to 25% [Weststrate and Meijer, 1998; Gylling et al., 1999; Hallikainen et al., 1999; Hendriks et al., 1999; Judd et al., 2002; Mensink et al., 2002; Hendriks et al., 2003]. In other cases no significant effects on plasma lipid-standardised concentrations of α- and β-carotene were reported [Hallikainen and Uusitupa, 1999; Sierksma et al., 1999; Christiansen et al, 2001; Raeini-Sarjaz et al., 2002]. Reduction of lipid adjusted lycopene was reported by Sierksma et al. [1999] and Admundsen et al. [2002]. Weststrate and Meijer reported that lycopene concentrations were reduced by 22% after an intake of 3 g plant sterols per day, but not when lycopene concentration was lipid adjusted.

**Table 2. Influence of Plant Sterols and Plant Stanols on Carotenoids and Fat Soluble Vitamins**

| Reference | Dosage | Parameters reported to be changed | Reported % change |
|---|---|---|---|
| Weststrate & Meijer, 1998 | 3 g/d sterol ester | lipid adjusted (alpha + beta) carotene | -19% |
| Hendriks et al., 1999 | 0.83 g/d sterol ester<br>1.61 g/d sterol ester<br>3.42 g/d sterol ester | lipid adjusted (alpha + beta) carotene | -8%<br>no change<br>-15% |
| Sierksma et al., 1999 | 0.8 g/d free sterols | lipid adjusted lycopene | -9.5% |
| Gylling et al., 1999 | 3 g/d stanol ester | lipid adjusted beta carotene | -25% |
| Hallikainen & Uusitupa, 1999 | 2.2 & 2.3 g/d stanol ester | Lipid adjusted beta carotene | No change |
| Christiansen et al., 2001 | 1.5 g/d free sterols<br>3.0 g/d free sterols | no changes in carotenoids and fat soluble vitamins | |
| Plat and Mensink, 2001 | 3.8 g/d stanol ester | beta carotenedelta tocopherolalpha tocopherollipid adjusted carotenoids were not significantly lower | -26.1%<br>-10.7%<br>-7.8% |
| Judd et al., 2002 | 3.6 g/d sterol ester | alpha carotenebeta carotenelycopene | -12.8%<br>-12.7%<br>-20% |
| Mensink et al., 2002 | 3 g/d plant stanol ester | lipid adjusted beta carotene | -12.9% |
| Raeini-Sarjaz et al., 2002 | 1.92 g/d sterol ester<br>1.76 g/d stanol ester | no changes in carotenoids and fat soluble vitamins | |
| Admundsen et al., 2002 | 1.6 g/d sterol ester | lipid adjusted lycopene | -8.1% |
| Hendriks et al., 2003 | 1.6 g/d sterol ester | lipid adjusted (alpha + beta) carotene | -15% to -25% |

In the meta analysis of Katan et al. [2003] 18 trials testing doses of 1.5 g/day or more reported plasma concentrations of fat soluble vitamins. Mean reductions across the trials were 9% for α carotene, 28% for ß-carotene, and 7% for lycopene. When adjusted for the change in cholesterol only ß-carotene was significantly reduced by plant stanols and plant sterols by 12.1% (6.8%-17.4%). The reduction in α-tocopherol was explained by the reduction in cholesterol [Katan et al., 2003]. The meta analysis of Katan et al. [2003] did not indicate that consumption of plant sterols and plant stanols would affect vitamin A, D or K status.

Carotenoids are not essential nutrients, but both α carotene and ß-carotene have provitamin A activity. They may be of importance in situations where vitamin A requirements are greater than normal as in pregnancy, lactation or infancy. The consequences of a persistent decrease of blood concentrations of carotenoids, specifically ß-carotene, as observed after consumption of plant sterols and plant stanols on human health are unknown. Dietary advice to consume an additional daily serving of a high-carotenoid vegetable or fruit when consuming spreads containing sterol or stanol esters may be effective to maintain plasma carotenoid concentrations [Noakes et al., 2002].

### Monitoring of Long-term Exposure

The introduction of new products containing plant sterols and plant stanols is proceeding. Margarines containing either plant stanol or plant sterol esters are marketed in the United Stated and several countries in Europe for more than 2 years and in Finland for over 5 years. More recently other formulations, including yoghurt, cream cheese spreads and cereal bars have been introduced in some countries, and cereals containing free (unesterified) plant sterols and stanols are being marketed in the United States. With the growing number of products enriched with plant sterols and stanols some consumers may reach high intake levels when consuming different enriched products. Safety of plant sterols and plant stanols has been extensively tested. Several GRAS notification dossiers are present. The scientific committee on food concluded that the use of plant sterols in yellow fat spread at a maximum level corresponding to 8% free plant sterols is safe for human use [SCF, 2000]. More recently the scientific committee on food [SCF, 2002] concluded that 'the available data do not provide a basis for setting a numerical upper level of daily intake of phytosterols'. However, the committee indicated that 'it is prudent to avoid plant sterol intakes exceeding a range of 1-3 g/day'. With the growing number of enriched foods the scientific committee on foods suggests that 'additional management measures may be needed to avoid excessive intakes' [SCF, 2002]. Although there is no major concern on adverse health effects, the lack of very long-term effects leaves a possibility of unforeseen effects. Therefore follow-up of samples from the general population eating these foods by post marketing surveillance techniques is important to monitor both the beneficial as well as the adverse effects on the very long term. This is underscored by the scientific committee on food [SCF 2003] in its most recent opinion in which 'the committee encourages the Commission to initiate a programme monitoring the total intake of phytosterols-enriched products'.

## Conclusion

Consumption of products enriched with plant sterols and plant stanols in dosages of 1.5-2.5 g/day is effective in lowering of total cholesterol and LDL cholesterol in normo- and mildly hypercholesterolaemic subjects as well as in hypercholesterolaemic subjects receiving cholesterol lowering therapies. Use of these dosages seems to be safe, although it results in a significant reduction in carotenoid levels and there is a lack of chronic exposure data. With the growing number of enriched products entering the market a follow-up of samples from the general population eating plant sterol and stanol enriched foods by post marketing surveillance techniques is important to evaluate both the beneficial as well as the adverse effects on the very long term.

# References


Amundsen, A. L., Ose, L., Nenseter, M. S. & Ntanios, F. Y. (2002). Plant sterol ester-enriched spread lowers plasma total and LDL cholesterol in children with familial hypercholesterolemia. *Am J Clin Nutr, 76*, 338-344.

Awad, A. B., Hernandez, A. Y., Fink, C. S. & Mendel S. L. (1997). Effect of dietary phytosterols on cell proliferation and protein kinase C activity in rat colonic mucosa. *Nutr Cancer, 27*, 210-215.

Awad, A. B., Hartati, M. S. & Fink, C. S. (1998). Phytosterol feeding induces alteration in testosterone metabolism in rat tissues. *J Nutr Biochem, 9*, 712-717.

Baker, V. A., Hepburn, P. A., Kennedy, S. J., Jones, P. A., Lea, L. J., Sumpter, J. P. & Ashby, J. (1999). Safety evaluation of phytosterol esters: Part 1. Assessment of oestrogenicity using a compination of *in vivo* and *in vitro* assays, *Food Chem Toxicol, 37*, 13-22.

Berges, R. R., Windeler, J., Trampisch, J. H. & Senge, T. (1995). Randomized, placebo-controlled, double-blind, clinical trial of beta sitosterol in patients with benign prostatic hyperplasia. *Lancet, 345,* 1529-1532.

Bhattacharyya, A. & Connor, W. E. (1974). β-sitosterolemia and xanthomatosis: A newly described lipid storage disease in two sisters. *J Clin Invest, 53*, 1033-1043.

Blair, S. N., Capuzzi, D. M., Gottlieb, S. O., Nguyen, T., Morgan, J. M. & Carter, N. B. (2000). Incremental reduction of serum total cholesterol and low density lipoprotein cholesterol with the addition of plant stanol ester-containing spread to statin therapy, *Am J Cardiol, 86*, 46-52.

Cerqueira, M. T., Fry, M. M. & Connor, W. E. (1979). The food and nutrient intakes of the Tamahumara Indians of Mexico. *Am J Clin Nutr, 32*, 905-915.

Christiansen, L.I., Lahteenmaki, P. L. A., Mannelin, M. R., Sppanen-Laakso, T. E., Hiltunen, R. V. K. & Yliruusi, J. K. (2001). Cholesterol lowering effect of spreads enriched with microcrystalline plant sterols in hypercholesterolemic subjects. *Eur J Clin Nutr, 40*, 66-73.

Cleghorn, C. L., Skeaff, C. M., Mann, J. & Chisholm, A. (2003). Plant sterol-enriched spread enhances the cholesterol-lowering potential of a fat reduced diet. *Eur J Clin Nutr, 57*, 170-176.

Clifton, P. M., Noakes, M., Sullivan, D., Erichsen, N., Ross, D., Annison, G., Fassoulakis, A., Cehun, M. & Nestel, P. (2004). Cholesterol-lowering effects of plant sterol esters differ in milk, yoghurt, bread and cereal. *Eur J Clin Nutr, 58*, 503-509.

Cohen, B. I. & Raicht, R. F. (1981). Effects of bile acids on colon carcinogenesis in rats treated with carcinogens. *Cancer Res, 41,* 3759-3760.

Connor, W. E. (1968). Plant sterols: their relationship to atherosclerosis. *J Am Diet Assoc, 52*, 202-208.

Davidson, M. H., Maki, K. C., Umporowicz, D. M., Ingramm, K. A., Dicklin, M. R., Schaefer, E. et al. (2001). Safety and tolerability of esterified phytosterols administered in reduced-fat spread and salad dressing to healthy adult men and women. *J Am Coll Nutr, 20*, 307-319.

De Graaf, J., de Sauvage Nolting P. R. W., Van Dam, M., Belsey, E. M., Kastelein, J. J. P., Pritchard, P. H. & Stalenhoef, A. (2002). Consumption of tall oil-derived phytosterols in a chocolate matrix significantly decreases plasma total and low density lipprotein cholesterol levels. *Br J Nutr*, *88*, 479-488.

De Jong, A., Plat, J. & Mensink, R. P. (2003). Metabolic effects of plant sterols and plant stanols (review). *J Nutr Biochem, 14*, 362-369.

Denke, M. A. (1995). Lack of efficacy of low-dose sitostanol therapy as an adjunct to a cholesterol-lowering diet in men with moderate hypercholesterolemia. *Am J Clin Nutr, 61*, 392-396.

Farquhar, J. W., Smith, R. E. & Dempsey, M. E. (1956). The effect of beta sitosterol on the serum lipids of young men with arteriosclerotic heart disease. *Circulation, 14*, 77-82.

Geelen, A., Zock, P. L., de Vries, J. H. & Katan, M. B. (2002). Apolipoprotein E polymorphism and serum lipid response to plant sterols in humans. *Eur J Clin Invest, 32*, 738-742.

Gould, A. L., Rossouw, J. E., Santanello, N. C., Heyse, J. F. & Furberg, C. D. (1998). Cholesterol reduction yields clinical benefits: impact of statin trials. *Circulation, 97,* 946-952.

Grundy, S. M. & Mok, H. Y. (1976). Effects of low phytosterols on cholesterol absorption in man; in Greten, *Lipoprotein metabolism*, 112-118, (Springer, Berlin).

Gylling, H. & Miettinen, T. A. (1994). Serum cholesterol lipoprotein metabolism in hypercholesterolemic NIDDM patients before and during sitostanol ester-margarine treatment', *Diabetologia*, *37*, 773-780.

Gylling, H. & Miettinen, T. A. (1996). Effects of inhibiting cholesterol absorption and synthesis on cholesterol and lipoprotein metabolism in hypercholesterolemic non-insulin-dependent diabetic men. *J Lipid Research*, *37*, 1776-1785

Gylling, H., Radhakrishnan, R. & Miettinen, T. A. (1997). Reduction of serum cholesterol in postmenopausal women with previous myocardial infarction and cholesterol malabsorption induced by dietary sitostanol ester margarine. *Circulation,12*, 4226-4231.

Gylling, H. & Miettinen, T. A. (1999). Cholesterol reduction by differnet plant stanol mixtures with variable fat intake. *Metabolism*, *48*, 575-580.

Gylling, H., Puska, P., Vartiainen, E. & Miettinen, T. A. (1999). Retinol, vitamin D, carotenes and alpha-tocopherol in serum of a moderately hypercholesterolemic population consuming sitostanol ester margarine, *Atherosclerosis*, *145*, 279-285.

Hallikainen, M. A. & Uusitupa, M. I. (1999). Effects of 2 low-fat stanol ester-containing margarines on serum cholesterol concentrations as part of a low-fat diet in hypercholesterolemic subjects. *Am J Clin Nutr*, *69*, 403-410.

Hallikainen, M. A., Sarkkinen, E. S. & Uusitupa, M. I. (1999). Effects of low-fat stanol ester enriched margarines on concentrations of serum carotenoids in subjects with elevated serum cholesterol concentrations. *Eur J Clin Nutr*, *53*, 966-969.

Hallikainen, M. A., Sarkkinen, E. S., Gylling, H., Erkkila, A. T. & Uusitupa, M. I. (2000). Comparison of the effects of plant sterol ester and plant stanol ester-enriched margarines in lowering serum cholesterol concentrations in hypercholesterolamic subjects on a low-fat diet. *Eur J Clin Nutr, 54*, 715-725.

Heinemann, T., Pietruck, B., Kullak-Ublick, G. & Von Bergmann, K. (1988). Comparison of sitosterol and sitostanol inhibition of intestinal cholesterol absorption. *Agents Actions (Suppl), 26*, 117-122.

Heinemann, T., Kullak-Ublick, G. A., Pietruck, B. & Von Bergmann, K. (1991). Mechanisms of action of plant sterols on inhibition of cholesterol absorption. Comparison of sitosterol and sitostanol. *Eur J Clin Pharmacol, 40 (Suppl 1)*, 59-63.

Heinemann, T., Axtmann, G. & Von Bergmann, K. (1993). Comparison of intestinal absorption of cholesterol with different plant sterols in man. *Eur J Clin Invest, 23*, 827-831.

Hendriks, H. F. J., Weststrate, J. A., Van Vliet, T. & Meijer, G. W. (1999). Spreads enriched with three different levels of vegetable oil sterols and the degree of cholesterol lowering in normocholesterolaemic and mildly hypercholesterolaemic subjects. *Eur J Clin Nutr, 53*, 319-327.

Hendriks, H. F. J., Brink, E. J., Meijer, G. W., Princen, H. M. G. & Ntanios, F. Y. (2003). Safety of long-term consumption of plant sterol esters-enriched spread. *Eur J Clin Nutr, 57*, 681-692.

Hepburn, P. A., Homer, S. A. & Smith, M. (1999). Safety evaluation of phytosterol esters: Part 2. Subchronic 90-day oral toxicity study on phytosterol esters: A novel functional food. *Food Chem Toxicol, 37*, 521-532.

Hirai, K., Shimazu, C., Takezoe, R. & Okezi, Y. (1986). Cholesterol, phytosterol and polyunsaturated fatty acid levels in 1982 and 1957 Japanese diets. *J Nutr Sci Vitaminol, 32*, 363-372.

Ikeda, I., Tanabe, Y. & Sugano, M. (1989). Effects of sitosterol and sitostanol on micellar solubility of cholesterol. *J Nutr Sci Vitaminol (Tokyo), 35*, 361-369.

Ishiwata, K., Homma, Y., Ishikawata, T., Nakamura, H. & Handa S (2002). Influence of apolipoprotein E phenotype on metabolism of lipids and apolipoproteins after plant stanol ester ingestion in Japanese subjects. *Nutrition, 18*, 561-565.

Janezic, S. A. & Rao, A. V. (1992). Dose-dependent effects of dietary phytosterol on epithelial cell proliferation of the murine colon. *Food Chem Toxicol, 30*, 611-616.

Jones, P. J. H., Ntanios, F. Y., Raeini-Sarjaz, M. & Vanstone, C. A. (1999). Cholesterol-lowering efficacy of a sitostanol-containing phytosterol mixture with a prudent diet in hyperlipidemic men. *Am J Clin Nutr, 69*, 1140-1150.

Jones, P. J., Raeini-Sarjaz, M., Ntanios, F. Y., Vanstone, C. A., Feng, J. Y. & Parsons, W. E. (2000). Modulation of plasma lipid levels and cholesterol kinetics by phytosterol versus phytostanol esters. *J Lipid Res, 41*, 697-705.

Jones, P. J. & Raeini-Sarjaz, M. (2001). Plant sterols and their derivatives: The current spread of results. *Nutr Rev, 59*, 21-24.

Jones, P. J. H., Vanstone, C. A., Raeini-Sarjaz, M. & St-Onge, M. P. (2003). Phytosterols in low- and nonfat beverages as part of a controlled diet fail to lower plasma lipid levels. *J Lipid Res, 44*, 1713-1719.

Judd, J. T., Baer, D. J., Chen, S. C., Clevidence, B. A., Muesing, R. A., Kramer, M. &

Meijer, G. W. (2002). Plant sterol esters lower plasma lipids and most carotenoids in mildly hypercholesterolemic adults. *Lipids, 37*, 33-42.

Katan, M. B., Zock, P. L. & Mensink, R. P. (1994). Effects of fats and fattya cids on blood lipids in humans: an overview. *Am J Clin Nutr, 60 (suppl)*, S1017-S1022.

Katan, M. B., Grundy, S. M., Jones, P., Law, M., Miettinen, T. & Paoletti, R. (2003). Efficacy and safety of plant stanols and sterols in the management of blood cholesterol levels. *Mayo Clin Proc, 78*, 965-978.

http://www.mayo.edu/proceedings/2003/aug/7808r1.pdf

Keys, A., Anderson, J. T. & Grande, F. (1965). Serum cholesterol response to changes in the diet. IV. Particular saturated fatty acids in the diet. *Metabolism, 14*, 776-787.

Law, M. R., Wald, M. J & Thompson, S. G. (1994). By how much and how quickly does a reduction in serum cholesterol concentrations lower risk of ischaemic heart disease? *BMJ, 308*, 367-373.

Ling, W. H. & Jones, P. J. H. (1995). Dietary phytosterols: a review of metabolism, benefits and and side effects. *Life Sciences, 57*, 195-206.

Maki, K. C., Davidson, M. H., Umporowicz, D. M., Schafer, E. J., Dicklin, M. R., Ingram, K. A., Chen, S., McNamara, J. R., Gebhart, B. W., Ribaya-Mercado, J. D., Perrone, G., Robins, S. J. & Franke, W. C. (2001). Lipid responses to plant-sterol-enriched reduced-fat spreads incorporated into a National Cholesterol Education Program Step I diet. *Am J Clin Nutr, 74*, 33-43.

Maki, K. C., Shinnick, F., Seeley, M. A., Veith, P. E., Quinn, L. C., Hallissey, P. J., Temer, A. & Davidson, M. H. (2003). Food products containing free tall oil-based phytosterols and oat beta-glucan lower serum total and LDL cholesterol in hypercholesterolemic adults (2003). *J Nutr, 133*, 808-813.

Matvienko, O. A., Lewis, D. S., Swanson, M., Arndt, B., Rainwater, D. L., Stewart, J. & Alekel, D. L. (2002). A single daily dose of soybean phytosterols in ground beef decreases serum total cholesterol and LDL cholesterol in young, mildly hypercholesterolemic men. *Am J Clin Nutr, 76*, 57-64.

Meguro, S., Higashi, K., Hase, T., Honda, Y., Otsuka, A., Tokimitsu, I. & Itakura, H. (2001). Solubiliation of phytosterols in diacylglycerol versus triacylglycerol improves serum cholesterol lowering effect. *Eur J Clin Nutr, 55*, 513-517.

Mensink, R. P. & Katan, M. B. (1992). Effect of dietary fatty acids on serum lipids and lipoproteins. *Arteriosclerosis and thrombosis, 12*, 912-919.

Mensink, R. P., Ebbing, S., Lindhout, M., Plat, J. & Heugten, M. M. A. (2002). Effects of plant stanol esters supplied in low-fat yoghurt on serum lipids and lipoproteins, non-cholesterol sterols and fat soluble antioxidant concentrations. *Atherosclerosis, 160*, 205-213.

Miettinen, T. A. & Vanhanen, H. (1994). Dietary sitostanol related to absorption, synthesis and serum level of cholesterol in different apolipoprotein E phenotypes. *Atherosclerosis, 105*, 217-226.

Miettinen, T. A., Tilvis, R. S., Kesaniemi, Y. A. (1990). Serum plant sterol and cholesterol precursors reflect cholesterol absorption and synthesis in volunteers of a randomly selected male population. *Am J Epidemiol, 131*, 20-31.

Miettinen, T. A., Puska, P., Gylling, H., Vanhanen, H. & Vartiainen E (1995). Reduction of serum cholesterol with sitostanol-ester margarine in a mildly hypercholesterolemic population. *N Engl J Med, 333*, 1308-1312.

Miettinen, T. A., Vuoristo, M., Nissinen, M., Jarvinen, H. & Gylling, H. (2000). Serum, biliary and fecal cholesterol and plant sterols in colectomized patients before and during consumption if stanol ester margarine. *Am J Clin Nutr, 71*, 1095-1102.

Morton, G. M., Lee, S. M., Buss, D. H. & Lawrence, P. (1995), 'Intakes and major dietary sources of cholesterols and phytosterols in the British diet', *J Hum Nutr Diet,* 8, 429-440.

Mussner, M. J., Parhofer, K. G., Von Bergmann, K., Schwandt, P., Broedl, U. & Otto, C. (2002). Effects of phytosterol ester-enriched margarine on plasma lipoproteins in mild to moderate hypercholesterolemia are related to basal cholesterol and fat intake. *Metabolism, 51*, 189-194.

Nair, P. P., Turjmna, N., Kessie, G., Culkins, B., Goodman, G. T., Davidovitz, H. & Nimmagadda, G. (1984). Diet, nutrition intake, and metabolism in populations at high and low risk for colon cancer. *Am J Clin Nutr, 40*, 927-930.

Naumann, E., Plat, J. & Mensink, R. P. (2003). Changes in serum concentrations of noncholesterol sterols and lipoproteins in healthy subjects do not depend on the ration of plant sterols to stanols in the diet. *J Nutr, 133*, 2741-2747.

Neil, H. A. W., Meijer, G. W. & Roe, L. S. (2001). Ranodomised controlled trial of use by hypercholesterolaemic patients of a vegetable oil sterol-enriched fat spread. *Atherosclerosis, 156*, 329-337.

Nestel, P., Cehun, M., Pomeroy, S., Abbey, M. & Weldon, G. (2001). Cholesterol-lowering effects of plant sterol esters and non esterified-stanols in margarine, butter and low-fat foods. *Eur J Clin Nutr, 55*, 1084-1090.

Nguyen, T. T., Dale, L. C., Von Bergmann, K. & Croghan, I. T. (1999). Cholesterol lowering effect of stanol ester in a US population of mildly hypercholesterolemic men and women: a randomized controlled trial. *Mayo Clin Proc, 74*, 1198-1206.

Nigon, F., Serfaty-Lacrosniere, C., Beucler, I., Chauvois, D., Neveu, C. et al. (2001). Plant sterol enriched margarine lowers plasma LDL in hyperlipidemic subjects with low cholesterol intake: Effect of fibrite treatment. *Clin Chem Lab Med, 39*, 634-640.

Noakes, M., Clifton, P., Ntanios, F., Shrapnel, W., Record, I. & McInerney, J. (2002). An increase in dietary carotenoids when consuming plant sterols or stanols is effective in maintaining plasma carotenoid concentrations. *Am J Clin Nutr, 75*, 79-86.

Normén, L., Dutta, P., Lia, A. & Andersson, H. (2000). Soy sterol esters and ß-sitostanol ester as inhibitors of cholesterol absorption in human small bowel. *Am J Clin Nutr, 71*, 903-913.

Normén, A. L., Brants, H. A. M., Voorrips, L. A., Andersson, H. A., Van den Brandt, P. A. & Goldbohm, R. A. (2001). Plant sterols intakes and colorectal cancer risk in the Netherlands Cohort Study on Diet and Cancer. *Am J Clin Nutr, 74*, 141-148.

Ntanios, F. & Jones, P. J. H. (1998). Effects of variable dietary sitostanol concentrations om plasma lipis profile and phytosterol metabolism in hamsters. *Biochim Biophys Acta, 1390*, 237-244.

Ntanios, F. Y., Homma, Y. & Ushiro, S. (2002). A spread enriched with plant sterol-esters lowers blood cholesterol and lipoproteins without affecting vitamins A and E in normal and hypercholesterolemic Japanese men and women. *J Nutr, 132*, 3650-3655.

Ostlund, R. E., McGill, J. B., Zeng, C. M., Covey, D. F., Stearns, J., Stenson, W. F. & Spilburg, C. A. (2002). Gastrointestinal absorption and plasma kinetics of soy delta(5)phytosterols and phytostanols in humans. *Am J Physiol Endocrinol Metabol, 282,* E911-E916.

Pelletier, X., Belbraouet, S., Mirable, D., Mordret, F., Perrin, J. L., et al. (1995). A diet moderatelt enriched in phytosterols lowers plasma cholesterol concentrations in normocholesterolemic humans. *Ann Nutr Metab, 39,* 291-295.

Plat, J. & Mensink, R. (1998). Safety aspects of dietary plant sterols and stanols. *Postgraduate Medicine -A Special Report: New developments in the dietary management of high cholesterol*, November 1998.

Plat, J., Van Onselen, E. N. M. & Mensink, R. P. (1999). Dietary plant stanol ester mixtures – Effects on safety parameters and erythrocyte membrane fatty acid composition in non-hypercholesterolaemic subjects. *European Heart Journal Supplements 1*, S58-S63.

Plat, J., Van Onselen, E. N. M., Van Heugten, M. M. A. & Mensink, R. P. (2000). Effects on serum lipids, lipoproteins and fat soluble anti-oxidant concentrations of consumption frequency of margarines and shortenings enriched with plant stanol esters. *Eur J Clin Nutr, 54*, 671-677.

Plat, J. & Mensink, R.P. (2000). Vegetable oil based versus wood based stanol ester mixtures: Effects on serum lipids and hemostatic factors in non hypercholesterolemic subjects. *Atherosclerosi, 148,* 101-112.

Plat, J. & Mensink, R. P. (2001). Effects of diets enriched with two different plant stanol ester mixtures on plasma ubiquinol-10 and fat-soluble antioxidant concentrations. *Metabolism, 20*, 520-529.

Plat, J. & Mensink, R. P. (2002). Increased intestinal ABCA1 expression contributes to the decrease in cholesterol absorption after plant stanol consumption', *FASEB J, 16*, 1248-1253.

Pollak, O. J. (1953). Reduction of blood cholesterol in man. *Circulation, 7,* 702-706.

Pollak, O. J. & Kritchevsky, D. (1981). *Monographs on atherosclerosis.* ISBN 3-8055-0568-X.

Raeini-Sarjaz, M., Ntanios, F. Y., Vanstone, C. A. & Jones, P. J. H. (2002). No changes in serum fat-soluble vitamin and carotenoid concentrations with the intake of plant sterol/stanol esters in the context of a controlled diet. *Metabolism, 51*, 652-656.

Richelle, M., Enslen, M., Hager, C., Groux, M., Tavazzi, I., et al. (2004) Both free and esterified plant sterols reducse cholesterol absorptiob and the bioavailability of beta-carotene and alpha-tocopherol in normocholesterolemic humans. *Am J Clin Nutr, 80,* 171-177.

Robinson, M., Wnorowski, G. & Dreher, M. (1998). Dietary stanols as anti-hypercholesterolemic agents: a 90-day sub-chronic feeding trial as a safety assessment in the rat. *#1202 Abstract from F.A.S.B. meeting in San Francisco. (Nabisco Inc, East Hanover, NJ 07936 and Product Safety Labs, East Brunswick, NJ 08816).*

Salen, G., Kwiterovich, P. O., Shefer, S., Tint, G. S., Horak, I., Shore, V., Dayal, B. & Horak, E. (1985). Increased plasma cholestanol and 5α-saturated plant sterol derivatives in subjects with sitosterolemia and xanthomatosis. *J Lipid Res*, *26*, 203-209.

SCF (Scientific Committee on Food) (2003). Opinion of the Scientific Committee on Food Applications for Approval of a Variety of Plant Sterol-Enriched Foods. General View expressed by the Scientific Committee on Food on 05 March 2003, available online at: *http://europa.eu.int/comm/food/fs/sc/scf/index_en.html*

SCF (Scientific Committee on Food) (2002). General view of the Scientific Committee on Food on the long-term effects of the intake of elevated levels of phytosterols from multiple dietary sources, with particular attention to the effects on β-carotene. Opinion adopted by the Scientific Committee on Food on 26 September 2002, available online at: *http://europa.eu.int/comm/food/fs/sc/scf/index_en.html*

SCF (Scientific Committee on Food) (2000). Opinion on a request for the safety assessment of the use of phytosterol esters in yellow fat spreads. Opinion adopted by the Scientific Committee on Food on 6 April 2000, available online at: *http://europa.eu.int/comm/food/fs/sc/scf/out56_en.pdf*

Sehayek, E. (2003). Genetic regulation of cholesterol absorption and plasma plan sterol levels: commonalities and differences. *J Lipid Res*, *44*, 2030-2038.

Shin, M. J., Rim, S. J., Jang, Y. S., Choi, D., Kang, S. M., Cho, S. Y., Kim, D. K., Song, K. J. & Chung, N. (2003). The cholesterol lowering effect of plant sterol-containing beverage in hypercholesterolemic subjects with low cholesterol intake. *Nutr Res, 23*, 489-496.

Shipley, R. E., Pfeiffer, R. R., Marsh, M. M. & Anderson, R. C. (1958). Sitosterol feeding: Chronic animal and clinical toxicology and tissue analysis. *Circulation Research, 6,* 373-382.

Sierksma, A., Weststrate, J. A. & Meijer, G. W. (1999). Spreads enriched with plant sterols, either esterified 4,4-dimethylsterols or free 4-desmethylsterols, and plasma total- and LDL-cholesterol concentrations. *Br J Nutr*, *82*, 273-282.

Slesinski, R. S., Turnbull, D., Frankos, V. H., Wolterbeek, A. P. M. & Waalkens-Berendsen, D. H. (1999). Developmental toxicity study in vegetable-oil derived stanol fatty acid esters. *Regulatory Toxicology and Pharmacology*, *29*, 227-233.

Spilburg, C. A., Goldberg, A. C., McGill, J. B., Stenson, W. F., Racette, S. B., et al. (2003). Fat-free foods supplemented with soy-stanol lecithin powder reduce cholesterol absorption and LDL cholesterol. *Am J Diet Assoc 103*, 577-581.

Stamler, J., Daviglus, M. L., Garside, D. B., Dyer, A. R., Greenland, P. & Neaton, J. D. (2000). Relationship of baseline serum cholesterol levels in 3 large cohorts of younger men to long-term coronary, cardiovascular, and all-cause mortality and to longevity. *JAMA, 284*, 311-318.

Subbiah, M. T. R. & Kuksis, A. (1973). Differences in metabolism of cholesterol and sitosterol following intravenous injection in rats. *Biochim et Biophys Acta, 306*, 95-105.

Tang, J. L., Armitage, J. M., Lancaster, T., Silagy, C. A., Fowler, G. H. & Neil H. A. W. (1998). Systematic review of dietary intervention trials to lower blood total cholesterol in free-living subjects. *BMJ, 316*, 1213-1220.

Temme, E. H., Van Hoydonck, P. G., Schouten, E. G. & Kesteloot, H. (2002). Effects of a plant sterol-enriched spread on serum lipids and lipoproteins in mildly hypercholesterolaemic subjects. *Acta Cardiol, 57*, 111-115.

Tikkanen, M. J., Hogstrom, P., Tuomilehto, J., Keinanen-Kiukaanniemi, S., Sundvall, J. & Karppanen, H. (2001). Effect of a diet based on low-fat foods enriched with nonesterified plant sterols and mineral nutrients on serum cholesterol. *Am J Cardiol*, *88*, 1157-1162.

Turnbull, D., Whittaker, M. H., Frankos, V. H. & Jonker, D. (1999a). 13-week oral toxicity study with stanol esters in rats. *Regulatory Toxicology and Pharmacology*, *29*, 216-226.

Turnbull, D., Frankos, V. H., Van Delft, J. H. M. & DeVogel, N. (1999b). Genotoxicity evaluation of wood-derived and vegetable-oil derived stanol esters. *Regulatory Toxicology and Pharmacology*, *29*, 205-210.

Turnbull, D., Frankos, V. H., Leeman, W. R. & Jonker, D. (1999c). Short-term tests of estrogenic potential of plant stanols and plant stanol esters. *Regulatory Toxicology and Pharmacology*, *29*, 211-215.

Vanhanen, H. T., Blomqvist, S., Ehnholm, C., Hyvonen, M., Jauhiainen, M., Torstila, I. & Miettinen, T. A. (1993). Serum cholesterol, cholesterol precursors, and plant sterols in hypercholesterolemic subjects with different apoE phenotypes during dietary sitostanol ester treatment. *J Lipid Res*, *34*, 1535-1544.

Vanstone, C. A., Raenini-Sarjaz, M., Parsons, W. E. & Jones, P. J. H. (2002). Unsterified plant sterols and stanols lower LDL-cholesterol concentrations equivalently in hypercholesterolemic persons. *Am J Clin Nutr, 76*, 1272-1278.

Vissers, M. N., Zock, P. L., Meijer, G. W. & Katan, M. B. (2000). Effect of plant sterols from rice bran oil and triterpene alcohols from sheanut oil on serum lipoprotein concrentrations in humans. *Am J Clin Nutr*, *72*, 1510-1515.

Volger, O. L., Van der Boom, H., De Wit, E. C. M., Van Duyvenvoorde, W., Hornstra, G., Plat, J., Havekes, L. M., Mensink, R. P. & Princen, H. M. G. (2001). Dietary plant stanol esters reduce VLDL cholesterol secretion and bile saturation in apolipoprotein E*3-Leiden transgenic mice. *Atheroscler Thromb Vasc Biol, 18*, 1046-1052.

Volpe, R., Niitynen, L., Korpela, R., Sirtori, C., Bucci, A. et al. (2001). Effects of yogurt enriched with plant sterols on serum lipids in patients with moderate hypercholesterolaemia. *Br J Nutr*, *86*, 233-239.

Vuori, A. F., Gylling, H., Turtola, H., Kontula, K., Ketonen, P. & Miettinen, T. A. (2000). Stanol ester margarine alone and with simvastatin lowers serum cholesterol in families with familial hypercholesterolemia caused by the FH-North Karelia Mutation. *Arterioscler Thromb Vasc Biol, 20*, 500-506

Wester, I. (2000). Cholesterol lowering effect of plant sterols. *Eur J Lipid Sci Technolo, 102*, 37-44.

Weststrate, J. A. & Meijer, G. W. (1998). Plant sterol-enriched margarines and reduction of plasma total and LDL-cholesterol concentrations in normocholesterolemic and mildly hypercholesterolemic subjects. *Eur J Clin Nutr, 52*, 334-343.

Wolfreys, A. M. & Hepburn, P. A. (2002). Safety evaluation of phytosterol esters. Part 7. Assessment of mutagenic activity of phytosterols, phytosterol esters and the cholesterol derivative, 4-cholesten-3-one. *Fd Chem Toxicol, 40*, 461-470.

In: Cholesterol in Atherosclerosis and Coronary Heart Disease ISBN 1-59454-302-X
Editor: Jean P. Kovala, pp.215-232 

*Chapter X*

# Homocysteine and Cardiovascular Risk

***Johann Auer,*[*] *Robert Berent and Bernd Eber***
General Hospital Wels, Austria

## Abstract

Homocysteine is a sulphydryl-containing aminoacid derived from demethylation of methionine and is metabolized either by remethylation or by transsulfuration. Nutritional deficiencies in the vitamin cofactors (folate, vitamin B12, and vitamin B6) required for homocysteine metabolism may promote hyperhomocysteinemia.

The prevalence of hyperhomocysteinaemia has been estimated to be about 5% in the general population, and 13-47% among patients with symptomatic atherosclerotic vascular disease. Multiple prospective and case-control studies suggested that a moderately elevated plasma homocysteine concentration is an independent risk factor for atherothrombotic vascular disease. Homocysteine concentrations are consistently higher in patients with peripheral, cerebrovascular, and coronary artery disease than in those without such diseases. Homocysteine seems to promote atherothrombogenesis by a variety of mechanisms; however, it is not yet clear whether homocysteine itself or a related metabolite or cofactor is primarily responsible for the atherothrombogenic effects of hyperhomocysteinemia in vivo. Before advocating widespread screening of patients with atherosclerotic vascular disease, we must have a clearer understanding of the clinical efficacy of potential therapeutic interventions. Vitamin supplementation decreases or even normalizes plasma homocysteine concentrations in most cases. Prospective, randomized clinical trials, however, will be necessary to determine the effect of vitamin supplementation on cardiovascular morbidity and mortality. The use of pills containing low dose B vitamins as a primary or secondary preventive measure against vascular disease remains unproved, although they are definitely cheap, probably innocuous, and may help prevent acute vascular episodes.

[*] Address of correspondence: Johann Auer, MD, II [nd] Medical Department, Division of Cardiology and Intensive Care, General Hospital Wels, Grieskirchnerstraße 42, 4600 Wels, Austria. Tel.:++43 7242 415 2215; Fax: ++43 7242 415 3992; e-mail: johann.auer@khwels.at

# What is Homocysteine?

Homocysteine is a sulfur-containing amino acid derived from the metabolic demethylation of dietary methionine, which is abundant in animal protein. Homocysteine is metabolized by one of two pathways: remethylation and transsulfuration It is present in plasma in four forms: as circulating free thiol (1%); disulphide-bound to plasma proteins, chiefly albumin (70-80%); and combinations with itself to form the dimer homocysteine or with other thiols, including cysteine, with which it forms the homocysteine-cysteine mixed disulphide (20-30%). The term "total plasma (or serum) homocysteine" (tHcy) refers to the combined pool of all four forms of homocysteine.

# Homocystein and Vascular Disease

In 1969, McCully[1] made the clinical observation linking elevated plasma homocysteine concentrations with vascular disease. Subsequent investigations have confirmed this hypothesis. For about two decades, moderately raised concentrations of total homocysteine (tHcy) have been correlated with an increased risk of atherothrombotic vascular events [2,3] but only recently has evidence mounted to suggest that the association may be causal. The association is independent of other known risk factors and it is consistent across many studies. Furthermore, it is strong and dose-related, and it is biologically plausible. Although the molecular mechanism by which homocysteine or a related metabolite promotes atherothrombosis is unknown, the epidemiologic evidence of the association of hyperhomocysteinemia with atherothrombotic vascular disease seems to be convincing. However, the evidence needs to be strengthened by the demonstration, in randomised trials, that lowering tHcy is followed by a significant reduction in atherothrombotic vascular disease. In addition, the measurement of tHcy needs to be standardised. If these can be achieved then tHcy measurement will become another useful marker of vascular risk, multivitamin therapy will be another therapeutic option for people at risk of atherothrombotic vascular disease, and fortification of food with folic acid will rise high on the political and public health agenda.

Only about two-thirds of all episodes of symptomatic atherothrombotic vascular disease in developed countries can be attributed to established genetic and environmental vascular risk factors [4]. An additional causal vascular risk factor may be raised plasma levels of homocysteine (hyperhomocysteinaemia). Mild hyperhomocysteinemia occurs in approximately 5 to 7 percent of the general population [5,6]. Patients with mild hyperhomocysteinemia are typically asymptomatic until the third or fourth decade of life when premature coronary artery disease develops, as well as recurrent arterial and venous thrombosis. Although 30 years have elapsed since hyperhomocysteinaemia were first associated with an increased risk of atherothrombotic vascular disease, it is only recently that sufficient evidence has mounted to suggest that the association is independent and dose-related, and it remains to be established whether it is causal and modifiable.

## Definition of Hyperhomocysteinaemia and Measurement of Plasma Homocysteine

An abnormal "total plasma (or serum) homocysteine" (tHcy) is defined by an arbitrary cut-off in the distribution of concentrations found in the "normal population", in much the same way as other more common vascular risk factors like hypertension and hypercholesterolaemia have been defined. For example, after methionine-loading, hyperhomocysteinaemia is defined as a tHcy of more than 2 standard deviations (SD) above the mean [7]. Among fasting individuals, "normal" tHcy commonly ranges from 5 to 15 μmol/L [8,9] and higher fasting values are classified as moderate (16-30), intermediate (31-100), and severe (>100 μmol/L) hyperhomocysteinaemia [10] on the basis of concentrations measured during fasting.

The majority of the clinical studies involving homocysteine have relied on the measurement of total plasma homocysteine, which includes homocysteine, mixed disulfides involving homocysteine, homocysteine thiolactone, free homocysteine, and protein-bound homocysteine. Protein-bound homocysteine accounts for 70 to 80 percent of the total pool. Data about the effect of acute occlusive vascular events on homocysteine levels are not consistent[11].

An oral dose of methionine (100 mg per kilogram of body weight) can be given to persons with suspected hyperhomocysteinemia who have normal homocysteine concentrations during fasting[12]. Plasma homocysteine concentrations are determined before the methionine challenge and between four and eight hours afterward. Hyperhomocysteinemia is considered to be present if the homocysteine concentration after methionine challenge is more than 2 SD above the mean [13]. The prognostic value of the methionine-challenge test has recently been discussed controversely [8]. In contrast to a weak association between plasma homocysteine concentrations after methionine challenge and premature coronary heart disease in persons with the thermolabile variant of N,N-methylenetetrahydrofolate reductase, there was a significant association between plasma homocysteine concentrations during fasting and premature coronary heart disease. In conclusion, this enzyme regulates basal homocysteine concentrations, and thus, its activity cannot be adequately assessed by a methionine-challenge test. By contrast however, enzymes in the transsulfuration pathway are responsible for reversing transient, postprandial increases in the homocysteine concentration, and their activities can be evaluated by a methionine-challenge test.

## Homocysteine Metabolism

Homocysteine is a sulphydryl-containing aminoacid derived from the metabolic demethylation of methionine. Homocysteine is metabolized by remethylation or transsulfuration. In the remethylation cycle, homocysteine is salvaged by the acquisition of a methyl group in a reaction catalyzed by methionine synthase. Vitamin B12 (cobalamin) is an essential cofactor for methionine synthase, N-methyl-tetrahydrofolate is the methyl donor in this reaction, and N,N-methylenetetrahydrofolate reductase acts as a catalyst in the remethylation process [14] (figure 1).

Under conditions with an excess of methionine or when cysteine synthesis is required, homocysteine enters the transsulfuration pathway. In this pathway, homocysteine condenses with serine to form cystathionine in a reaction catalyzed by the vitamin B6-dependent enzyme cystathionine (beta)-synthase.

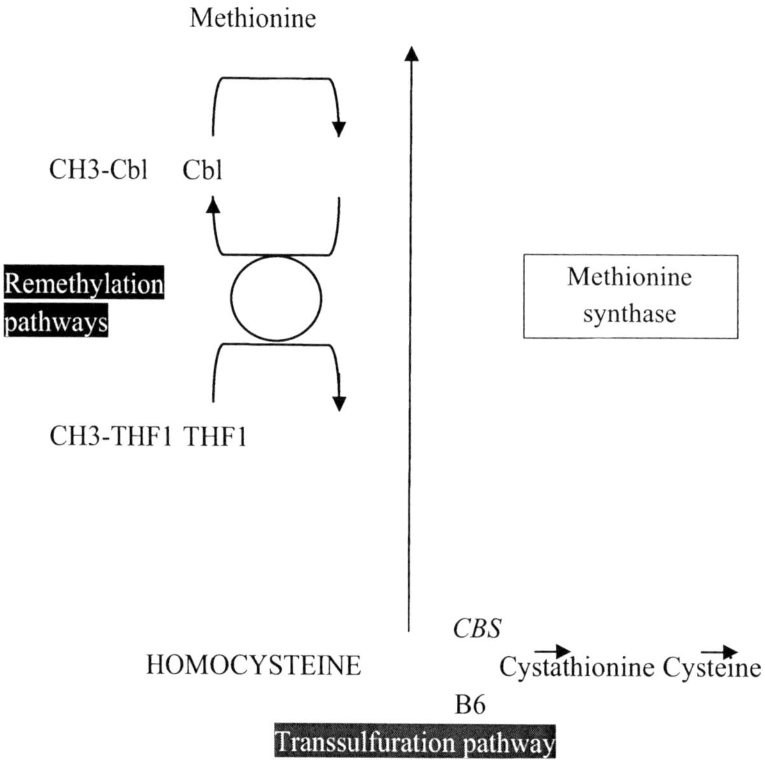


Figure 1. Pathways of homocysteine metabolism. (CBS=cystathionine-ß-synthase; Cbl=cobalamin; THF1 = monoglutamated form of tetrahydrofolate; B6=vitamin B6; CH3=Mythyl-)
Homocysteine is metabolized either by transsulfuration to cysteine (in a reaction catalyzed by cystathionine-ß-synthase [CBS] with vitamin B6 as cofactor) or by remethylation to methionine. Remethylation is catalyzed by methionine synthase (and 5, 10 methylenetetrahydrofolate reductase). Methionine synthase is dependent upon cobolamin (vitamin B 12) as cofactor and folate as cosubstrate. An alternative remethylation pathway (not shown in the figure) uses the cobolamin independent betain-homocysteine methyltransferase.

## Nutritional Factors and Homocysteine Metabolism (Table 1)

Nutritional deficiencies in the vitamin cofactors (folate, vitamin B12, and vitamin B6) required for homocysteine metabolism may promote hyperhomocysteinemia. Markedly elevated homocysteine concentrations have been observed in patients with nutritional deficiencies of the essential cofactor vitamin B12 [15] and the cosubstrate folate [16]. It has been suggested that about two-thirds of hyperhomocysteinaemia is due to inadequate blood levels of one or more of these vitamin cofactors [17,18].

Inadequate plasma concentrations of one or more B vitamins are contributing factors in approximately two thirds of all cases of hyperhomocysteinemia. Vitamin supplementation can normalize high homocysteine concentrations, however, it remains to be determined whether normalizing homocysteine concentrations will improve cardiovascular morbidity and mortality.

**Table 1. Factors Influencing Homocysteine Metabolism (Factors Increasing Homocysteine Levels)**

| |
|---|
| Nutritional deficiencies in vitamin cofactors |
| Folate |
| Vitamin $B_6$ (pyridoxine) |
| Vitamin $B_{12}$ (cobalamin) |
| Genetic defects in homocysteine metabolism |
| CßS |
| MTHFR |
| Methionine synthase |
| Medications/toxins |
| Folate antagonists (methotrexate, phenytoin, carbamazepine) |
| Vitamin $B_6$ antagonists (theophylline, azarabine, oestrogen-containing oral contraceptives, cigarette smoking) |
| Age/sex |
| Increasing age |
| Male sex |
| Menopause |
| Diseases |
| Malignancy: acute lymphoblastic leukaemia; carcinoma of the breast, ovary and pancreas |
| Severe psoriasis |
| Pernicious anaemia |
| Renal impairment |
| Hypothyroidism |

## Hyperhomocysteinemia caused by Other Factors

Renal impairment commonly causes hyperhomocysteinaemia. Fasting tHcy rises as serum creatinine rises, not because of impaired urinary excretion but because of impaired metabolism of homocysteine by the kidney, the major route by which homocysteine is cleared from plasma. In contrast, urinary excretion is a very minor route for direct homocysteine clearance [19].

Total homocysteine levels are considerably higher in patients with chronic renal disease than the moderately raised concentrations commonly found in patients with atherothrombotic vascular disease, and this may contribute to the high incidence of vascular complications in patients with chronic renal failure. Values are higher in patients undergoing haemodialysis compared to peritoneal dialysis. The exact mechanisms for the raised levels of the amino acid seen in these patients remain unclear but reduced systemic clearance of homocysteine, lower circulating folate, and folate inhibition are probably major determinants.

A number of reports have linked hyperhomocysteinemia to hypothyroidism, suggesting a potential mechanism for the higher incidence of vascular disease observed in patients with hypothyroidism. Hyperhomocysteinemia has also been reported in patients with pernicious anemia and It is unclear whether these patients are at increased risk for vascular events.

Elevated homocysteine concentrations have been reported in association with several types of carcinoma, including breast, ovarian, and pancreatic cancer [20].

Several drugs and toxins increase plasma homocysteine concentrations. Methotrexate depletes folate, the cosubstrate for methionine synthase, and causes a transient increase in plasma homocysteine concentrations. Phenytoin, Theophylline (interference with the synthesis of pyridoxal phosphate) and cigarette smoking interact with homocysteine metabolism. Cyclosporin may impair renal function and it has been associated with hyperhomocysteinaemia.

It has been reported that smokers have significantly lower pyridoxal phosphate concentrations than nonsmokers [21]. These results suggest another important mechanism whereby smoking may promote atherogenesis.

Homocysteine concentrations rise with age in both sexes. Women in general have lower concentrations than men, and concentrations rise after menopause. a high intake of caffeine or alcohol, and a sedentary lifestyle are associated with raised homocysteine.

## Pathophysiologic Mechanisms of Association between Hyperhomocysteinemia and Atherosclerosis

Clinical and experimental studies suggest that high homocysteine concentrations may cause the atherogenic and thrombotic tendencies of homocystinuric and hyperhomocysteinaemic patients. Experimental evidence suggests that the atherogenic propensity associated with hyperhomocysteinemia results from endothelial dysfunction and injury followed by platelet activation and thrombus formation. Studies in humans and animals demonstrate that homocysteine-induced atherosclerosis is characterized by substantial platelet accumulation and platelet-rich thrombus formation in areas of endothelial injury [22,23]. It has been proposed that homocysteine-induced endothelial injury exposes the subendothelial matrix, which in turn leads to platelet activation [24]. Diet-induced hyperhomocysteinemia in primates leads to impaired vasomotor regulation in vivo and endothelial antithrombotic function ex vivo [25]. Endothelial anticoagulant function is impaired in young patients with hyperhomocysteinemia and peripheral vascular disease [26]. Although the exact mechanism of endothelial dysfunction is unknown, there is growing evidence that homocysteine exerts its effects by promoting oxidative damage.

Homocysteine is rapidly auto-oxidized when added to plasma, forming homocystine, mixed disulfides, and homocysteine thiolactone [27]. Potent reactive oxygen species, including superoxide and hydrogen peroxide, are produced during the auto-oxidation of homocysteine, and hydrogen peroxide, in particular, has been implicated in the vascular toxicity of hyperhomocysteinemia [28]. There is extensive evidence that homocysteine-induced endothelial-cell injury in vitro is largely due to the generation of hydrogen peroxide [29]. Homocysteine-induced endothelial-cell injury mediated by hydrogen peroxide exposes the underlying matrix and smooth-muscle cells, which in turn proliferate and promote the activation of platelets and leukocytes [22]. Superoxide-dependent formation of the hydroxyl radical has been shown to initiate lipid peroxidation [30], an effect that occurs at the level of the endothelial plasma membrane and within lipoprotein particles [31]. Homocysteine auto-oxidation has been shown to support the oxidation of low-density lipoprotein through the generation of the superoxide anion radical [32].

Although the precise molecular mechanism is unknown, homocysteine causes endothelial dysfunction at several levels. Homocysteine alters the normal antithrombotic phenotype of the endothelium by enhancing the activities of factor XII and factor V and depressing the activation of protein C [33]. Homocysteine also inhibits the expression of thrombomodulin, induces the expression of tissue factor, and suppresses the expression of heparan sulfate by the endothelium [34]. All of these effects ultimately facilitate the formation of thrombin and create a prothrombotic environment.

The production of endothelial-derived nitric oxide is also adversely affected by homocysteine [35]. Normal endothelial cells detoxify homocysteine by releasing nitric oxide, which combines with homocysteine in the presence of oxygen to form S-nitroso-homocysteine. Nitrosation of the sulfhydryl group of homocysteine inhibits sulfhydryl-dependent generation of hydrogen peroxide. S-nitroso-homocysteine is also a potent platelet inhibitor and vasodilator. This protective effect of nitric oxide is eventually compromised as long-term exposure to hyperhomocysteinemia damages the endothelium sufficiently to limit nitric oxide production. Impaired endothelial production of nitric oxide leaves the endothelium vulnerable to unopposed homocysteine-mediated oxidative injury [36].

Homocysteine promotes lipid peroxidation, which may subsequently decrease the expression of endothelial nitric oxide synthase and directly degrade nitric oxide [37].

In addition to promoting atherosclerosis through endothelial injury or dysfunction, homocysteine is also a potent mitogen for vascular smooth-muscle cells. Exposure to homocysteine leads to a marked increase in vascular smooth-muscle proliferation in vitro, an effect that is due in part to an increase in the expression of messenger RNA of cyclin D1 and cyclin A [38].

Homocysteine increases nitric oxide production in vascular smooth-muscle cells by activating the transcription factor NF-(kappa)B [39]. Homocysteine-mediated activation of NF-(kappa)B seems to contribute to the mitogenic effect of homocysteine.

Homocysteine also directly damages the vascular matrix by affecting the biochemical and biosynthetic functions of vascular cells. Homocysteine thiolactone, a highly reactive anhydrous byproduct of homocysteine oxidation, combines with low-density lipoprotein to form aggregates that are taken up by intimal macrophages and incorporated into foam cells within nascent atheromatous plaques [40]. Homocysteine-induced disturbance in oxidative metabolism also leads to overproduction of oxidative radicals that subsequently induce intimal injury, activate elastase, and increase calcium deposition [41].

The recently observed multiplicative increase in the risk of vascular disease in the presence of traditional risk factors and hyperhomocysteinemia may in part be related to the effect of homocysteine on lipid peroxidation [42]. The vascular cytotoxicity of oxidized low-density lipoprotein has been linked to its content of lipid peroxidation products [43]. Homocysteine increases the formation of highly atherogenic oxycholesterols, increases lipid peroxidation, and increases the oxidation of low-density lipoprotein in vitro [44]. These observations suggest a potential role for antioxidant therapy in ameliorating homocysteine-dependent oxidative vascular injury; however, this therapeutic approach has not yet been tested in prospective clinical trials.

In conclusion, it is clear that there is no one unifying hypothesis of the mechanism, if any, of homocysteine induced vascular damage although at present the endothelium is the most likely candidate.

# Homocysteine as a Risk Factor for Vascular Disease

In a European multicentre investigation of 750 cases and a similar number of controls, a high homocysteine concentration conferred a risk equal to that of hypercholesterolaemia, smoking or hypertension [45]. Some, but not all, prospective (or nested case control) studies have confirmed these findings. In the multiple risk factor intervention trial (MRFIT), for example, the homocysteine concentrations in serum samples from men who subsequently suffered a myocardial infarction were no different from those in controls [46,47].

In another recent prospective study by Folsom and colleagues higher homocysteine concentrations added to the risk of incident coronary artery disease in women but not in men [48]. In patients with coronary disease, higher homocysteine concentrations are related to lower circulating B vitamin concentrations. Indeed, in one study, as the concentration of folate fell, the levels of both homocysteine and cardiovascular risk rose [49]. Similarly, there is an increased vascular risk associated with lower levels of vitamin B6 [50].

## Prospective Cohort Studies

The strongest epidemiological evidence for an association between hyperhomocysteinaemia and vascular risk comes from large prospective observational cohort studies. The studies are not consistent [51,52,53,54,55,56,57,58,59,60,61]. The unequivocally positive studies-with relative risks (RR) whose lower 95% confidence interval is above 1-are the Physicians' Health Study, the British United Provident Association study, the Tromso study, the British Regional Heart Study, and the study of Nygard and colleagues [61]. A strong graded relation has been reported between increasing tHcy and overall mortality in individuals with angiographically demonstrated coronary heart disease [61]. However, other prospective studies, including further reports from the Physicians' Health Study [55], have not found a significant association between hyperhomocysteinaemia and myocardial infarction or stroke.

## Retrospective Case-control and Cross-sectional Studies

Retrospective and cross-sectional designs are methodologically less rigorous than cohort designs but most of them strongly support an association between tHcy and vascular disease risk. A meta-analysis of 27 observational studies (23 cross-sectional or retrospective case-control and four nested case-control studies based on prospective cohorts), including about 4000 patients reported that a raised tHcy (usually defined as above the 90th or 95th percentile of controls) was associated with an increased risk of fatal and nonfatal atherosclerotic vascular disease in the coronary (odds ratio 1,7; 95% CI 1,5-1,9), cerebral (OR 2,5 [2,0-3,0]), and peripheral (OR 6,8 [2,9-15,8]) circulations [62]. The magnitude of risk was similar to that for other risk factors, such as hypercholesterolaemia and smoking, and it was estimated that about 10% of coronary heart disease in the general population might be attributable to homocysteine. A graded, linear relation between homocysteine levels and vascular risk has been estimated, with a 5 μmol/L increase in tHcy to be associated with an increase in vascular risk of about one-third, which is of similar magnitude to an increase in plasma cholesterol of 0·5 mmol/L.

Most of the studies published [42,63,64,65,66,67,68] support the conclusions of the meta-analysis by Boushey and colleagues [62]. The large European Collaborative Study concluded that tHcy was an independent risk factor for atherosclerotic disease, and calculated that a 5 μmol/L increment in fasting basal tHcy was associated with a relative risk (RR) of atherosclerotic vascular disease of 1,35 (1,1-1,6) in men and 1·42 (0,99-2,55) in women [42].

## Interpretation of Clinical Data

There is a large body of epidemiological evidence that links increasing tHcy with an increasing risk of atherothrombotic vascular disease. There is not complete consistency but there hardly ever is, even for well-established relationships, usually because of differences in study design, statistical power, and chance. Whilst it is possible that the abundance of published studies that show a positive association could reflect publication bias it is just as likely that the negative studies are falsely negative because of a lack of methodological or statistical power or random error. A systematic review of studies with the same types of patients and controls and the same methods and outcome events could provide a more accurate estimate of the true association between tHcy and vascular risk.

Assuming that a strong, dose-dependent, and positive association does exist, there is reasonable evidence, from regression analyses, that the association is independent of other factors known to be associated with raised tHcy (eg, age, sex, smoking, low physical activity, blood pressure, and cholesterol) [69]. Furthermore, homozygotes for the three distinct autosomal-recessive inborn errors of homocysteine metabolism (CßS deficiency, MTHFR deficiency, and the cobalamin metabolic defects that impair methionine synthase activity) have tHcy concentrations that are 10-50 times higher than those in the general population and a very high risk of premature atherothrombotic vascular disease. This suggests that the only biochemical change these metabolic errors have in common (ie, a high circulating tHcy or homocysteine metabolite concentration) is the cause of the premature atherothrombotic vascular disease that is shared by all three disorders. However, the conclusion that tHcy is an independent risk factor for atherothrombotic vascular disease should be tempered by the variable findings of prospective cohort studies, and the failure to demonstrate a clear association between genetic markers of raised tHcy (notably, the thermolabile MTHFR genotype), and vascular disease despite a significant relation between genotype and tHcy. Furthermore, the more positive results of retrospective studies may reflect a consistent bias resulting from homocysteine levels measured after the acute vascular event, which may be higher than levels measured beforehand [70], but data about the effect of acute occlusive vascular events on homocysteine levels are not consistent [11]. Finally, it is also possible that tHcy is simply a marker of another causal risk factor such as folate status or some other, unknown factor which could explain the higher rates of coronary artery disease among people with lower intakes of folate and vitamin B6 (eg, folate-depleted diets may be prothrombotic).

## Venous Thromboembolism and Hyperhomocysteinemia

Most retrospective case-control and cross-sectional studies have demonstrated a positive association between raised tHcy and an increased risk of initial and recurrent venous thrombosis, and this has been confirmed by a meta-analysis (RR=2,95 [2,08-4,17]) in patients with fasting hyperhomocysteinaemia [71]. Supporting data comes from the Physicians' Health Study cohort (RR=3,38 [1,57-7,25] in patients with a tHcy above the 95th percentile of controls) [72]. However, an association was not found between tHcy and risk of venous thrombosis in a prospectively studied cohort of patients with systemic lupus erythematosus [73]. Thus, data of association between raised tHcy and an increased risk of venous thrombosis are not consistent.

## Therapeutic Considerations of Hyperhomocysteinemia

The treatment of hyperhomocysteinemia varies with the underlying cause; however, vitamin supplementation (with folic acid, pyridoxine (vitamin $B_6$), and vitamin $B_{12}$) is generally effective in reducing homocysteine concentrations. The minimal effective doses of folic acid and pyridoxine have not yet been determined. In most patients, small doses of folate (0,4 to 5 mg per day) rapidly decrease homocysteine concentrations [74]. Thus far, most studies have focused on the homocysteine-lowering effects of folates. However, recently, benefits of folates independent of homocysteine lowering have also been reported. Potential mechanisms include antioxidant actions, effects on cofactor availability, or direct interactions with the enzyme endothelial NO synthase. Obviously, beneficial effects of folates on cardiovascular risk would have important clinical and dietary consequences. However, for definite conclusions, the completion of ongoing randomized controlled trials will have to be awaited [75]. Whether doses lower than 400 μg are effective has not been adequately explored. Patients with renal impairment require much higher doses. A meta-analysis of data from 1114 individual participants in 12 randomised controlled trials of the effects of folic-acid-based supplements on basal tHcy found that the proportional and absolute reductions in tHcy produced by folic acid were greater at higher pretreatment tHcy and at lower pretreatment blood folate levels [76]. Folic acid alone, folic acid combined with vitamins $B_{12}$ and $B_6$, and vitamins $B_6$ and $B_{12}$ have all been shown to reduce homocysteine concentrations [77]. Because the response to homocysteine-lowering therapy is not uniform, and is dependent on factors such as genotype for enzymes involved in the metabolism of homocysteine, vitamin status, and nutritional needs [14], multivitamin doses required for the treatment of hyperhomocysteinaemia may vary according to individual patient requirements.

Normalization of the plasma homocysteine concentration usually occurs within four to six weeks after the initiation of therapy, but may occur in as little as two weeks. Interestingly, the reduction in mortality from cardiovascular causes since 1960 has been correlated with the increase in vitamin $B_6$ supplementation in the food supply.

A potential hazard of folic acid therapy is progressive neurological damage (subacute combined degeneration of the spinal cord) in people with subclinical vitamin $B_{12}$ deficiency in whom folic acid therapy may mask the development of the haematological manifestations of the $B_{12}$ deficiency. This can be avoided by either excluding $B_{12}$ deficiency before starting folic acid or by supplementing folic acid therapy with vitamin $B_{12}$. At least 400 μg per day of vitamin $B_{12}$ is suggested as a supplement because the recommended daily intake of this vitamin is about 2 μg per day but only 1-3% of oral vitamin $B_{12}$ is absorbed by simple diffusion.

The major potential hazard of vitamin $B_6$ is a sensory peripheral neuropathy with use over months to years at doses of vitamin $B_6$ usually at least 400 mg daily. However, most doses for the treatment of moderate hyperhomocysteinaemia are only 10-50 mg per day.

In patients with severe hyperhomocysteinaemia due to CßS deficiency effective homocysteine-lowering therapy does reduce the risk of cardiovascular disease during long-term follow-up [78]. However, although the combination of folic acid 2·5 mg, vitamin $B_6$ 25 mg, and vitamin $B_{12}$ 250 μg per day reduces the progression of atherosclerosis, as measured by carotid plaque area [79], it remains to be confirmed that homocysteine-lowering therapy will prevent important atherosclerotic vascular events in patients with moderate hyperhomocysteinaemia. Several large randomised clinical trials are addressing this issue (table 2).

Meta-analyses of observational studies suggests that elevated homocysteine is at most a modest independent predictor of ischemic heart disease and stroke risk in healthy populations. Studies of the impact on disease risk of genetic variants that affect blood homocysteine concentrations will help determine whether homocysteine is causally related to vascular disease, as may large randomized trials of the effects on ischemic heart disease and stroke of vitamin supplementation to lower blood homocysteine concentrations [80]. A recently published meta-analysis suggests that „genetic" studies and „prospective" studies do not share the same potential sources of error, but both yield similar highly significant results, that is strong evidence that the association between homocysteine and cardiovascular disease is causal. On this basis, lowering homocysteine concentrations by 3 µmol/l from current levels (achievable by increasing folic acid intake) would reduce the risk of ischaemic heart disease by 16% (11% to 20%), deep vein thrombosis by 25% (8% to 38%), and stroke by 24% (15% to 33%) [81]. However, data have to be interpretated with caution, since a recent cohort study with follow up of 29 years investigating 1419 men and 1531 women aged 20 to 90 years found no independent association between folate and B-12 concentrations and death from coronary heart disease or cardiovascular disease in the full cohort or the subcohort with no cardiovascular disease at baseline. Thus, these findings do not support the hypothesis that lower folate and B-12 concentrations increase the risk of fatal cardiovascular disease in a general population. The routine use of these vitamins for preventing cardiovascular disease should await evidence from clinical trials [82].

**Table 2. Trials of Homocysteine-lowering Therapy in Vascular Disease**

- Vitamins in Stroke Prevention (VISP) Trial; Bowman Gray School of Medicine, USA
- Norwegian Study of Homocysteine Lowering with B-vitamins in Myocardial Infarction (NORVIT); University of Tromso, Norway
- Study of the Effectiveness of Additional Reductions in Cholesterol and Homocysteine (SEARCH); Clinical Trial Service Unit, Oxford, UK
- Women's Antioxidant and Cardiovascular Disease Study (WACS); Harvard Medical School, USA
- Bergen Vitamin Study, University of Bergen, Norway
- Cambridge Heart Antioxidant Study (*Chaos*-2); University of Cambridge, UK
- Heart Outcomes Prevention Evaluation (*Hope-2*) Study; McMaster University, Canada
- Prevention with A Combined Inhibitor and Folate in Coronary Heart Disease (PACIFIC) Study; University of Sydney, Australia
- Vitamins to Prevent Stroke (VITATOPS) Study; Stroke Unit, Royal Perth Hospital, Western Australia

# Remaining Questions

Many important questions remain – for example, is a high circulating homocysteine concentration causal in the pathogenesis of coronary disease, and other atherosclerotic and thrombotic vascular diseases, or is it merely an epiphenomenon? Is the high homocysteine level a reflection of lower B vitamin status which is itself directly (or indirectly) linked to atherosclerosis? Or is it a reflection of diminished renal function so often seen in patients with vascular disease [83,84]?

What, if any, is the mechanism by which homocysteine may induce atherosclerosis? In other clinical circumstances such as following organ transplantation, or in the presence of hypothyroidism or inflammatory bowel disease, does high homocysteine predict increased vascular risk?

# Conclusion

Multiple prospective and case-control studies suggested that a moderately elevated plasma homocysteine concentration is an independent risk factor for atherothrombotic vascular disease. Homocysteine concentrations are consistently higher in patients with peripheral, cerebrovascular, and coronary artery disease than in those without such diseases. Homocysteine seems to promote atherothrombogenesis by a variety of mechanisms; however, it is not yet clear whether homocysteine itself or a related metabolite or cofactor is primarily responsible for the atherothrombogenic effects of hyperhomocysteinemia in vivo. Before advocating widespread screening of patients with atherosclerotic vascular disease, we must have a clearer understanding of the clinical efficacy of potential therapeutic interventions. Vitamin supplementation decreases or even normalizes plasma homocysteine concentrations in most cases. Prospective, randomized clinical trials, however, will be necessary to determine the effect of vitamin supplementation on cardiovascular morbidity and mortality. The use of pills containing low dose B vitamins as a primary or secondary preventive measure against vascular disease remains unproved, although they are definitely cheap, probably innocuous, and may help prevent acute vascular episodes.

# References


[1] McCully KS. Vascular pathology of homocysteinemia: implications for the pathogenesis of arteriosclerosis. *Am J Pathol* 1969;56:111-28.

[2] Ueland PM. Homocysteine species as components of plasma redox thiol status. *Clin Chem* 1995; 41: 340-42.

[3] Kang SS, Wong PW, Malinow MR. Hyperhomocysteinemia as a risk factor for occlusive vascular disease. *Ann Rev Nutr* 1992;12:279-98.

[4] Stampfer MJ, Malinow MR, Willett WC, et al. A prospective study of plasma homocysteine and risk of myocardial infarction in US physicians. *J Am Med Assoc* 1992;268:877-81.

[5] Whisnant JP. Modeling of risk factors for ischemic stroke: the Willis lecture. *Stroke* 1997; 28: 1839-43.

[6] Ueland PM, Refsum H. Plasma homocysteine, a risk factor for vascular disease: plasma levels in health, disease, and drug therapy. *J Lab Clin Med* 1989; 114:473-501.

[7] Ueland PM, Refsum H, Stabler SP, Malinow MR, Andersson A, Allen RH. Total homocysteine in plasma or serum: methods and clinical applications. *Clin Chem* 1993;39:1764-79.

[8] Dudman NP, Wilcken DE, Wang J, Lynch JF, Macey D, Lundberg P. Disordered methionine/homocysteine metabolism in premature vascular disease: its occurrence, cofactor therapy, and enzymology. *Arterioscler Thomb Vasc Biol* 1993; 12: 1253-60.

[9] Still RA, McDowell IF. Clinical implications of plasma homocysteine measurement in cardiovascular disease. *J Clin Pathol* 1998; 51: 183-88.

[10] Refsum H, Fiskerstrand T, Guttormsen AB, Ueland PM. Assessment of homocysteine status. *J Inherit Metab Dis* 1997; 20: 286-94.

[11] Auer J, Eber B 1999 Homocystein and fibrinolysis in acute occlusive coronary events. *Lancet* 354: 1474-1475.

[12] Auer J, Berent R, Eber B. Homocysteine and dementia. *N Engl J Med* 2002;346:2007.

[13] Kang SS, Wong PW, Malinow MR. Hyperhomocysteinemia as a risk factor for occlusive vascular disease. *Ann Rev Nutr* 1992;12:279-98.

[14] McCully KS. Homocysteine and vascular disease. *Nat Med* 1996;2:386-9.

[15] Malinow MR, Nieto FJ, Kruger WD, et al. The effects of folic acid supplementation on plasma total homocysteine are modulated by multivitamin use and methylenetetrahydrofolate reductase genotypes. *Arterioscler Thromb Vasc Biol* 1997; 17: 1157-62.

[16] Brattstrom L, Israelsson B, Lindgarde F, Hultberg B. Higher total plasma homocysteine in vitamin B12 deficiency than in heterozygosity for homocystinuria due to cystathionine (beta)-synthase deficiency. *Metabolism* 1988;37:175-8.

[17] Stabler SP, Marcell PD, Podell ER, Allen RH, Savage DG, Lindenbaum J. Elevation of total homocysteine in the serum of patients with cobalamin or folate deficiency detected by capillary gas chromatography-mass spectrometry. *J Clin Invest* 1988;81:466-74.

[18] Selhub J, Jacques PF, Wilson PW, Rush D, Rosenberg IH. Vitamin status and intake as primary determinants of homocysteinemia in an elderly population. *J Am Med Assoc* 1993; 270: 2693-98.

[19] Bostom AG, Lathrop L. Homocysteinemia in end-stage renal disease: prevalence, etiology, and potential relationship to arteriosclerotic outcomes. *Kidney Int* 1997; 52: 10-20.

[20] Mayer EL, Jacobsen DW, Robinson K. Homocysteine and coronary atherosclerosis. *J Am Coll Cardiol* 1996;27:517-27.

[21] Vermaak WJ, Ubbink JB, Barnard HC, Potgieter GM, van Jaarsveld H, Groenewald AJ. Vitamin B6 nutrition status and cigarette smoking. *Am J Clin Nutr* 1990;51:1058-61.

[22] Harker LA, Slichter SJ, Scott CR, Ross R. Homocystinemia: vascular injury and arterial thrombosis. *N Engl J of Med* 1974; 291: 537-543.

[23] James TN. The spectrum of diseases of small coronary arteries and their physiologic consequences. *J Am Coll Cardiol* 1990; 15: 763-774.

[24] Malinow MR, Duell PB, Hess DL. Reduction of plasma homocysteine levels by breakfast cereal fortified with folic acid in patients with coronary heart disease. *N Engl J Med* 1998; 338: 1009-1015.

[25] Lentz SR, Sobey CG, Piegors DJ. Vascular dysfunction in monkeys with diet-induced hyperhomocysteinemia. *J Clin Invest* 1996; 98: 24-29.

[26] Van den Berg M, Boers GH, Franken DG. Hyperhomocysteinaemia and endothelial dysfunction in young patients with peripheral arterial occlusive disease. *European J Clin Invest* 1995; 25: 176-181.

[27] Andersson A, Lindgren A, Hultberg B. Effect of thiol oxidation and thiol export from erythrocytes on determination of redox status of homocysteine and other thiols in plasma from healthy subjects and patients with cerebral infarction. *Clin Chem* 1995;41: 361-366.

[28] Welch GN, Upchurch GR Jr, Loscalzo J. Hyperhomocysteinemia and atherothrombosis. *Ann N Y Acad Sci* 1997; 811: 48-58.

[29] Starkebaum G, Harlan JM. Endothelial cell injury due to copper-catalyzed hydrogen peroxide generation from homocysteine. J Clin Invest 1986; 77: 1370-1376.

[30] Rowley DA, Halliwell B. Superoxide-dependent formation of hydroxyl radicals in the presence of thiol compounds. *FEBS Lett* 1982;138:33-6.

[31] Loscalzo J. The oxidant stress of hyperhomocyst(e)inemia. J Clin Invest 1996;98:5-7.

[32] Heinecke JW, Rosen H, Suzuki LA, Chait A. The role of sulfur-containing amino acids in superoxide production and modification of low density lipoprotein by arterial smooth muscle cells. *J Biol Chem* 1987;262:10098-103.

[33] Rodgers GM, Conn MT. Homocysteine, an atherogenic stimulus, reduces protein C activation by arterial and venous endothelial cells. *Blood* 1990;75:895-901.

[34] Nishinaga M, Ozawa T, Shimada K. Homocysteine, a thrombogenic agent, suppresses anticoagulant heparan sulfate expression in cultured porcine aortic endothelial cells. *J Clin Invest* 1993; 92:1381-1386.

[35] Stamler JS, Osborne JA, Jaraki O. Adverse vascular effects of homocysteine are modulated by endothelium-derived relaxing factor and related oxides of nitrogen. J *Clin Invest* 1993; 91: 308-318.

[36] Stamler JS, Simon DI, Osborne JA. S-nitrosylation of proteins with nitric oxide: synthesis and characterization of biologically active compounds. *Proc Nat Acad Sci USA* 1992; 89: 444-448.

[37] Liao JK, Shin WS, Lee WY, Clark SL. Oxidized low-density lipoprotein decreases the expression of endothelial nitric oxide synthase. *J Biol Chem* 1995; 270: 319-324.

[38] Tsai J-C, Perrella MA, Yoshizumi M. Promotion of vascular smooth muscle cell growth by homocysteine: a link to atherosclerosis. *Proc Natl Acad Sci USA* 1994; 91: 6369-6373.

[39] Welch GN, Upchurch GR Jr, Farivar RS. Homocysteine-induced nitric oxide production in vascular smooth muscle cells by NF-(kappa) B dependent transcriptional activation of NOS-2. *Proc Am Assoc Phys* 1998; 110: 22-31.

[40] Naruszewicz M, Mirkiewicz E, Olszewski AJ. Thiolation of low-density lipoprotein by homocysteine thiolactone causes increased aggregation and altered interaction with cultured macrophages. *Nutr Metabolism Cardiovasc Dis* 1994; 4: 70-77.

[41] McCully KS. Homocysteine metabolism in scurvy, growth and arteriosclerosis. Nature 1971; 231: 391-2.

[42] Graham IM, Daly LE, Refsum HM. Plasma homocysteine as a risk factor for vascular disease: the European Concerted Action Project. *J Am Med Assoc* 1997; 277: 1775-1781.

[43] Hughes H, Mathews B, Lenz ML, Guyton JR. Cytotoxicity of oxidized LDL to porcine aortic smooth muscle cells is associated with the oxysterols 7-ketocholesterol and 7-hydroxycholesterol. *Arteriosclerosis Thromb* 1994; 14: 1177-1185.

[44] Heinecke JW, Kawamura M, Suzuki L, Chait A. Oxidation of low density lipoprotein by thiols: superoxide-dependent and -independent mechanisms. *J Lipid Res* 1993; 34: 2051-2061.

[45] Graham IM, Daly LE, Refsum HM, et al. Plasma homocysteine as a risk factor for vascular disease. The European concerted action project. J Am Med Assoc 1997;277:1775-1781.

[46] Evans RW, Shaten BJ, Hempel JD, et al. Homocysteine and risk of cardiovascular disease in the multiple risk factor intervention trial. *Arterioscler Thromb Vasc Biol* 1997;17:1947-1953.

[47] Auer J, Berent R, Eber B. Lack of association of increased C-reactive protein and total plasma homocysteine. *Circulation*. 2001;104:E164.

[48] Folsom AR, Nieto FJ, McGovern PG. Prospective study of coronary heart disease incidence in relation to fasting total homocysteine, related genetic polymorphisms, and B vitamins: the atherosclerosis risk in communities (ARIC) study. *Circulation* 1998;98:204-210.

[49] Pancharuniti N, Lewis CA, Sauberlich HE. Plasma homocysteine, folate, and vitamin B-12 concentrations and risk for early-onset coronary artery disease. *Am J Clin Nutr* 1994;59:940-948.

[50] Robinson K, Arheart K, Refsum H. Low circulating folate and vitamin B6 concentrations: risk factors for stroke, peripheral vascular disease, and coronary artery disease. European COMAC Group. *Circulation* 1998;97:437-443.

[51] Kang SS, Zhou J, Wong PWK, Kowalisyn J, Strokosch G. Intermediate homocysteinemia: a thermolabile variant of methylenetetrahydrofolate reductase. *Am J Hum Genetics* 1988; 43: 414-421

[52] Frosst P, Blom HJ, Milos R. A candidate genetic risk factor for vascular disease: a common mutation in methylenetetrahydrofolate reductase. *Nat Genetics* 1995; 10: 111-113.

[53] Malinow MR, Nieto FJ, Kruger WD. The effects of folic acid supplementation on plasma total homocysteine are modulated by multivitamin use and methylenetetrahydrofolate reductase genotypes. *Arteriosclerosis Throm Vasc Biol* 1997; 17: 1157-1162.

[54] Selhub J, Jacques PF, Wilson PW, Rush D, Rosenberg ICH. Vitamin status and intake as primary determinants of homocysteinemia in an elderly population. *J Am Med Assoc* 1993; 270: 2693-1698.

[55] Kang SS, Wong PWK, Norusis M. Homocysteinaemia due to folate deficiency. *Metabolism* 1987; 36: 458-462.

[56] Bostom AG, Lathrop L. Homocysteinemia in end-stage renal disease: prevalence, etiology, and potential relationship to arteriosclerotic outcomes. *Kidn Internat* 1997; 52: 10-20.

[57] Frantzen F, Faaren AL, Alfheim I, Nordhei AK. Enzyme conversion immunoassay for determining total homocysteine in plasma or serum. Clin Chem 1998; 44: 311-316.

[58] Guttormsen AB, Scheede J, Fiskerstrand T, Ueland PM, Refsum HM. Plasma concentrations of homocysteine and other aminothiol compounds are related to food intake in healthy human subjects. *J Nutr* 1994; 124: 1934-1941.

[59] Savage DG, Lindenbaum J, Stabler SP, Allen RH. Sensitivity of serum methylmalonic acid and total homocysteine determinants for diagnosing cobalamin and folate deficiencies. *Am J Med* 1994 96: 239-246.

[60] Folsom AR, Nieto J, McGovern PG. Prospective study of coronary heart disease incidence in relation to fasting total homocysteine, related genetic polymorphisms, and B vitamins: the Atherosclerosis Risk in Communities (ARIC) study. *Circulation* 1998; 98: 204-210.

[61] Nygard O, Nordrehaug JE, Refsum H, Ueland PM, Farstad M, Vollset SE. Plasma homocysteine levels and mortality in patients with coronary artery disease. *N Engl J Med* 1997; 337: 230-236.

[62] Boushey CJ, Beresford SAA, Omenn GS, Motulsky AG. A quantitative assessment of plasma homocysteine as a risk factor for vascular disease: probable benefits of increasing folic acid intake. *J Am Med Assoc* 1995; 274: 1049-1057.

[63] Lindgren A, Brattstrom L, Norrving B, Hultberg B, Anderson A, Johansson BB. Plasma homocysteine in the acute and convalescent phases of stroke. *Stroke* 1995 26: 796-800.

[64] Hopkins PN, Wu LL, Hunt SC. Higher plasma homocysteine and increased susceptibility to adverse effects of low folate in early familial coronary artery disease. *Arteriosclerosis Thromb Vasc Biol* 1995; 15: 1314-1320.

[65] Dalery K, Lussier-Cacan S, Selhub J, Davignon J, Latour Y, Genest J. Homocysteine and coronary artery disease in French Canadian subjects: relation with vitamins $B_{12}$, $B_6$, pyridoxal phosphate, and folate. *Am J Cardiol* 1995; 75: 1107-1111.

[66] Robinson K, Meyer EL, Miller DP. Hyperhomocysteinaemia and low pyridoxal phosphate: common and independent reversible risk factors for coronary artery disease. *Circulation* 1995; 92: 2825-2830.

[67] Malinow MR, Ducimetiere P, Luc G. Plasma homocyst(e)ine levels and graded risk for myocardial infarction: findings in two populations at contrasting risk for coronary heart disease. *Atherosclerosis* 1996; 26: 27-34.

[68] Markus HS, Nadira A, Swaminathan R, Sankaralingam A, Molloy J, Powell J. A common polymorphism in the methylenetetrahydrofolate reductase gene, homocysteine, and ischaemic cerebrovascular disease. *Stroke* 1997; 28: 1739-1743.

[69] Nygard O, Vollset SE, Refsum H. Total plasma homocysteine and cardiovascular risk profile. *J Am Med Assoc* 1995; 274: 1526-1533.

[70] Hankey GJ, Eikelboom JW. Homocysteine and vascular disease. *Lancet* 1999; 354: 407-413.

[71] Ray JG. Meta-analysis of hyperhomocysteinemia as a risk factor for venous thromboembolic disease. *Arch Int Med* 1998; 158: 2101-2116.

[72] Ridker PM, Hennekens CH, Selhub J, Miletich JP, Malinow MR, Stampfer MJ. Interrelation of hyperhomocyst(e)inaemia, factor V Leiden, and risk of future venous thromboembolism. *Circulation* 1997; 95: 1777-1782.

[73] Petri M, Roubenoff R, Dallal GE, Nadeau MR, Selhub J, Rosenberg ICH. Plasma homocysteine as a risk factor for atherothrombotic events in systemic lupus erythematosus. *Lancet* 1996; 348: 1120-1124.

[74] Brattstrom LE, Israelsson B, Jeppsson JO, Hultberg BL. Folic acid - an innocuous means to reduce plasma homocysteine. *Scand J Clin Lab Invest* 1988;48:215-21.

[75] Verhaar MC, Stroes E, Rabelink TJ. Folates and cardiovascular disease. *Arteriosclerosis Thromb Vasc Biol* 2002;22:*6-14.*

[76] Den Heijer M, Brouwer IA, Bos GMJ, et al. Vitamin supplementation reduces blood homocysteine levels: a controlled trial in patients with venous thrombosis and healthy volunteers. *Arterioscler Thromb Vasc Biol* 1998; 18: 356-61.

[77] Saltzman E, Mason JB, Jacques PF, et al. B vitamin supplementation lowers homocysteine levels in heart disease. *Clin Res* 1994;42:172A.

[78] Wilcken DEL, Wilcken B. The natural history of vascular disease in homocystinuria and the effects of treatment. *J Inher Metab Dis* 1997;20:295-300.

[79] Peterson JC, Spence JD. Vitamins and progression of atherosclerosis in hyperhomocysteinaemia. *Lancet* 1998; 351:263.

[80] Homocysteine studies collaboration. Homocysteine and Risk of Ischemic Heart Disease and Stroke A Meta-analysis. *J Am Med Assoc* 2002;288:2015-2022.

[81] Wald DS, Law M, Morris JK. Homocysteine and cardiovascular disease: evidence on causality from a meta-analysis *BMJ* 2002; 325:1202-1212.

[82] Hung J, Beilby JB, Knuiman MW, Divitini M. Folate and vitamin B-12 and risk of fatal cardiovascular disease: cohort study from Busselton, Western Australia. *BMJ* 2003; 326:131- 142.

[83] Robinson K. Homocysteine, B vitamins, and risk of cardiovascular disease. *Heart* 2000;83:127-130.

[84] Auer J, Berent R, Eber B. Homocysteine: a novel risk factor in vascular disease. *Coron Health Care* 2001;5:89-99.

In: Cholesterol in Atherosclerosis and Coronary Heart Disease ISBN 1-59454-302-X
Editor: Jean P. Kovala, pp.233-254 

*Chapter XI*

# Infection, Dyslipidemia and Early Atherosclerosis: Interaction and Causation

***Petru Liuba****

Division of Pediatric Cardiology, University Hospital Lund, 22185 Lund, Sweden

## Abstract

One of the earliest steps in the development of atherosclerosis involves a complex interaction between the vascular endothelium and various circulating components such as inflammatory cells, acute-phase proteins, and proatherogenic lipids. This initiates a cascade of endothelial injury and response-to-injury events, which, perhaps depending on the genetic vulnerability and the burden of risk factors, could have important implications for the clinical outcome of the vascular disease. Mounting epidemiological, experimental and microbiological evidence suggests that a wide spectrum of microbes could modulate the interaction between lipids & inflammation and the vascular endothelium, and influence the development of atherosclerosis. Accumulating studies support the view that pediatric population might represent a more fertile ground for the noxious effects of infection, possibly, in part, due to more sustained inflammatory and lipid-related mechanisms set by infection. In light of the multifactorial etiology of atherosclerosis, an interdisciplinary approach is important when establishing strategies aimed to retard atherosclerosis in order to attain gratifying benefit on the clinical outcome later in life.

**Key-words**: infection, dyslipidemia, oxidized lipoproteins, endothelium, early atherosclerosis

# Atherosclerosis: From Myth to an Evidence-based Concept

Atherosclerosis was for many decades regarded as a disease of elderly, being thought to occur as a result of blank accumulation of lipids into arterial intima. The observations that, already in childhood, inflammatory cells and lipids accumulate hand in hand within the vessel wall [1] have set a reorientation to studies focusing on the inflammatory mechanisms of early atherosclerosis in order to understand to what extent these mechanisms may influence the development of this disease. Gradually, the mythic view of atherosclerosis as an aging-related, lipid-based disease has been replaced by a new, evidence-supported concept that atherosclerosis is a multifactorial, response-to-injury disease that begins early in life, and owes a strong inflammatory component acting at all stages of its development [2]. Indeed, it is now established that inflammation drives a number of cardinal features of atherosclerosis, such as endothelial cell activation and dysfunction, lipid infiltration and oxidation, smooth muscle cell proliferation and foam cell formation, matrix degradation, and, at a later stage, plaque destabilization, rupture, and thrombosis [3]. In addition, important interactions between inflammatory and lipid-related mechanisms have been described, both systemically and intravascular. Nowadays, comprehensive reviews on the pathogenesis of atherosclerosis unequivocally agree upon the view that inflammation and dysregulation of lipid metabolism *a)* represent the main protagonists of atherosclerosis development, and *b)* could be key-targets for interventions aimed at retarding the development of atherosclerosis or reducing the prevalence of its clinical manifestations such as unstable angina, myocardial infarction, and stroke. Notably, the view that atherosclerosis prevention should be initiated already in childhood is becoming a desideratum for epidemiologists dealing with cardiovascular diseases. Thus far, the tools to achieve this goal remain however insufficiently defined, partly due to incomplete elucidation of the entire spectrum of risk factors and their interactions in early life.

The recognition of the inflammatory nature of atherosclerosis along with epidemiological observations indicating that many patients with coronary or cerebrovascular arterial disease lack traditional risk factors (ie, diabetes mellitus, hypertension, hypercholesterolemia, aging, and smoking) have rekindled efforts to identify other conditions, which, through inflammatory and lipid-related pathways, could contribute to the formation of atherosclerotic plaque. Mounting evidence supports the association between infection and atherosclerotic arterial disease [4], although solid proofs for a causative link remain unveiled. From the mechanistic point of view, two major lines of evidence render conceivable the atherogenic potential of infection. First, infection is an important stimulus of systemic inflammation, which, correlates with, and could even predict the development of atherosclerosis and its clinical manifestations [5]. Second, pro-atherogenic disturbances in lipid and lipoprotein metabolism may occur during infection.

# Infection and Atherosclerosis: An Overview

The possibility that infectious organisms could concur to the development of atherosclerosis was first raised by Sir William Osler in 1908 [6]. Osler's hypothesis that "experimental production of arteriosclerosis by various bacterial toxins afford an explanation of this gradual production of sclerosis in the chronic infections" received consistent support in the late 1970s, when Fabricant and colleagues managed to induce atherosclerosis-like intimal thickening and lipid accumulation in coronary arteries and aortas from pathogen-free chicken infected with an avian herpes virus called Marek's disease herpes virus [7]. Importantly, the authors observed greater lesions in the infected animals receiving a hypercholesterolemic diet compared with those animals placed on ordinary diet. Fabricant extended the studies *in vitro*, showing that incubation of avian smooth muscle cells with herpes virus led to 7-10-fold increase in the accumulation of free and esterified cholesterol and a 2-fold increase in phospholipids [8]. Nearly one decade later, considerable support to a contributive role of infection to cardiovascular disease was furnished by studies of Saikku and colleagues, who found in a rather small cohort of myocardial infarction patients a greater prevalence of serology-assessed infectivity with Chlamydia pneumoniae (C. pneumoniae) than in control subjects [9]. These studies were followed by numerous epidemiologic, pathogenic, and intervention studies in the attempt to elucidate the relationship between infectious pathogens and atherosclerotic artery disease.

Thus, some seroepidemiologic studies suggest that adults with serological markers of chronic infections with, for instance, C. pneumoniae, Helicobacter pylori (H. pylori), cytomegalovirus and herpes simplex virus (HSV)-1, might be at increased risk for coronary artery disease [10-13]. In several studies, subclinical measures of atherosclerosis, such as carotid intima-media thickening and impairment of brachial artery endothelium-dependent dilatation, were associated with positive serology for C. pneumoniae [14], cytomegalovirus [15], or B hepatitis [16]. The association of infection with atherosclerosis appears to be stronger in individuals presenting both markers of infection and conventional risk factors such as hypercholesterolemia (17], or in those with signs of co-infection with multiple pathogens [18]. One fascinating hypothesis is that macrolide antibiotic treatment of some infections (eg, C. pneumoniae) might retard the development of atherosclerosis [19] or lower the risk for atherosclerosis-related cardiovascular events [20]. In some trials, the observed cardiovascular benefit attained with antibiotics was suggested to be partly mediated by improvement in lipid profile, inflammation, and oxidant status [21]. However, a significant number of epidemiological studies and antibiotic trials could not confirm these findings [22-27], illustrating the complexity of factors that could influence the possible association between infection and atherosclerosis. Detection of pathogens such as C. pneumoniae [28] and herpes viruses [29] especially in diseased arteries from CHD patients was advocated to support the hypothesis of infection participation in atherosclerosis, although these findings cannot rule out the possibility that these pathogens might be ubiquitous bystanders, carried by inflammatory cells from a distant infection into the plaque.

Animal studies have, however, suggested that the ability of infection to contribute to atherosclerosis does not necessarily implicate endovascular infection [30]. Infection can initiate a variety of systemic changes involving inflammation, auto-immunity, and metabolic disturbances including alterations in lipid and lipoprotein metabolism [4]. Perhaps depending on the genetic vulnerability of the arterial wall, nutrition, life-style, and presence of additional risk factors, these systemic changes promoted by infection could influence the progression of atherosclerosis. Some studies on atherosclerosis-susceptible mice have also suggested that the impact of infection on atherosclerosis might be significant at young ages [31], and could positively correlate with the number of pathogen inoculations [32]. These experimental observations might be of relevance for the initial stages of atherosclerosis in childhood, as children are commonly exposed to a high number of recurrent infections. In addition, most of the pathogens suggested to contribute to atherosclerosis (eg, C. pneumoniae, herpes viruses, H. pylori) are actually acquired in childhood.

At present, there is only a scanty number of pediatric studies that have surveyed possible atherogenic effects of infections. Autopsy studies revealed that children with signs of acute infections at their death were more susceptible to intima thickenings of fibroproliferative nature in their coronary arteries compared to those lacking evidence for infection [33]. The structural changes appeared to be more prominent in those with viral infections. More recently, we conducted studies on children admitted at our hospital for severe acute systemic infections, and carotid intima-media thickness was measured with aid of external high-resolution ultrasound [34]. We observed that infection children displayed significantly greater carotid intima-media thickness 3 months after the cessation of the infectious disease than during the acute illness and controls. A greater susceptibility of LDL to oxidative modification along with a decreased HDL-to-total cholesterol ratio was noted in infection patients during the infectious illness, suggesting, thus, their possible implications in the development of intimal thickening following infection. Our results are in keeping with recent studies suggesting that children with preceding viral respiratory infections could have persistent arterial endothelial dysfunction many weeks [35] or even one year [36] after the infectious illness. How these findings could influence the development of atherosclerosis is discussed in chapter 6.

## Dyslipidemia and Infection: Possible Synergistic Interactions in Atherosclerosis

Although attractive, a possible causal relationship between singular infection and atherosclerosis remains debatable. Moreover, only sparse or no evidence for such an association has been observed in prospective clinical studies, and one highly illustrative example in this regard is H. pylori. In keeping with the paradigmatic view of atherosclerosis as a disease with multifactorial etiology, several lines of evidence indicate that the adverse effects of infection on arterial wall might be augmented by other cardiovascular risk factors such as hypercholesterolemia and diabetes. For instance, experimentally induced infection of LDL receptor–deficient mice with the C. pneumoniae AR39 strain significantly exacerbated the atherosclerotic lesions only in those animals receiving in addition a cholesterol-rich diet [37], suggesting that, at least in this animal model, a hypercholesterolemic condition is a prerequisite for C. pneumoniae to accelerate atherogenesis. When the same group conducted similar studies using a different species of Chlamydia (ie, a trachomatis strain that cause mouse pneumonitis), the augmentation of atherosclerosis by infection was no longer observed even though the animals were maintained on identical hyper-cholesterolemic diet, and the pathogen was also detected in the vessel wall. Based on this observation, the authors concluded that the ability of infectious pathogens to interact with hypercholesterolemia in atherogenesis might be pathogen-specific. Additive atherogenic interactions of C. pneumoniae and hypercholesterolemia were also noted in C57BL/6J mice [38], apoE-knockout mice [39], and rabbits [40]. Other pathogens have been shown to elicit similar effects in presence of hypercholesterolemia in both mice and rabbits. Atherosclerosis was further potentiated when infection and hypercholesterolemia were induced in a diabetic milieu [41]. Studies by Sunnemark et al showed that even infection Trypanosoma cruzi, a protozoan parasite with known tropism to the heart (causing Chagas' disease), led to accumulation of macrophages, T lymphocytes, and lipids into the intimal layer of aortas from CBA/J mice when these animals were fed a high-cholesterol diet [42]. At the same time, neither the noninfected animals nor the "diet alone"-treated animals displayed any signs of atherosclerosis.

A hypercholesterolemic milieu could increase the susceptibility to or the virulence of infection, rendering thus favourable circumstances for an additive interaction between pathogens and hypercholesterolemia in atherosclerosis. Studies by Laurila et al on LDL receptor- knockout mice showed that a high-cholesterol diet stimulated inflammatory changes in gastric mucosa [43]. H. pylori might mediate in part the diet-induced inflammation of the gastro-duodenal mucosa, as suggested by studies showing that the incidence of duodenal ulcer is higher in Hp-positive than in Hp-negative people [44]. Decreased serum levels of HDL-C seem to be associated with increased risk of nosocomial (surgical-site and respiratory tract) infection in post-surgery patients [45]. Even abnormally increased or decreased levels of total cholesterol may predispose to respiratory tract infections in these patients. Of note, respiratory tract infections have been proposed to increase the risk for coronary events [46].

One condition that has been shown to pose significant cardiovascular risk through accelerated atherosclerosis is the so-called metabolic syndrome, which is characterized by dyslipidemia, abdominal obesity, insulin resistance/hyperinsulinemia, type 2 diabetes mellitus, and hypertension. The epidemiologists estimate that by 2010, there could be nearly 75 millions people affected by this complex syndrome in the United States. Although the clinical manifestations occur in adults, perinatal nutritional disturbances emerge as an important risk factor. In a case-control study by Saikku, the risk of a cardiac event was increased 4.6-fold when markers of the metabolic syndrome (obesity, lowered HDL cholesterol, elevated systolic blood pressure and blood glucose) were all combined with markers of chronic C. pneumoniae infection [47] as compared to the risk posed by infection alone. However, the risk was significantly reduced when only one or two of the metabolic syndrome markers were associated with infection, a finding consistent with the concept that the risk for atherosclerosis increases with the burden of risk factors.

What are the mechanisms underlying the exacerbation of infection-related vascular effects by dyslipidemia? First, infection may promote metabolic abnormalities of the lipoprotein profile (see below), which may add to those related to primary dyslipidemia (eg, decreased HDL or increased LDL), with subsequent increase of the atherogenic risk. Second, infection and dyslipidemia could each cause systemic inflammation, which is, therefore, enhanced when these two conditions act together. For instance, adipocytes of obese patients release increased amounts of interleukin (IL)-6, which stimulates hepatic synthesis of C-reactive protein [48]. C-reactive protein (CRP) may in turn promote as such endothelial damage in a dose-dependent manner [49], and, according to recent prospective studies, might even predict the risk for cardiovascular events [50]. Third, antigens (eg, lipopolysaccharide) of infectious agents may form with lipoprotein particles (eg, LDL and lipoprotein(a)) circulating immune complexes with atherogenic properties [51, 52]. All of these systemic abnormalities could, via vascular endothelium, initiates a cascade of intravascular processes that ultimately lead to atherosclerosis.

## Chronic Infection Promotes Dislipidemic Disturbances, which could Increase Predisposition to Atherosclerosis

Chronic infections could promote disturbances of lipid and lipoprotein metabolism, and these have been speculated to mediate in part the putative atherogenic effects of infection [53]. Decreased plasma levels of HDL and elevated levels of triglyceride, which are known to independently increase the risk for atherosclerosis, have been documented in humans with signs of chronic C. pneumoniae infection [54, 55]. Scharnagl et al conducted studies on 87 patients with duodenal ulcer, and noticed that eradication of H. pylori in these patients led to 25 % increase of HDL [56]. One study on healthy adults found a significant association between markers of active chronic infection with H. pylori and atherogenic changes consisting of decreased HDL and increased apolipoprotein B levels, whilst no such pattern could be observed in connection to C. pneumoniae and cytomegalovirus [57 Hoffmeister, ATVB 2001). Paradoxically, to date, H. pylori has been only inconsistently associated with atherosclerosis, and one possible explanation could be that only virulent types of H. pylori could play a role in atherosclerosis [58]. Although CMV is mainly discussed in context of post-transplant atherosclerotic vasculopathy, where this pathogen is supposed to impart a significant contribution, it is of interest to mention that seropositivity to CMV was associated with decreased HDL levels in otherwise healthy children [59]. HDL was also found to be reduced in asymptomatic children with human immunodeficiency virus (HIV) infection [60]. HIV infection has recently been connected to accelerated atherosclerosis in carotid arteries [61]. Studies on 991 patients with coronary artery disease (CAD) pointed out that patients simultaneously seropositive for a high ($\geq$ 4) number of pathogens had significantly lower HDL and higher LDL/HDL ratio than those with low (< 4) or no seropositivities [62]. Eight pathogens were screened altogether (C. pneumoniae, H. pylori, Mycoplasma pneumoniae, Haemophilus influenzae HSV-1, HSV-2, cytomegalovirus, and Epstein-Barr virus). The findings are consistent with the emerging concept that the risk for atherosclerosis may increase with increasing number of pathogens [63].

Although total levels of LDL tend to decrease during chronic infections, increase of circulating small dense LDL particles have been reported particularly in HIV-infected patients [64]. This subclass of LDL is highly atherogenic due to its ability to cross the endothelial barrier and to infiltrate the subendothelial space, where it binds to proteglycans, a process coincident with intravascular retention [65]. Here, these LDL particles are most susceptible to oxidation, a process with major implications for the initiation and exacerbation of atherosclerosis (se below). The accumulation of small dense LDL in circulation during infection appears to be largely induced by hypertriglyceridemia, but elevated concentrations of fibrinogen might have a similar effect. Indeed, studies by Halle showed that plasma fibrinogen values > 2.90 g/L in adults were associated with twofold higher concentrations of small, dense LDL particles than in those with fibrinogen levels < 2.55 g/L [66]. Of note, this correlation was obtained in clinically healthy men with no evidence for acute or chronic inflammatory disease, rendering thus unlikely the possibility that an underlying inflammatory disease might have accounted for the increase in small dense LDL. Because fibrinogen, a component of acute-phase reaction, increases during inflammatory conditions and infection, it is likely that the stimulatory effect of infection-induced hypertriglyceridemia on the small dense LDL formation would be further augmented by fibrinogen.

An additional lipid-related mechanism speculated to link infection and atherosclerosis involves alteration of proteins incorporated in LDL. One such protein is platelet-activating factor acetylhydrolase, which may be upregulated by bacterial lipopolysaccharide (LPS), leading to increased levels of lysophosphatidylcholine [67]. The latter owes important atherogenic actions, such as endothelial cell activation and dysfunction, smooth muscle cell and macrophage proliferation [68].

The lipidemic disturbances during chronic infections are seemingly a consequence of systemic release of inflammatory mediators such as cytokines, and of intravascular accumulation of microbial products. In support to this theory, similar dyslipidemic phenotype occurs during chronic inflammatory states accompanying various conditions, such as diabetes mellitus [69] and chronic renal failure [70], in which levels of inflammatory cytokines are also elevated.

Most of the cytokines-induced effects on lipid and lipoprotein metabolism during infection are probably mediated by tumor necrosis factor-alpha (TNF-α), which was shown to decrease plasma levels of total cholesterol, mainly due to a reduction in HDL and LDL fractions [71]. Cytokines, especially TNF-α and IL-1, may also inhibit lipoprotein lipase activity with subsequent decreased conversion of VLDL to low-density lipoprotein, leading thus to hypertriglyceridemia [72].

E. coli, but also C. pneumoniae, H. pylori, and other gram-negative bacteria, may release endotoxins such as lipopolysaccharyde (LPS). LPS is a glycolipid component of bacterial outer membranes, being responsible for many of the directly or indirectly induced symptoms of infection. The majority of experimental studies have used E. coli LPS to investigate its detrimental effects *in vivo* or *in vitro*. LPS can induce *per se* atherogenic alterations in cholesterol metabolism similar to cytokines [71]. HDL inactivate LPS through binding the bioactive lipid-A portion of LPS to its surface, thereby acting as a humoral detoxification mechanism [73]. A decrease of HDL during infectious or inflammatory illness is therefore thought to impair this clearance mechanism, and to facilitate further accumulation of endotoxin. Kitchens et al found, however, that phospholipids-related compensatory mechanisms might develop during inflammation and infection, and these mechanisms tend to maintain the LPS-binding ability of lipoproteins despite reduced HDL levels [74]. Moreover, binding of LPS to HDL has been speculated to stimulate atherogenesis via inhibition of lecithin:cholesterol acyltransferase, one of the key enzymes mediating the reverse cholesterol transport function of HDL [51]. This could be one way by which HDL may lose its anti-atherogenic properties and become atherogenic [75]. Lipoteichoic acid, an immunostimulatory component of Gram-positive bacteria, may also induce similar dislipidemic changes as LPS [76].

## Intravascular Effects of Infection: Oxidized LDL Could Link Chronic Infection to Atherosclerosis

LDL particles had been earlier believed to be directly involved in the occurrence of foam cells, one of the most characteristic features of atherogenesis. Subsequent studies have, however, demonstrated that vascular environments enriched with native LDL display down-regulation of LDL scavenger receptors on the surface of macrophages, the precursors to foam cells. These findings have suggested that a LDL-derived product could instead serve as a driving mechanism of foam cell formation [77]. Over the last two decades, a number of experimental studies have shown that intravascular oxidative modification of LDL particles could be a crucial link in the formation of atherosclerotic plaque [78]. LDL oxidation occurs in macrophages, endothelial and smooth muscle cells, leading to bioactive products that exert a number of atherogenic effects including expression of pro-inflammatory adhesion molecules on endothelial cell surface, induction of monocyte and lymphocyte chemoattractant proteins, smooth-muscle-cell proliferation and foam-cell formation [79]. Oxidized LDL (ox-LDL) also stimulates induction of the pro-inflammatory nuclear factor kappa B (NF-kappaB) in endothelial cells, an important mechanism in atherogenesis [80]. It is therefore of interest that disturbances in vascular endothelial function or upregulation of NF-kappaB pathway were demonstrated to occur in response to infectious pathogens such as C. pneumoniae [81, 82], Epstein-Barr virus [83], and cytomegalovirus [84], or H. pylori [85], rendering, therefore, plausible the hypothesis that these effects might have been mediated by ox-LDL. In support to this, previous studies by Kalayoglu et al showed that exposure of C. pneumoniae-infected monocytes & macrophages to LDL promoted accumulation of LDL oxidation products in a C. pneumoniae-dose-dependent manner [86], and transformation of infected macrophages into foam cells ([87]; Figure 1). When human fibroblasts were subjected to the generated products of LDL oxidation important cytotoxic effects were observed, suggesting that similar damage to endothelial cells could occur *in vivo* following intimal infiltration of arterial wall with circulating monocytes carrying C. pneumoniae. In the same experiments, treatment of C. pneumoniae organisms with heat nearly abolished the capacity of C. pneumoniae to induce LDL oxidation, suggesting that chlamydial heat shock proteins (HSP) 60 were main mediators of the LDL oxidation by Chlamydiae. The findings deserve attention since Chlamydial HSP, as well as other bacterial HSP, have been correlated with atherosclerosis in a number of clinical and experimental studies [88]. In a subsequent set of experiments, Kalayoglu showed that C. pneumoniae-infected monocytes displayed increased capacity to adhere to vascular endothelial cells [89].

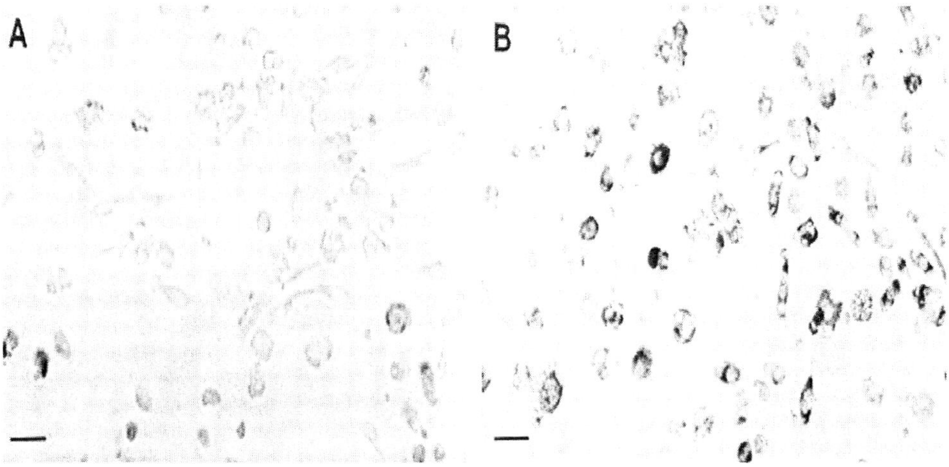


Figure 1: Foam cell formation by uninfected (A) and infected (B) human monocyte-derived macrophages. Cells were infected or not infected for 2 h and incubated with 100 mg/mL low-density lipoprotein for 24 h. Micrographs show Oil-Red O–stained macrophages (horizontal bar = 50 μm).
*From Kalayoglu et al, J Infect Dis; with permission.*

The results of these studies have reinforced the view that oxidized LDL could be an important mechanistic link between chronic infection and atherosclerosis. As other microbes, such as viruses and H. pylori, may as well contaminate the vascular wall via monocytes, one could speculate that enhanced lipoprotein oxidation could be accomplished by a wide variety of pathogens causing chronic infection. *In vitro* studies by Zhou et al found that infection of human smooth muscle cells with cytomegalovirus resulted in increased uptake of ox-LDL (Figure 2) via upregulation of specific scavenger receptors [90]. Of note, upregulation of ox-LDL scavenger receptors on the surface of smooth muscle cells is a ubiquitous finding in atherogenesis. It has, as consequence, increased uptake of oxidized lipoproteins by smooth muscle cells that migrate into intima, leading to foam cell formation.

Endovascular infection is not a prerequisite for oxidative modification of LDL during chronic infection. Indeed, ox-LDL have been associated with several chronic inflammatory diseases, such as diabetes mellitus [91] and rheumatoid arthritis [92]. It is therefore reasonable to assume that inflammatory components that are released during chronic infection could also modulate the process of LDL oxidation. Bacterial LPS could also amplify this process. Important mechanistic support to these hypotheses were provided by studies by Memon and colleagues, who found that induction of systemic inflammation in hamsters inoculated with zymosan led to elevated amounts of circulating products of lipid oxidation (ie, conjugated dienes in the LDL fraction) at comparable levels to those occurring after administration of E. coli LPS [67]. The LDL particles extracted from LPS-treated animals displayed further increased susceptibility to oxidation *in vitro*. Importantly, inflammatory cytokines mediate many of the metabolic effects of LPS, and previous studies from the same laboratory have demonstrated that both LPS and IL-1 enhances LDL`s content of ceramide, glucosylceramide, and sphingomyelin [93]. Ceramid, in particular, favours LDL aggregation and oxidation. Based on these findings, the authors suggested that the host response to infection may play an important role in LDL oxidation.

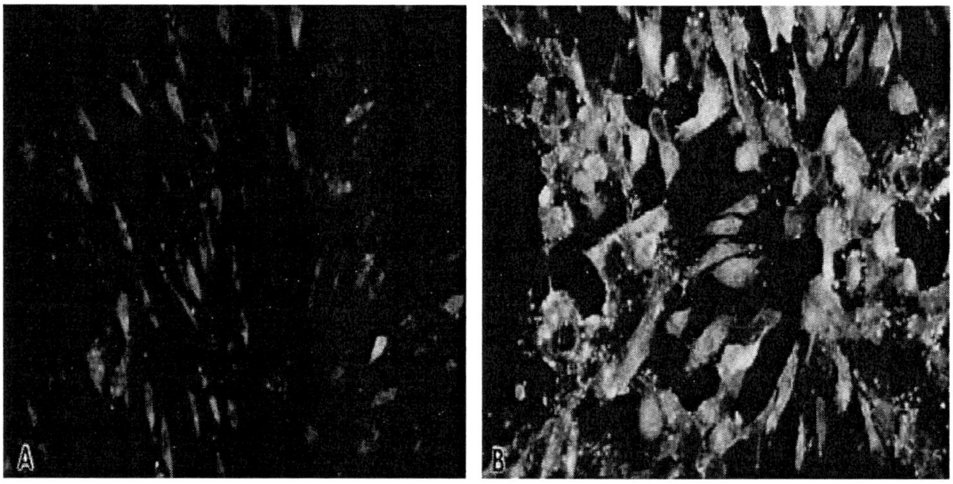

Figure 2: Acetylated LDL uptake of human aortic SMCs: (A) Fluorescent micrography of uninfected human SMCs incubated with DiI-Ac-LDL; (B) Fluorescent micrography of human SMCs infected 4 d earlier with HCMV and incubated with DiI-Ac-LDL.
*From Zhou et al, J Clin Invest. 1996; with permission*

## Dyslipidemia during Acute Infection: Possible Implications in Atherosclerosis

Although the host response to an acute infection is transitory, tending to resolve after the cessation of the infectious insult, the inflammatory changes are of much higher magnitude than those occurring during a chronic infection. This could have a major impact on the lipid and lipoprotein disturbances, which may exceed in intensity the corresponding changes accompanying chronic infection.

Kerttula [94] reported significant rise in triglyceride and decrease in HDL cholesterol in both pneumococcal pneumonia and ornithosis, thereby strengthening the view that the acute-phase response to infection rather than microbes is largely responsible for the lipid disturbances during acute infection. Nonetheless, in some cases, the type of pathogen might further influence the magnitude of lipid disturbances as suggested by studies accomplished by Leinonen [95], who found more profound changes in serum triglycerides and HDL in patients with C.pneumoniae-induced pneumonia than in those with viral and pneumococcal pneumonia.

Studies from our center indicated that a wide variety of acute infections (eg, respiratory, urinary tract, gastrointestinal, and skin infections), associated with elevation of inflammatory markers (C-reactive protein and fibrinogen) in children aged 0 to 16 years, elicited transitory reduction in HDL-to-total cholesterol ratio, and, most importantly, increase in anti-ox-LDL antibody levels [34]. Since no differences in these changes were observed in relation to the microbial pattern, we speculated that the observed lipid disturbances were caused by the inflammatory response to infection. Children with Kawasaki disease, a disorder with strong inflammatory component being increasingly suggested to predispose to accelerated atherosclerosis, may present a similar pro-atherogenic profile [96]. However, we could not find any correlation between CRP and the lipidemic changes, suggesting that multiple mechanisms may be implicated. Somewhat surprisingly, ultrasound investigation furnished evidence of carotid artery intima-media thickening in these children 3 months after the infectious illness, although no signs of infection or inflammation (as illustrated by normal values of CRP and fibrinogen) were present at this time point (Figure 3). We therefore inferred that the observed disturbances in HDL and ox-LDL, in tandem with inflammation, could have set in motion intravascular processes of possible atherogenic nature. Of note, even short exposure of arterial wall to ox-LDL could lead to intimal thickening consisting of both inflammatory and proliferative intimal changes [97]. CRP may bind to ox-LDL, thereby increasing the intravascular retention and toxicity of ox-LDL [98]. Decrease in HDL further exacerbates the vascular damage by lessening the protective vascular mechanisms. Additional analyses of blood samples from these children showed an increase in plasma soluble CD40 ligand (CD40L) at 3 months [99]. Upregulation of CD40L is a primary mechanism in the cell-mediated inflammatory reaction underlying plaque formation, and elevation of this marker in circulation has been associated with carotid atherosclerosis [100]. Recent *in-vitro* studies by Li and colleagues indicated that exposure of cultured human coronary endothelial cells to ox-LDL increased expression of CD40 and CD40L in a concentration and time-dependent manner [101]. These effects appeared to be mediated by upregulation of Lectin-like receptor (LOX-1) for ox-LDL.

Taken these findings together, the hypothesis of ox-LDL participation in the development of post-infection arterial thickening is conceivable. However, the possibility that this residual thickening could progress as such toward atherosclerosis is unlikely. Instead, subsequent episodes of acute infectious/inflammatory insults might pose additional burden on the arterial wall, thereby increasing the susceptibility to atherosclerosis (Figure 4). Our view is in keeping with findings from serial angiography studies [102] suggesting that atherosclerosis follows a stepwise rather than a linear progression, with periodic spurts of vascular growth followed by incomplete resolution. Results of an autopsy study emphasized that children with clinical signs of acute infection prior to death could have greater risk for intimal thickening in their coronary artery than those without evidence for acute infection [33]. Animal studies have shown that atherosclerosis or functional vascular abnormalities predisposing to it was more likely to develop in animals that receive repeated rather than single pathogen inoculation [82].

# Vascular Endothelium Could Link Infection-Related Lipid and Inflammatory Disturbances to Atherosclerosis

Abnormalities in vascular endothelial function play a critical role in the initiation and progression of atherosclerosis, being also a central mechanism in the occurrence of ischemic events [103]. Measures of endothelial dysfunction, such as impaired endothelium-dependent dilatation and soluble fractions of pro-inflammatory adhesion molecules, were shown to correlate with the development of atherosclerosis [104, 105]. Impaired bioactivity of nitric oxide, which is normally produced by endothelial cells via activation of the constitutive form of nitric oxide synthase (eNOS), is an important component of endothelial dysfunction as most of the anti-atherogenic properties of vascular endothelium are mediated by NO [106]. Endothelial dysfunction was demonstrated in a large number of studies on animals and humans with conventional risk factors for atherosclerosis. Infection or administration of bacterial endotoxin may also cause arterial endothelial dysfunction, and the risk for endothelial injury positively may correlate with the number of pathogens an individual is exposed to [82, 107].

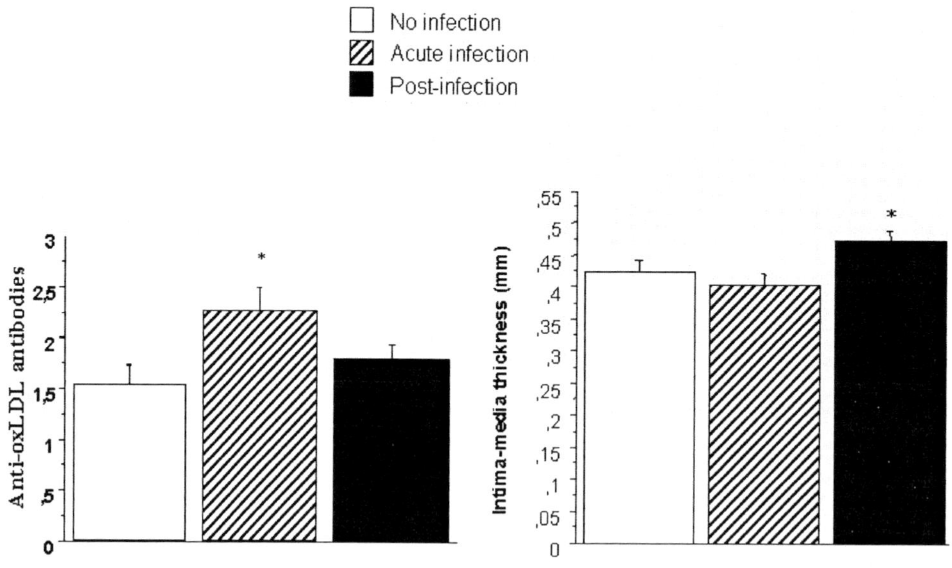


Figure 3: Levels of antibodies against ox-LDL (A) and carotid artery intima-media thickness (B) in healthy controls ("no infection), and in children with infection during the acute infectious illness ("acute infection") and 3 months after ("post-infection").
*From Liuba et al, Eur Heart J 2003; with permission*

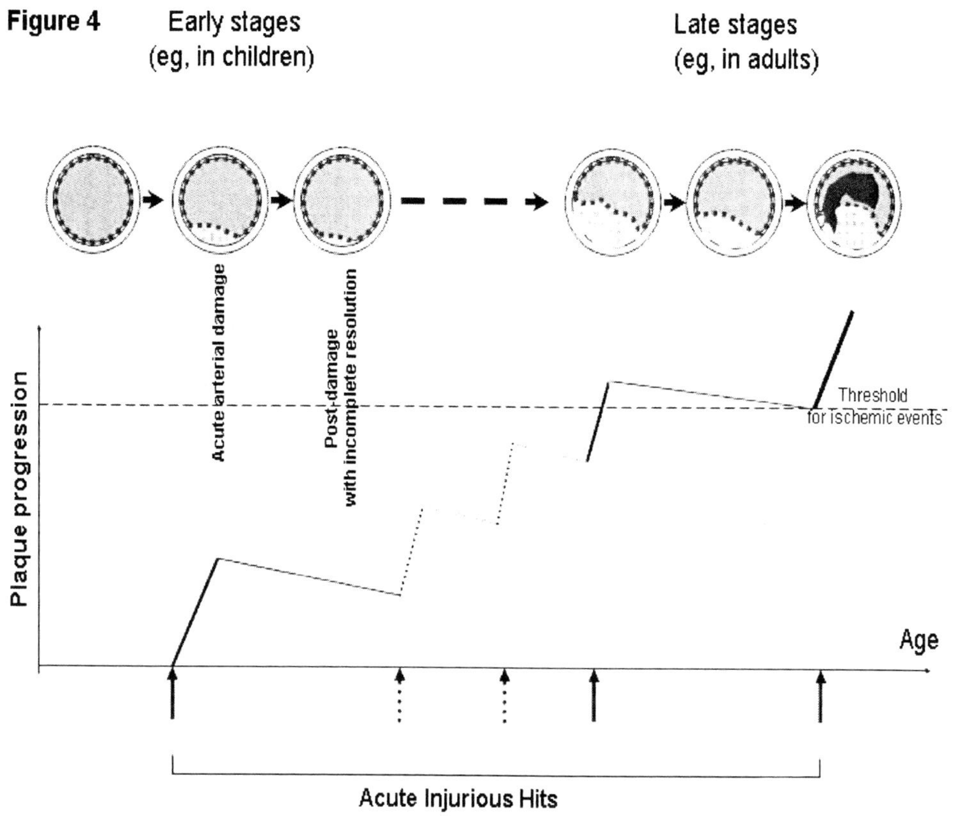


Figure 4: The development of atherosclerosis could be a result of cumulative arterial injuries by short-lasting hits, e.g., acute infections. Intima lesions in response these hits are highly rich in ox-LDL. The disease severity could increase with the number of hits, ultimately leading to a mature plaque at risk for rupture and thrombosis.

*From Liuba P, Acta Paed. 2004 (in press); adapted, with permission*

One attractive hypothesis is that infection, via systemic inflammation, could "switch on" the pro-atherogenic potential of vascular endothelium through activation of nuclear factor NF-kappa B [108]. This promotes induction of pro-inflammatory mechanisms, with subsequent activation and dysfunction of endothelial cells, decreased NO production, intimal infiltration with inflammatory cells, and smooth muscle cell proliferation [109]. Activation of NF-kappaB could be achieved via ox-LDL [80], which, as mentioned above, is increased by infection. Ox-LDL may also inhibit eNOS by inducing dephosphorylation of Akt pathway, which contributes to the normal function of eNOS [110]. Decreased levels of HDL during infection could facilitate adhesion of circulating monocyte to TNF-alpha-activated endothelial cells via increased expression of vascular cell adhesion molecule-1, with subsequent increased accumulation of these cells into intimal layer [111]. This effect seems to be independent of the cholesterol reverse transport function of HDL, but could in part relate to a decreased HDL-dependent activity of eNOS. Indeed, recent work in both cell culture and in mice indicates that HDL normally causes robust activation of eNOS, a process that takes place in endothelial cell caveolae and requires apoA-I binding [112].

Dyslipidemia might also be important modulator of the interaction between infectious pathogens and endothelial cells. Thus, incubation of human arterial endothelial cells with C. pneumoniae led to increased lipid peroxidation products, as determined by thiobarbituric acid-reacting substances assay [113]. Shimaoka et al demonstrated that the scavenger receptor for ox-LDL, LOX-1, supports adhesion of Gram-positive and Gram-negative bacteria to endothelial cells, and this is enhanced by cytokines such as TNF-alpha [114].

## Conclusion

Accumulating evidence suggests that infection could be implicated in the development of atherosclerosis through a number of mechanisms including inflammatory, metabolic, autoimmune, and pathogen-related mechanisms. Alterations in lipid and lipoprotein metabolism induced by infection, such as increase in triglycerides and in small, dense LDL and decrease in HDL, are proatherogenic, thereby purporting a mechanistic role of these disturbances in the eventual association of infection with atherosclerosis. Oxidative modification of LDL during infection could be one key-event in the development of arterial injury promoted by infection, and vascular endothelium could be a major target. The pathogenic implications of lipoprotein oxidation in the arterial disease could be more significant in young populations. In children, repeated acute infections might cause cumulative fibroproliferative changes in the arterial wall, which, probably depending on the genetic vulnerability, could increase predisposition to atherosclerosis. In addition, the lipid and lipoprotein alterations during infection could modulate the interaction of infection and associated inflammation with the arterial wall.

To date, proofs for a definite causative link between infection and atherosclerosis remain unveiled. Most likely, infectious agents may act in concert with known risk factors, such as hypercholesterolemia, to accelerate atherogenesis. This view is gaining increasing support from both scientists and clinicians, and accords with the paradigm of multifactorial etiology of atherosclerosis. Therefore, an interdisciplinary approach is important when establishing strategies aimed to retard atherosclerosis in order to attain gratifying benefit on the clinical outcome later in life.

## Acknowledgments

Research grants were received from The Swedish Royal Physiographic Society, The Swedish Medical Association, The Heart-Lung Foundation, Anna-Lisa and Sven-Eric Lundgren's Foundation for Medical Research, Lund University, and Lund University Hospital.

# References


[1] Ross R. Atherosclerosis--an inflammatory disease. *N Engl J Med.* 1999;14;340:115-126.

[2] Ross R. The pathogenesis of atherosclerosis: a perspective for the 1990s. *Nature.* 1993;362:801-809.

[3] Libby P, Maseri A, Ridker P. Inflammation and atherosclerosis. *Circulation.* 2002;105:1135-1143.

[4] O'Connor S, Taylor C, Campbell L, Epstein S, Libby P. Potential infectious etiologies of atherosclerosis: a multifactorial perspective. *Emerg Infect Dis.* 2001;7:780-788.

[5] Blake G, Ridker P. Inflammatory bio-markers and cardiovascular risk prediction. *J Intern Med.* 2002;252:283-294.

[6] Osler W. Diseases of the arteries. Modern Medicine: Its Practice and Theory. Philadelphia: Lea and Febiger. 1908:429–447.

[7] Fabricant C, Fabricant J, Litrenta M, Minick C. Virus-induced atherosclerosis. *J Exp Med.* 1978;148:335-340.

[8] Hajjar D, Falcone D, Fabricant C, Fabricant J. Altered cholesteryl ester cycle is associated with lipid accumulation in herpes virus-infected arterial smooth muscle cells. *J Biol Chem.* 1985.260:6124-6128.

[9] Saikku P, Leinonen M, Mattila K, Ekman M, Nieminen M, Makela P, et al. Serological evidence of an association of a novel Chlamydia, TWAR, with chronic coronary heart disease and acute myocardial infarction. *Lancet.* 1988;29:983-986.

[10] Saikku P, Leinonen M, Tenkanen L, Linnanmaki E, Ekman MR, Manninen V, et al. Chronic Chlamydia pneumoniae infection as a risk factor for coronary heart disease in the Helsinki Heart Study. *Ann Intern Med.* 1992;116:273–278.

[11] Loebe M, Schuler S, Zais O, Warnecke H, Fleck E, Hetzer R. Role of cytomegalovirus infection in the development of coronary artery disease in the transplanted heart. *J Heart Transplant.* 1990;9:707–711.

[12] Siscovick D, Schwartz S, Corey L, Grayston J, Ashley R, Wang S, et al. Chlamydia pneumoniae, herpes simplex virus type 1, and cytomegalovirus and incident myocardial infarction and coronary heart disease death in older adults: the Cardiovascular Health Study. *Circulation.* 2000;102:2335-2340.

[13] Ossei-Gerning N, Moayyedi P, Smith S, et al. Helicobacter pylori infection is related to atheroma in patients undergoing coronary angiography. *Cardiovasc Res.*1997;35:120-124.

[14] Schmidt C, Hulthe J, Wikstrand J, Gnarpe H, Gnarpe J, Agewall S, et al. Chlamydia pneumoniae seropositivity is associated with carotid artery intima-media thickness. *Stroke.* 2000;31:1526-1531.

[15] Human cytomegalovirus seropositivity is associated with impaired vascular function. *Circulation.* 2003;108:678-683.

[16] Ishizaka N, Ishizaka Y, Takahashi E, Toda Ei E, Hashimoto H, Ohno M, Nagai R, Yamakado M. Increased prevalence of carotid atherosclerosis in hepatitis B virus carriers. *Circulation.* 2002 Mar 5;105(9):1028-30.

[17] Kinjo K, Sato H, Sato H, Ohnishi Y, Hishida E, Nakatani D, et al. Joint effects of Chlamydia pneumoniae infection and classic coronary risk factors on risk of acute myocardial infarction. *Am Heart J.* 2003;146:324-330.

[18] Espinola-Klein C, Rupprecht H-J, Blankenberg S, Bickel C, Kopp H, Victor A, et al. Impact of Infectious Burden on Progression of Carotid Atherosclerosis *Stroke.* 2002;33:2581-2586.

[19] Sander D, Winbeck K, Klingelhofer J, et al. Reduced progression of early Carotid Atherosclerosis after antibiotic treatment and C. pneumoniae seropositivity. *Circulation.* 2002;106:2428–2433.

[20] Sinisalo J, Mattila K, Valtonen V, Anttonen O, Juvonen J, Melin J, et al. Effect of 3 months of antimicrobial treatment with clarithromycin in acute non–Q-wave coronary syndrome. *Circulation.* 2002;105:1555-1560.

[21] Muhlestein J. Antibiotic treatment of atherosclerosis. *Curr Opin Lipidol.* 2003;14:605-614.

[22] Hirashima Y, Kuwayama N, Kubo M, et al. Chlamydia pneumoniae infection is not involved in carotid artery stenosis. *Atherosclerosis.* 2002;163:165-168.

[23] Coles K, Plant A, Riley T, Smith D, McQuillan B, Thompson P. Lack of association between seropositivity to Chlamydia pneumoniae and carotid atherosclerosis. *Am J Cardiol.* 1999;84:825-828.

[24] Adler S, Hur J, Wang J, Vetrovec G. Prior infection with cytomegalovirus is not a major risk factor for angiographically demonstrated coronary artery atherosclerosis. *J InfectDis.* 1998;177:209-212.

[25] Zhu J, Quyyumi AA, Muhlestein JB, Nieto FJ, Horne BD, Zalles-Ganley A, Anderson JL, Epstein SE. Lack of association of Helicobacter pylori infection with coronary artery disease and frequency of acute myocardial infarction or death. *Am J Cardiol.* 2002;89:155-158.

[26] Sander D, Winbeck K, Klingelhofer J, Etgen T, Conrad B. Progression of early carotid atherosclerosis is only temporarily reduced after antibiotic treatment of Chlamydia pneumoniae seropositivity. *Circulation.* 2004;109:1010-1015.

[27] Cercek B, Shah PK, Noc M, Zahger D, Zeymer U, Matetzky S, et al. Effect of short-term treatment with azithromycin on recurrent ischaemic events in patients with acute coronary syndrome in the Azithromycin in Acute Coronary Syndrome (AZACS) trial: a randomised controlled trial. *Lancet.* 2003;361:809-813.

[28] Kuo C, Shor A, Campbell L, et al. Demonstration of Chlamydia pneumoniae in atherosclerotic lesions of coronary arteries. *J Infect Dis.* 1993;167:841-849.

[29] Shi Y, Tokunaga O. Herpesvirus (HSV-1, EBV and CMV) infections in atherosclerotic compared with non-atherosclerotic aortic tissue. *Pathol Int.* 2002;52:31-39.

[30] Zhou Y, Shou M, Guetta E, Guzman R, Unger E, Yu Z, et al. Cytomegalovirus infection of rats increases neointimal response to vascular injury without consistent evidence of direct infection of the vascular wall. *Circulation.* 1999;100:1569-1575.

[31] Saikku P, Laitinen K, Leinonen M. Animal models for Chlamydia pneumoniae infection. *Atherosclerosis.* 1998;140:S17-19.

[32] Moazed T, Kuo C, Grayston, Campbell L. Murine models of Chlamydia pneumoniae infection and atherosclerosis. *J Infect Dis.* 1997;175:883-890.

[33] Pesonen E, Paakkari I, Rapola J. Infection-associated intimal thickening in the coronary arteries of children. *Atherosclerosis.* 1999;142:425-429.

[34] Liuba P, Persson J, Luoma J, Ylä-Herttuala S, Pesonen E. Acute infections in children are accompanied by oxidative modification of LDL and decrease of HDL cholesterol, and are followed by thickening of carotid intima-media. *Eur Heart J.* 2003;24:515-521.

[35] Aburawi E, Liuba P, Pesonen E, Ylä-Herttuala-S, Sjöblad S. Acute respiratory viral infections aggravate arterial endothelial dysfunction in children with type I diabetes mellitus. *Diabetes Care* (in press).

[36] Charakida M, Donald A, Halcox J, Terese M, Ness A, Friberg P, et al. Acute infection in children is associated with endothelial dysfunction. Abstract presented at the *Scientific Session of the American Heart Association*, Orlando, Florida, 2003.

[37] Hu H, Pierce GN, Zhong G. The atherogenic effects of Chlamydia are dependent on serum cholesterol and specific to Chlamydia pneumoniae. *J Clin Invest.* 1999;103:747–753.

[38] Blessing E, Campbell L, Rosenfeld M, Chough N, Kuo C. Chlamydia pneumoniae infection accelerates hyperlipidemia induced atherosclerotic lesion development in C57BL/6J mice. *Atherosclerosis.* 2001;158:13-17.

[39] Moazed T, Campbell L, Rosenfeld M, Grayston J, Kuo C. Chlamydia pneumoniae infection accelerates the progression of atherosclerosis in apolipoprotein E-deficient mice. *J Infect Dis.* 1999;180:238-241.

[40] Muhlestein JB, Anderson JL, Hammond EH, et al. Infection with Chlamydia pneumoniae accelerates the development of atherosclerosis and treatment with azithromycin prevents it in a rabbit model. *Circulation.* 1998;97:633–636.

[41] Sung M-T, Tsun-Mei Lin T-M, Wang Y-Z, Eng H-L. Accelerated atherogenesis in BHN-4 infected rabbit model of diabetes mellitus. Abstract presented at *ICB symposium*, October 2002.

[42] Sunnemark D, Harris R, Frostegard J, Orn A. Induction of early atherosclerosis in CBA/J mice by combination of Trypanosoma cruzi infection and a high cholesterol diet. *Atherosclerosis.* 2000;153:273-282.

[43] Laurila A, Cole S, Merat S, Obonyo M, Palinski W, Fierer J, Witztum J. High-fat, high-cholesterol diet increases the incidence of gastritis in LDL receptor-negative mice. *Arterioscler Thromb Vasc Biol.* 2001;21:991-996.

[44] Archimandritis AJ, Chronaki M, Kalogeras D, Galanopoulos G, Grigoriadis P, Tzivras M.The incidence of Helicobacter pylori is not increased in obese people, but the risk of duodenal ulcer is higher in H. pylori-positive people of high obesity. *J Clin Gastroenterol.* 2003;36:184-185.

[45] Delgado-Rodriguez M, Medina-Cuadros M, Martinez-Gallego G, Sillero-Arenas M. Total cholesterol, HDL-cholesterol, and risk of nosocomial infection: a prospective study in surgical patients. *Infect Control Hosp Epidemiol.* 1997;18:9-18.

[46] Meier C, Jick S, Derby L, Vasilakis C, Jick H. Acute respiratory-tract infections and risk of first-time acute myocardial infarction. *Lancet.* 1998;351:1467-1471.

[47] Leinonen M, Toivanen P, Tenkanen L, et al. Chlamydia pneumoniae and metabolic syndrome as risk factors for coronary events in the Helsinki heart Study. In: Abstracts

of the *38th Interscience Conference on Antimicrobial Agents and Chemotherapy*, San Diego, Calif, 1998.

[48] Heilbronn L, Clifton P. C-reactive protein and coronary artery disease: influence of obesity, caloric restriction and weight loss. *J Nutr Biochem*. 2002;13:316-321.

[49] Glader C, Boman J, Saikku P, Stenlund H, Weinehall L, Hallmanns G, et al. The proatherogenic properties of lipoprotein(a) may be enhanced through the formation of circulating immune complexes containing Chlamydia pneumoniae-specific IgG antibodies. *Eur Heart J*. 2000;21:639-646.

[50] Koenig W, Lowel H, Baumert J, Meisinger C. C-reactive protein modulates risk prediction based on the Framingham Score: implications for future risk assessment: results from a large cohort study in southern Germany. *Circulation*. 2004;109:1349-1353.

[51] Schwartz Y, Dushkin M. Endotoxin-Lipoprotein Complex Formation as a Factor in Atherogenesis: Associations with Hyperlipidemia and with Lecithin:Cholesterol Acyltransferase Activity. *Biochemistry*. 2002;67:747-753.

[52] Tarnacka B, Gromadzka G, Czlonkowska A. Increased circulating immune complexes in acute stroke: the triggering role of Chlamydia pneumoniae and cytomegalovirus. *Stroke*. 2002;33:936-40.

[53] Khovidhunkit W, Kim M, Memon RA, Shigenaga J, Moser A, Feingold K, et al. Effects of infection and inflammation on lipid and lipoprotein metabolism: mechanisms and consequences to the host. *J Lipid Res*. 2004;45:1169-1196.

[54] Laurila A, Bloigu A, Nayha S, Hassi J, Leinonen M, Saikku P. Chronic Chlamydia pneumoniae infection is associated with a serum lipid profile known to be a risk factor for atherosclerosis. *Arterioscler Thromb Vasc Biol*. 1997;17:2910-2913.

[55] Laurila A, Bloigu A, Nayha S, Hassi J, Leinonen M, Saikku P. Chlamydia pneumoniae antibodies and serum lipids in Finnish men: cross sectional study. *BMJ*. 1997;314:1456-1457.

[56] Scharnagl H, Kist M, Grawitz AB, Koenig W, Wieland H, Marz W. Effect of Helicobacter pylori eradication on high-density lipoprotein cholesterol. *Am J Cardiol*. 2004;93:219-220.

[57] Hoffmeister A, Rothenbacher D, Bode G, Persson K, Marz W, Nauck M, et al. Current infection with Helicobacter pylori, but not seropositivity to Chlamydia pneumoniae or cytomegalovirus, is associated with an atherogenic, modified lipid profile. *Arterioscler Thromb Vasc Biol*. 2001;21:427-432.

[58] Mayr M, Kiechl S, Mendall MA, Willeit J, Wick G, Xu Q. Increased risk of atherosclerosis is confined to CagA-positive Helicobacter pylori strains: prospective results from the Bruneck study. *Stroke*. 2003;34:610-615.

[59] Szkaradkiewicz A, Bogaczynska-Staniewicz J, Torlinski L, Wal M. Cytomegalovirus infection and atherogenesis. *Med Sci Monit*. 2002;8:104-107.

[60] Jahoor F, Abramson S, Heird WC. The protein metabolic response to HIV infection in young children. *Am J Clin Nutr*. 2003;78:182-189.

[61] Georges J, Rupprecht H, Blankenberg S, Poirier O, Bickel C, Hafner G, et al. Impact of pathogen burden in patients with coronary artery disease in relation to systemic

inflammation and variation in genes encoding cytokines. *Am J Cardiol.* 2003;92:515-521.

[62] Hsue P, Lo J, Franklin A, Bolger A, Martin J, Deeks S, Waters D. Progression of atherosclerosis as assessed by carotid intima-media thickness in patients with HIV infection. *Circulation.* 2004;109:1603-1608.

[63] Epstein S, Zhu J, Burnett M, Zhou Y, Vercellotti G, Hajjar D. Infection and atherosclerosis: potential roles of pathogen burden and molecular mimicry. *Arterioscler Thromb Vasc Biol.* 2000;20:1417-1420.

[64] Badiou S, De Boever C, Dupuy A, Baillat V, Cristol J, Reynes J. Decrease in LDL size in HIV-positive adults before and after lopinavir/ritonavir-containing regimen: an index of atherogenicity? *Atherosclerosis* 2003;168:107–113.

[65] Packard C, Shepherd J. Lipoprotein heterogeneity and apolipoprotein B metabolism. *Arterioscler. Thromb. Vasc. Biol.* 1997;17:3542–3556.

[66] Halle M, Berg A, Keul J, Baumstark M. Association between serum fibrinogen concentrations and HDL and LDL subfraction phenotypes in healthy men. *Arterioscler Thromb Vasc Biol.* 1996;16:144-148.

[67] Memon R, Staprans I, Noor M, Holleran W, Uchida Y, Moser A, et al. Infection and inflamation induce LDL oxidation in vivo. *Arterioscler Thromb Vasc Biol.* 2000;20:1536–1542.

[68] Nishi E. Lysophosphatidylcholine increases expression of heparin-binding epidermal growth factor-like growth factor in human T lymphocytes. *Circ Res.* 1997;80:638-644.

[69] Yoshino G, Hirano T, Kazumi T. Dyslipidemia in diabetes mellitus. *Diabetes Res Clin Pract.* 1996;33:1-14.

[70] Prichard S. Impact of dyslipidemia in end-stage renal disease. *J Am Soc Nephrol.* 2003;14:S315-320.

[71] Ettinger W, Miller L, Albers J, Smith T, Parks J. Lipopolysaccharide and tumor necrosis factor cause a fall in plasma concentration of lecithin: cholesterol acyltransferase in cynomolgus monkeys. *J. Lipid Res.* 31:1099–1107.

[72] Feingold K, Marshall M, Gulli R, Moser A, Grunfeld C. Effect of endotoxin and cytokines on lipoprotein lipase activity in mice. *Arterioscler. Thromb.* 1994;14:1866–1872.

[73] Munford R, Andersen J, Dietschy J. Sites of tissue binding and uptake in vivo of bacterial lipopolysaccharide-high density lipoprotein complexes: studies in the rat and squirrel monkey. *J Clin Invest.* 1981;68:1503-1513.

[74] Kitchens R, Thompson P, Munford R, O'Keefe G. Acute inflammation and infection maintain circulating phospholipid levels and enhance lipopolysaccharide binding to plasma lipoproteins. *Crit Care Med.* 2003;31:1647-53.

[75] Durrington P. HDL in risk prediction and its direct and indirect involvement in atherogenesis. *Atherosclerosis.* 2002;3:S3-12.

[76] Grunfeld C, Marshall M, Shigenaga J, Moser A, Tobias P, Feingold K. Lipoproteins inhibit macrophage activation by lipoteichoic acid. *J. Lipid Res.* 1999;40:245-252.

[77] Klinkner A, Waites C, Kerns W, Bugelski P. Evidence of foam cell and cholesterol crystal formation in macrophages incubated with oxidized LDL by fluorescence and electron microscopy. *J Histochem Cytochem.* 1995;43:1071-1078.

[78] Boullier A, Bird D, Chang M, Dennis E, Friedman P, Gillotre-Taylor K, Horkko S, et al. Scavenger receptors, oxidized LDL, and atherosclerosis. *Ann N Y Acad Sci.* 2001;947:214-222.

[79] Kita T, Kume N, Minami M, Hayashida K, Murayama T, Sano H, et al. Role of oxidized LDL in atherosclerosis. *Ann N Y Acad Sci.* 2001;947:199-205.

[80] Heermeier K, Leicht W, Palmetshofer A, Ullrich M, Wanner C, Galle J. Oxidized LDL suppresses NF-kappaB and overcomes protection from apoptosis in activated endothelial cells. *J Am Soc Nephrol.* 2001;12:456-63.

[81] Kol A, Bourcier T, Lichtman AH, Libby P. Chlamydial and human heat shock protein 60s activate human vascular endothelium, smooth muscle cells, and macrophages. *J Clin Invest.* 1999;103:571-577.

[82] Liuba P, Karnani P, Pesonen E, Paakkari I, Forslid A, Johansson L, et al. Endothelial dysfunction after repeated Chlamydia pneumoniae infection in apolipoprotein E-knockout mice. *Circulation.* 2000;29;102:1039-1044.

[83] Xiong A, Clarke-Katzenberg R, Valenzuela G, Izumi K, Millan M. Epstein-Barr virus latent membrane protein 1 activates nuclear factor-kappa B in human endothelial cells and inhibits apoptosis. *Transplantation.* 2004;78:41-49.

[84] Grahame-Clarke C, Chan N, Andrew D, Ridgway G, Betteridge D, Emery V, et al. Human cytomegalovirus seropositivity is associated with impaired vascular function. *Circulation.* 2003;108:678-683.

[85] Liuba P, Pesonen E, Paakkari I, Batra S, Andersen L, Forslid A, et al. Co-infection with Chlamydia pneumoniae and Helicobacter pylori results in vascular endothelial dysfunction and enhanced VCAM-1 expression in apoE-knockout mice. *J Vasc Res.* 2003;40:115-122.

[86] Kalayoglu M, Hoerneman B, LaVerda D, Morrison S, Morrison R, Byrne G. Cellular oxidation of low-density lipoprotein by Chlamydia pneumoniae. *J Infect Dis.* 1999;180:780–790.

[87] Kalayoglu M, Byrne G. Induction of macrophage foam cell formation by Chlamydia pneumoniae. *J Infect Dis.* 1998;177:725–729.

[88] Xu Q. Infections, heat shock proteins, and atherosclerosis. *Curr Opin Cardiol.* 2003;18:245-252.

[89] Kalayoglu M, Perkins B, Byrne G. Chlamydia pneumoniae-infected monocytes exhibit increased adherence to human aortic endothelial cells. *Microbes Infect.* 2001;3:963-969.

[90] Zhou Y, Guetta E, Yu Z, Finkel T, Epstein S. Human cytomegalovirus increases modified low density lipoprotein uptake and scavenger receptor mRNA expression in vascular smooth muscle cells. *J Clin Invest.* 1996;98:2129-2138.

[91] Makimattila S, Luoma J, Yla-Herttuala S, Bergholm R, Utriainen T, Virkamaki A, Autoantibodies against oxidized LDL and endothelium-dependent vasodilation in insulin-dependent diabetes mellitus. *Atherosclerosis.* 1999;147:115-122.

[92] Cvetkovic J, Wallberg-Jonsson S, Ahmed E, Rantapaa-Dahlqvist S, Lefvert A. Increased levels of autoantibodies against copper-oxidized low density lipoprotein, malondialdehyde-modified low density lipoprotein and cardiolipin in patients with rheumatoid arthritis. *Rheumatology.* 2002;41:988-995.

[93] Memon R, Holleran W, Moser A, Seki T, Uchida Y, Fuller J, et al. Endotoxin and cytokines increase hepatic sphingolipid biosynthesis and produce lipoproteins enriched in ceramides and sphingomyelin. *Arterioscler Thromb Vasc Biol.* 1998;18:1257-1265.

[94] Kerttula Y, Weber T. Serum lipids in pneumonia of different aetiology. *Ann Clin Res* 1988;20:184-188.

[95] Leinonen M, Kerttula Y, Weber T. Acute phase response in Chlamydia pneumoniae pneumonia. Presented at the *5th European Congress on Clinical Microbiology and Infectious Diseases*, Oslo, Norway, 1991.

[96] Cabana V, Gidding S, Getz G, Chapman J, Shulman S. Serum amyloid A and high density lipoprotein participate in the acute phase response of Kawasaki disease. *Pediatr Res.* 1997;42:651-655.

[97] Matthys K, Van Hove C, Kockx M, Andries L, Van Osselaer N, Herman A, et al. Local application of LDL promotes intimal thickening in the collared carotid artery of the rabbit. *Arterioscler Thromb Vasc Biol.* 1997;17:2423–2429.

[98] Taskinen S, Kovanen P, Jarva H, Meri S, Pentikäinen M. Binding of C-reactive protein to modified low-density-lipoprotein particles: identification of cholesterol as a novel ligand for C-reactive protein. *Biochem. J.* 2002;367:403–412.

[99] Liuba P, Truedsson L. Soluble CD-40 ligand is elevated in children with carotid intima-media thickening following acute infection. *Cardiovasc Pathol.* 2004;13:100.

[100] Blake G, Ostfeld R, Yucel E, Varo N, Schonbeck U, Blake M, et al. Soluble CD40 ligand levels indicate lipid accumulation in carotid atheroma: an in vivo study with high-resolution MRI. *Arterioscler Thromb Vasc Biol.* 2003;23:11-14.

[101] Li D, Liu L, Chen H, Sawamura T, Mehta J. LOX-1, an oxidized LDL endothelial receptor, induces CD40/CD40L signaling in human coronary artery endothelial cells. *Arterioscler Thromb Vasc Biol.* 2003;23:816-821.

[102] Bruschke A, Kramer J Jr., Bal E, Haque I, Detrano R, Goormastic M. The dynamics of progression of coronary atherosclerosis studied in 168 medically treated patients who underwent coronary arteriography three times. *Am Heart J.* 1989;117:296–305.

[103] Gimbrone M. Vascular endothelium: an integrator of pathophysiologic stimuli in atherosclerosis. *Am J Cardiol.* 1995;75:67-70.

[104] Prasad A, Zhu J, Halcox J, Waclawiw M, Epstein S, Quyyumi A. Predisposition to atherosclerosis by infections: role of endothelial dysfunction. *Circulation.* 2002;106:184-190.

[105] Ikata J, Wakatsuki T, Oishi Y, Oki T, Ito S. Leukocyte counts and concentrations of soluble adhesion molecules as predictors of coronary atherosclerosis. *Coron Artery Dis.* 2000;11:445-449.

[106] Gewaltig M, Kojda G. Vasoprotection by nitric oxide: mechanisms and therapeutic potential. *Cardiovasc Res.* 2002;55:250-260.

[107] Berman RS, Frew J, Martin W. Endotoxin-induced arterial endothelial barrier dysfunction assessed by an in vitro model. *Br J Pharmacol.* 1993;110:1282-1284.

[108] Naumann M. Nuclear factor-kappa B activation and innate immune response in microbial pathogen infection. *Biochem Pharmacol.* 200060:1109-1114.

[109] Thurberg B, Collins T. The nuclear factor-kappa B/inhibitor of kappa B autoregulatory system and atherosclerosis. *Curr Opin Lipidol.* 1998;9:387-396.

[110] Chavakis E, Dernbach E, Hermann C, Mondorf U, Zeiher A, Dimmeler S. Oxidized LDL inhibits vascular endothelial growth factor-induced endothelial cell migration by an inhibitory effect on the Akt/endothelial nitric oxide synthase pathway. *Circulation.* 2001;103:2102-2107.

[111] Park S, Park J, Kang J, Kang Y. Involvement of transcription factors in plasma HDL protection against TNF-alpha-induced vascular cell adhesion molecule-1 expression. *Int J Biochem Cell Biol.* 2003;35:168-182.

[112] Mineo C, Shaul P. HDL stimulation of endothelial nitric oxide synthase: a novel mechanism of HDL action. *Trends Cardiovasc Med.* 2003;13:226-231.

[113] Dittrich R, Dragonas C, Mueller A, Maltaris T, Rupp J, Beckmann M, et al. Endothelial Chlamydia pneumoniae infection promotes oxidation of LDL. *Biochem Biophys Res Commun.* 2004;319:501-505.

[114] Shimaoka T, Kume N, Minami M, Hayashida K, Sawamura T, Kita T, Yonehara S. LOX-1 supports adhesion of Gram-positive and Gram-negative bacteria. *J Immunol.* 2001;166:5108-5114.

# Index

## A



## B

## D



## E

## K



## L



## M

## Q



## R



## S

## W



## Y